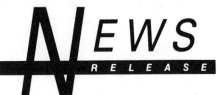
Embargoed by Metabolism
until August 15, 1994

Contact: Jennifer O'Brien

"Essential Fatty Acid Deficiency Identified
As Key Heart Disease Risk Factor"

Characterizing their discovery as the critical "missing link" in understanding the role of fat in heart disease, a team of Boston University Medical Center (BUMC) researchers has reported in the August issue of the journal *"Metabolism"* that *insufficient* levels of essential fatty acids are a key risk factor for coronary artery disease.

This finding, the researchers say, indicates that the current clinical emphasis on restricting saturated fat and cholesterol in the diet to reduce the risk of coronary artery disease is misplaced. It is a sufficient level of essential fatty acids, which, the researchers propose, *regulates* the correct balance of saturated fat in cells and blood cholesterol, that is most important for reducing the risk of coronary artery disease.

"The amounts of dietary saturated and monounsaturated fats and cholesterol are not as important as achieving optimal levels of essential fatty acids," says Edward N. Siguel, MD, PhD, co-principal investigator of the study, and a senior scientist at BUMC. "Sufficient levels of essential fatty acids," he says, "will help to regulate the correct balance of saturated fats and cholesterol in cells."

In the 1960s, researchers suspected that a deficiency of essential fatty acids was the most significant risk factor for coronary artery disease, but they were unable to identify biochemical evidence of essential fatty acids deficiency in coronary artery disease patients. With millions of people in the U.S. having heart disease, the thinking went, essential fatty acids abnormalities should have been found easily if they existed. But for more than 20 years researchers did not detect the biochemical evidence. Reflecting this state of the science, the 1988 U.S. Surgeon General's report stated that essential fatty acids deficiency is practically non-existent in the United States. As a result, U.S. nutritional policy has focused on diets low in saturated fat and cholesterol and on drugs to lower cholesterol.

Now, however, using a new and highly sensitive biochemical test, Siguel and co-principal investigator Robert H. Lerman, MD, PhD, have found evidence of essential fatty acids deficiency in patients with coronary artery disease, what they call "the missing link in the nutrition-heart

-more-disease hypothesis." Identifying this deficiency should lead to fundamental changes in clinical care and nutrition policy, the researchers say.

Essential fatty acids, along with saturated and monounsaturated fatty acids, are the principal components of fats. The balance of these three types of fatty acids plays a key role in determining the consistency of the walls of the cells lining the arteries supplying blood to the heart.

Experts agree that maintaining the proper consistency of the cell walls is a crucial factor for avoiding hardening of the arteries, or atherosclerosis, which causes coronary artery disease. However, they have disagreed about the role each type of fatty acid plays in the body and how imbalances should be corrected.

Given their finding, the BUMC researchers say, it's imperative that essential fatty acids levels be taken into account in the diagnosis and treatment of patients with coronary artery disease. Moreover, they call for an overhaul of the current U.S. Public Health Service and USDA guidelines for a healthy diet, in order to emphasize the importance of eating foods with substantial amounts of essential fatty acids in them.

Essential fatty acids are the only fatty acids that the body does not manufacture on its own and that must therefore be consumed in food. The body can synthesize the other major types of fatty acids--monounsaturated and saturated fatty acids--from proteins and carbohydrates, which people eat.

The USDA guidelines currently advocate a low fat diet, as represented by the "food pyramid," which advises people to obtain the bulk of their calories from pasta and grains, which contain few, if any, essential fatty acids, and to use fats and oils sparingly.

"Unfortunately," explains Siguel, "essential fatty acids are difficult to obtain in processed foods, as food manufacturers generally remove essential fatty acids from plant products because they shorten their shelf-life."

"When viewed in light of our findings, the USDA recommendations are misleading," says Siguel. "A low fat diet is counterproductive if it is low in essential fatty acids. Foods containing saturated fat and essential fatty acids, such as Tofu and some types of pizza, are to be preferred to foods high in carbohydrate and low in saturated fat and essential fatty acids, such as processed breads, cereals and pasta."

Instead of eating foods low in fat and cholesterol, people should strive to reach their ideal weight and to achieve an optimal balance of essential fatty acids, says Siguel. He points out that excess calories--from any source--are stored as saturated fat. Thus it is calories, rather than the intake of saturated fat and cholesterol in the diet, that controls levels of saturated fat in the *body*.

"Avoiding cholesterol and saturated fats in the diet and replacing those calories with carbohydrates will not decrease blood levels of saturated fat and cholesterol," Siguel says. "The body simply makes more cholesterol and saturated fat from carbohydrates. Eating more essential fatty acids increases the body levels of essential fatty acids because essential fatty acids are an essential nutrient that the body cannot make."

Ideally, says Siguel, people should eat natural, unprocessed foods that are low in fat, low in cholesterol and high in essential fatty acids and that provide fiber, vitamins and minerals.

In their study, the BUMC researchers compared the fatty acid patterns of 47 patients with

ESSENTIAL FATTY ACIDS IN

HEALTH AND DISEASE

✳✳✳✳✳

Using the essential fats Omega -3 and Omega-6 to improve your health, lower your cholesterol and prevent cardiovascular disease

by Edward N. Siguel, M.D., Ph.D.

What the FDA and USDA failed to tell you about Essential and Trans Fatty Acids

Contains a discussion of US guidelines on fat, cholesterol, cardiovascular disease, cancer and diabetes.

Includes advice on how to lower dangerous blood levels of Trans fatty acids

Eat meals rich in essential fatty acids (EFAs) and take control of your health. Replace saturated fat with essential fats for a healthier, trimmer body, and younger-looking skin.

Based on scientific findings by the author

This book is provided solely for informational purposes. Please read the disclaimer in the acknowledgments section. No representations, either express or implied, are made or given regarding the medical consequences of opinions herein presented. This book contains only the opinions of the author. Please consult a physician and nutritionist who can interpret test results and provide the appropriate treatment for you in accordance with the entire clinical evaluation and other test results.

Nutrek Inc., Nutrek Press.   SAN 298-3567

P.O. Box 1269, Brookline, MA 02146.

ESSENTIAL FATTY ACIDS IN HEALTH AND DISEASE

Copyright © 1994, Edward N. Siguel, M.D., Ph.D.

ISBN   0-9642534-0-2

Library of Congress Catalog Card Number: 94-

Library of Congress Catalog ing in Publication Data

Essential Fatty Acids in Health and Disease: Edward Siguel. ---1st ed.

1. Essential Fatty acids. 2. Trans fatty acids. 3. Cardiovascular disease treatment. 4. Essential Fatty Acid Deficiency. 5. Fat metabolism. I. Title

Library of Congress Catalog Card Number 94-67872

First Edition, First printing.

Printed in the United States of America.

TABLE OF CONTENTS

Acknowledgments, Disclaimer x
Foreword xii
Preface xiv
Introduction..xxi
Book Summary xxxvi

I.1. DIET AND NUTRITION   **1**
You can prevent heart disease 1
The basic nutrients...2
Nutrition vs. diet; Nutritional Status 3
What constitutes optimal nutrition?...4
The body as a "machine"...5
Cells and enzymes; How nutrients are used 6
What keeps a cell alive ; Good health; Disease.........................7
How long can you live?...8
Balance is the key 8
Nutrients, nutrient needs and interrelations 9
How to determine what your body needs 11

I.2 FAT: SATURATED, MONOUNSATURATED, POLYUNSATURATED   16
Lipids, liquid and hard fat 17
Saturated fatty acids (SFA)
Saturated (hard) fat hardens the arteries 18
Monounsaturated fatty acids (MUFA).....................................18
Polyunsaturated fatty acids (PUFA) 19
PUFAs soften arteries..19
Essential (EFAs) vs. non essential fatty acids.........................19
Energy vs. Drive..20

I.3 ESSENTIAL FATTY ACIDS   23
Essential Fats: The ω3 and ω6 families 24
Precursors and Derivatives..25
The omega-3 (ω3) family...25
Sources of ω3: vegetables and fish; Fish and fish oils.............26
The omega-6 (ω6) family..26
Sources of ω6: vegetables, cattle and poultry........................26
The role of fat in good health 27
People should eat more EFAs..27
The need for precursors and derivatives................................28
Some people need fish oils 29
Consequences of ω6 deficiency...29

Consequences of ω3 deficiency 30
Isomers and *Trans fatty acids(TFAs)*...32
Hydrogenated, processed fat contains TFAs..32
Popular misconceptions...34
Essential Oils vs. Essential Fatty Acids (**EFAs**) 35
Differences with other authors 38
USDA **Food Pyramid**..38
Which is better, butter or margarine. Use oils instead 39
For health professionals 40
Description and Names; Biochemical characteristics....................40, 41
Functions 43
Diagnosis of EFA abnormalities aids in the prevention and treatment of:47
Treatment & management of EFA abnormalities 48
Technical issues on fatty acids 49

I.4 CARBOHYDRATES AND PROTEIN   55
Carbohydrates 56
We need a minimum of 3 ounces per day..56
Extra carbohydrate is stored as fat; it does not burn fat 56
Complex carbohydrates contain many nutrients 57
Proteins 58
We need to eat 2-4 ounces of protein every day...................................59

I.5 VITAMINS AND MINERALS   62
What are vitamins and minerals 62
Most people may be eating the wrong mixtures of vitamins and
minerals...63
Effects of deficiencies 64
Practical guidelines 64
Do we need fortified foods? 66
Most likely deficiencies..67

I.6 FIBER, WATER AND OTHER NUTRIENTS   68
Fiber or roughage 69
Some fibers prevent constipation; others lower cholesterol 69
Too much fiber can interfere with mineral absorption..............................69
Water...70
Lecithin and choline; Phytochemicals..71

I.7 CHOLESTEROL   72
Cholesterol; Most people eat too many calories which are converted to
hard saturated fat 73
We need cholesterol. Only in combination with excess saturated fat in the
body does it become dangerous. 74

It is the type of fat and total calories you eat that matters, not just
cholesterol or saturated fat 75
Animal fat is high in cholesterol and low in PUFA 76
Why lower cholesterol; "Good" vs. "Bad" cholesterol 76
High cholesterol and high blood pressure are not diseases: They are
indicators of health status 77

I.8   NORMAL AND ABNORMAL CHOLESTEROL LEVELS   78
Normal means average in medicine 78
You want a healthy, not average, cholesterol level 79
Healthy levels are under 150 mg/dl for all ages 81

I.9   NOTHING BUT THE BEST   83
Excess protein or carbohydrate equals excess fat 84
Regulation and equilibrium 85
Exceptions: When you are sick 86
Corrections for a lifetime of poor eating habits 86

II.1   BLOOD TESTS   89
Why you need to know about tests; The use of tests 89, 90
No one can have all tests done 91
Blood tests: general indications 91

II.2   USE OF FAT BY THE BODY   83
Lipoproteins are blood vehicles that carry fat 93
Increased HDL particles suggest low risk 95
Cardiovascular disease and hardening of the arteries 96

II.3   TESTS FOR CARDIOVASCULAR DISEASE   98
Cholesterol tests; High cholesterol is a sign, not a disease 98
Total Cholesterol; **HDL** Cholesterol; **LDL** cholesterol. 100
VLDL Cholesterol; Total Cholesterol divided by HDL cholesterol 100
The risk of Coronary Artery Disease vs. **Total Cholesterol/HDL** ... 101
Triglycerides 101
Coagulation tests (tests for **clots**) 102
A long **bleeding time** may help people with hardening of the arteries. 102
A very long bleeding time can give you anemia 102
Platelet Aggregation 103
Apoproteins 103
The **fatty acid profile EFA-SR** 104
Assessing the risk of coronary artery disease (**CAD**) 104

III.1   CARDIOVASCULAR DISEASE   107
Aspects of cardiovascular disease 107

Table of Contents   v

Atherosclerosis, arteriosclerosis and thrombosis.....................................108
Heart attack or **myocardial infarction** 112
Hypertension; **Stroke**; **Diabetes**; Combined Effects.........113, 114, 115, 116
Warning signs of heart disease or stroke   117

III.2   PEOPLE WITH CORONARY ARTERY DISEASE   119
Case histories...119
Factors that increase and decrease the risk of cardiovascular disease...121
Doctors who used essential fats to treat heart disease and high cholesterol124
Sudden death is often predictable and preventable 126
Heart disease is a silent killer 129
Physicians and dentists have heart disease and high cholesterol...........129
You are never too old or too sick to improve your health 130
A man with prostate cancer and heart disease....................................131
A diabetic patient with high cholesterol 132

III.3   RISK FACTORS FOR CORONARY ARTERY DISEASE   134
Risk Factors; Smoking; **High blood pressure** (Hypertension)......134, 135
Elevated cholesterol/ HDL cholesterol 135
High glucose levels and Diabetes; Overweight.....................................136
Stress; Alcohol; Genetics (family factors)......................................137, 138

III.4   BASIC PREVENTION PROGRAM   140
How you can improve your health; treatment is simple.........................141
Do not smoke; achieve ideal (not normal) weight 143
A big body burdens your heart 144
Exercise maintains your muscle tone and weight......................................144
Change your fat: 147

III.5   CURRENT AMERICAN DIET   151
What is wrong with our usual diet 152
Where do you stand 153
Natural complex carbohydrates contain EFAs 153
What you can do: hints to eat better...154
Easily lose 25 pounds and 50 units of cholesterol 156

III.6   MODERN PREVENTION DIET   157
The basic food groups 161
Vegetables, Grains, Fruits, Seeds, nuts 161
Fish, Poultry, Pork, Cattle, Dairy..162
Plan your meals using foods, not nutrients 162
Excess calories are converted to saturated fat 163
Eat more **Essential Fats**...166

Precursor (parent) or EFAs; Derivatives (daughter) of EFAs 168
How essential fats have evolved 170
Prevention vs. Treatment 175

III.7 WEIGHT LOSS   180

What is overweight?; How to make a diet work 180, 181
Steps to follow; Other hints to change your eating habits 181, 183
The secret to weight loss: scientific basis 186
Lose fat, not water or protein 186
Losing weight means eating better foods 187
Typical plan (weight loss) 188
Foods to eat: low calorie, high volume, high fiber 189
The Boston Egg White Diet: A diet for weight loss 189
Example of a typical day 193
Are low fat diets dangerous for you? 195
Do you have enough EFAs in your body? 195
Are you eating foods without EFAs? 196
The future of overweight and obesity 196
Is there hope in the new fats and fat substitutes? 199
Eating more carbohydrates does not help you burn more fat 202
EFAs do not make you burn more fat but can make you less hungry 202

V.1 FATS THAT LOWER CHOLESTEROL AND PREVENT HEART DISEASE

Treatment Objectives 206
Make your blood less likely to form clots 206
Reducing your blood fat 207
Softening your vessels and normalizing blood pressure 207
Normalizing blood sugar (glucose) 207
Creating healthy blood cells 208
Improving organ function 208
Symptoms vs. Disease; Drugs vs. Nutrition 209
Case studies: The care of two patients with signs of heart disease 212

IV.2 OILS AND FATS   215

Essential fat content of common fats and oils 215
How to use oils; Fatty acid composition of common foods 217, 218
Oil Effects: what EFAs do 218

IV.3 FISH OILS   220

Fish versus Fish Oils; Desirable effects 221
Why fish oils instead of fish; Types of fish oils; Purchasing fish oil 225

IV.4   PUTTING IT ALL TOGETHER   229
When to use fish and vegetable oils...231

General rules about fatty acid treatment.................................232
Start with a mixture high in ω3 233
How much oil should you take? What type of diet should you follow?235
ω3 vs. ω6: General guidelines...235
General steps to correct EFA abnormalities.............................236
Most people also need more ω6 fatty acids..............................242
Other conditions that respond to fatty acid mixtures..................242
General comments about oil use 243
Case study: A 71 year old with heart disease 244
How to lower *trans* fatty acid (**TFAs**) levels 245

IV.5   DIETS FOR SPECIFIC DISEASES   247
Severe Heart disease; bypass surgery 248
Clot obstruction is the final event 249
How to achieve proper clot formation......................................249
Fish oils rapidly decrease clot formation 249
Less oil with bleeding, more with narrow vessels 250
Poor circulation...251
Case Study: Coronary Artery Disease with hyperlipidemia and high *trans*
plasma levels 251
What causes **hypertension**?; About blood pressure.......................253
Stroke..255
Hyperlipidemia and dyslipidemia; Treatment.............................258
Diabetes Mellitus; Kidney Disease; **Arthritis**..............259, 260, 261
Allergies and Asthma; Dry and itchy skin 263, 264
Cholesterol and fat in Cancer 266
Neurological Disorders..269
Inflammatory Bowel Disease (Crohn's Disease and Ulcerative Colitis) .269
Diarrhea; Inflammation; Obstruction; Malabsorption271, 272,.273, 274
Malnutrition; Treatment of Crohn's disease..................274, 277
Short bowel syndromel **Cystic Fibrosis** (CF)..............279, 280
Case study: Cystic Fibrosis and Crohn's disease with EFA Deficiency..281
Infection - AIDS 281
Adrenoleukodystrophy (ALD) and related disorders.....................282
Sickle Cell disease 283

IV.6   THE EFFECT OF AGE, GENES AND TEMPERATURE   286
Children; Infants and very young children.....................287, 289
Late adolescents and adults; Middle age; Elderly 290, 291

If you eat few calories per day (under 1,500), you may need vitamin and
mineral supplements 292
Your ancestry or genes; Your environment: cold or warm climate 293

IV.7   OTHER POPULATION GROUPS   295
Men and women...295
Premenstrual syndrome; Pregnant women 298
Active vs. passive physical activity...299
Anemia, bleeding, burns, disease 299

V.1   HOW TO EVALUATE A DIET   301
Which diets to select and why 302
A problem with most diets 302
Most common diets produce only mild improvements 302
The American Heart Association diet (AHA) 303
The US Department of Agriculture recommendations for a "healthy diet"..304
Vegetarian Diets; Macrobiotic Diets; 306, 308; The Living Foods Diet...310

V.2   MORE DIETS   313
Weight Watchers (WW) 314
The New American Diet 315
The Scarsdale Diet..316
The Pritikin Program of Diet and Exercise 316
The Setpoint Diet..317

V.3   THE EFA DIET IN THIS BOOK   319
The approach of this book 319
The role of the essential fats and natural, raw foods 320
Prevention vs. Treatment...323

V.4   SHOPPING FOR THE RIGHT FOODS; RECIPES   325
Where to buy 325; Fatty acid related products 326
Fat replacements...328
How to prepare meals using oils.; You can make your own mayonnaise 330
Recipes for chocolate lovers..330
Where there is a will, there is a way...334
Glossary..335
Appendix 338
Tables and Figures, 368 (A1-A16), Tables of Fatty Acids, 384 (C1-C6);
NIH Cholesterol recommendations, 391 (E1-E8), Food Pyramid 398, (D1)
INDEX 399

ACKNOWLEDGMENTS

Thanks to my parents, who provided continued support during many difficult years (in sickness and in health, in poverty and in wealth, without ever demanding too much from myself). Without the help of my parents I would not have been able to attend college and complete Medical School. My father spent many days sitting in front of a computer entering data for my research, and helping me with paperwork and other related tasks. My mother helped me with household tasks so that I could have more time for my research. My parents and my child were there when I needed them. To M, who supported me when I needed it. To my teachers and colleagues who felt that increased emphasis should be placed on nutritional therapy and EFAs, and who asked me to write this book. To JEB, and to numerous colleagues, who spent countless hours helping to make this book more readable. To those who gave me a hard time and made life miserable for me and in the mysterious ways of life contributed to my being here and writing this book.

DISCLAIMER

This book will help you communicate more effectively with your physicians. It will teach you how to ask them intelligent questions and understand their recommendations and instructions. You must keep in mind that many suggestions made here require sophisticated medical tests in order to be implemented. They therefore require the continuous advice and guidance of a physician, nutritionist or individual with similar expertise. They are in no way intended to replace your doctor or to teach you how to treat yourself. All medical issues, including those dealing with circulation and heart disease, are extremely complex. There are too many hidden factors involved for it to be safe for lay people to attempt to treat themselves without an expert physician. But the wrong diagnosis and the wrong treatment, however well intended, could make the disease worse, and would ultimately make it more difficult to diagnose the correct disorder.

To make complex topics available to the general public we have simplified the material presented. Therefore, some of the statements made are incomplete from a scientific point of view. We[1] have included scientific references for those who want to learn more about the science of nutrition. Because each person is different it is impossible for us to provide advice that is appropriate for each and every person who may read this book. I can tell you what I do, and what is good for humans, but I cannot tell you what is best for you. Your decision requires a balance of risks, benefits, inconvenience, time and money. Your physician or nutritionist will help you tailor the ideas of this book to your unique needs.

Warning/disclaimer. This is only a book. It is not intended to provide diagnosis or treatment advice. All the statements made in this book represent only the personal opinion of the author. Comments, reviews and criticisms of diets or writings by other people are only the author's opinions and beliefs and are intended only to review and discuss the opinions of the author of this book. No representations, either express or implied, are made or given regarding the medical consequences of opinions herein presented. Please consult a physician and nutritionist who can interpret test results and provide the appropriate treatment for you in accordance with the entire clinical evaluation and other test results. Do not self-diagnose or treat. Ask your physician to analyze your blood to determine whether or not you have insufficient amounts of essential fats (EFAs).

All cases presented describe composites of people and have been created for this book. Any similarities to actual individuals or institutions is circumstantial and fictitious. No criticism is intended of any particular person or institution.

---

[1] The word "I" and "we" are used interchangeably throughout this book.

FOREWORD

This is not "just another book on nutrition" written by someone who has read a number of articles and said again what has been said in a hundred other books. Dr. Siguel has synthesized years of his original research into a readable book with a unique message and practical recommendations. Just a glance at the footnotes at the end of each chapter will provide the reader with evidence that Dr. Siguel is a prolific researcher. I have had the unique opportunity of working closely with Dr. Siguel for the last five years. I can attest that his mind works very fast, that his ideas are original. He has focused all his energies on the "obscure" area of fatty acid metabolism and in this book crystallizes his ideas in a readable fashion so that both health practitioners and the general public will be able to understand and apply the fruit of his labor. He has developed new, far reaching concepts about the role of fatty acids in health and disease, challenging the established medical community on many fronts. Understanding this, I predict that this text will stir controversy and hopefully will lead to greater emphasis in furthering research in this most important area of medicine.

Dr. Siguel presents his credentials in the introduction. Therefore, I will not repeat them. However, I would like to emphasize that his mathematical expertise and medical knowledge have been combined with a driving interest in fatty acids that have led him to develop theoretical models and expand our understanding of the role of fatty acids. He has refined methods of fatty acid analysis, increasing ten-fold the sensitivity of detecting fatty acid insufficiency. We expect to continue publishing articles in scientific journals, providing further evidence of the extent (prevalence) and importance of essential fatty acids and *trans* fatty acids.

My foreword would be incomplete if I did not mention Dr. Siguel's style of writing. He uses analogies widely and these keep the reader's interest. He has a biting sarcasm and sense of humor which can be noted as early as his initial Acknowledgments. He provides a list of "excuses for dieters" and recommendations on "how to die sooner". These tongue-in-cheek segments keep the reader awake and allow the real message to permeate.

I recommend this landmark book to you. Once read, you will have a greater understanding of the role of fats in disease prevention and management.

Robert H. Lerman, M.D, Ph.D.

Robert H. Lerman M.D., Ph.D.   **July 10, 1994**

Director, Clinical Nutrition, Boston University Medical Center Hospital.

Director, Clinical Nutrition, Jewish Memorial Hospital and Rehabilitation Center.

Assistant Professor of Medicine, Boston University School of Medicine

Assistant Professor of Nutritional Sciences, Goldman School of Graduate Dentistry.

Past Chief of Medicine at US Army Hospitals.

Medical Degree from Jefferson Medical College, Philadelphia, PA.

Ph.D. in Nutritional Biochemistry from MIT.

Board Certified in Internal Medicine. Cardiovascular Research Fellow. Fellow in Nephrology.

Acting Chief of Nephrology, Soroka Medical Center, Beer Sheba, Israel.

Chairman, Nutrition Committee, Boston University Medical Center Hospital.

Consultant to the Park Plaza Hotel to develop and design their Lifestyle Cuisine (meals that are nutritionally balanced and contain essential fats)

Member of Mass. Medical Society and American Society for Parenteral and Enteral Nutrition.

Invited speaker on nutrition, heart disease, renal disease, and obesity at Harvard-affiliated Hospitals.

Author of several articles and book chapters on Nutrition and the Medical Management of Obesity.

Director, Evans Nutrition Clinic, Boston Univ. Medical Center.

PREFACE

Why I wrote this book

I wrote this book to answer the questions that patients, friends and physicians ask me at parties, lectures and consultations. In my research, I have discovered that many Americans are deficient in essential fats. Correcting these deficiencies with dietary change, and sometimes with fish and vegetable oil supplements, leads to improved health and well-being.

At the end of my lectures on nutrition to health professionals, usually several people from the audience, all specialists in some field of medicine, come and ask me for personal advice. I cannot provide good advice, even to a physician, in 5 minutes or less. In addition, many physicians and friends call me and want to know what to eat, what blood tests to have done, or have questions about a specific food. I am asked questions such as: What blood tests should I have? Should I use safflower oil? Sunflower oil? Canola oil? Which one is best? Why? How should I use the oil? What about saturated fat? Butter? Margarine? Is my calcium level OK? Should I take more magnesium? Is it really dangerous to eat hydrogenated oils and *trans* fatty acids?

Over the years I have prepared lists of tests, guidelines for test interpretation, foods to eat, etc. for physicians. I expanded on these ideas while I prepared the 1986 and 1987 Nutrition and Cholesterol Exhibits for the Annual Meeting of the Massachusetts Medical Society. There, we distributed several handouts, but they only covered a few of the critical issues. A little information leads to more questions. In the 1990's I lectured at professional meetings. The response is always the same: People ask me where they can find information about my research. After I appeared on TV, radio and various magazines, I was deluged with questions and requests for copies of my articles and notes.

In 1994, the American College of Cardiology called a press conference to announce my research linking the types of fat that people eat to abnormal cholesterol levels and heart disease.[1] In the Fall of 1994, the journal *Metabolism* published my study where I presented data to support my view that the balance of Essential Fatty Acids (**EFAs**) are the most significant nutritional factor influencing whether people get coronary artery disease. In that article I explain the science behind the concept that EFAs and total calories are the major nutritional factors in cardiovascular disease. Eating more or less saturated fat, cholesterol or monounsaturated fatty acids are far less significant.

The Surgeon General's report identifies the type of fat that people eat as one of the most significant factors in health and disease. However, the US Surgeon General's report states that EFA deficiencies are reported rarely in the United States[2] (p. 58). The idea that Essential Fatty Acid deficiency (**EFAD**) is a major cause in cardiovascular disease was proposed by two scientists, Dr. Sinclair and Dr. Ahrens in the 1970's. A major problem with Dr. Sinclair's theory was the lack of evidence of EFA deficiency in people with coronary artery disease. Given the high prevalence of coronary artery disease in the USA, if it is associated with EFA deficiencies, biochemical evidence of EFA deficiency should be widespread in the general population. Unfortunately, researchers were not able to find evidence of EFA deficiency in the general population, except for a few rare patients with severe malabsorption of fats. As a result, the hypothesis linking EFAs to heart disease became discredited and forgotten. Instead, the emphasis was shifted to lowering saturated fat and cholesterol. For food companies, increasing the amount of EFAs in foods is expensive (because the EFAs are unstable). However, it is relatively easy to eliminate saturated fat and cholesterol and replace it with monounsaturated and *trans* fatty acids. Because many enzymes and steps are involved in the making of cholesterol by the body, companies can develop many drugs to lower blood's cholesterol. Everybody was happy with these events.

While I was in medical school I proposed that abnormalities of EFA metabolism and EFAD cause alterations of cell membrane fluidity and other biochemical changes that cause disease. These alterations in turn cause abnormal levels of cholesterol. I developed a method to measure EFA deficiency which is about 10 times more sensitive than methods used by previous researchers. In the 1980's I published several studies with my new methods. I proposed that EFA deficiencies were highly prevalent in the US. Unfortunately my theories were not taken seriously, and in fact my research funds ended up being practically eliminated.

With personal funds and some government support I continued my research. My results supported the hypothesis by Sinclair that the ratio of PUFA/NoPUFA, that is, the ratio of all polyunsaturated fat to other types of fat, is "the most important factor in atherosclerotic disease and in coronary thrombosis".[3] Like Sinclair and Ahrens,[4] I proposed that *a diet low in fat, which is likely to be deficient in EFAs, may not lead to a reduced risk of coronary artery disease, but may actually increase the risk*. This increase in risk is because excess carbohydrates and protein are converted by the body to saturated fat. I now have found that EFA abnormalities are quite prevalent in the USA. According to my research, they are the most significant nutritional factor in abnormal levels of cholesterol, in coronary artery disease and in high blood pressure. Other researchers are finding that EFA abnormalities are a major factor in the complications of diabetes, brain function, arthritis, child growth and development, PMS, immune system function and a wide range of body functions in health and disease.[5]

I have learned a sad lesson on the politics of nutrition research; it has been a tremendous financial strain for me to research the role of EFAs in nutrition and health. This should not be surprising, since my research has shown that huge amounts of government money are wasted on useless research, aimed at testing old hypotheses about saturated fat and cholesterol while avoiding the fundamental role of EFAs in human nutrition. My research indicates that current recommendations encourage people to eat foods low in EFAs and high in *trans* fatty acids, and therefore contribute to the premature death of hundreds of thousands of Americans. Companies that have invested hundreds of millions of dollars to prepare foods very low in fat, saturated fat and cholesterol would not like people to know that low fat, low EFA foods are not necessarily healthy. It is my position that current food labeling encourages companies to develop unhealthy products low in EFAs and total fat. A company who develops a food product with an excellent balance of EFAs would probably be ignored because it is high in fat. Furthermore, products high in EFAs may need to contain some saturated fats (for stability and texture). A product with an excellent EFA balance may appear less desirable than one high in dangerous *trans* fatty acids because it contains more saturated fat.

Drug companies that target their research to drugs that lower cholesterol would need to change their strategy when people realize that cardiovascular disease is in great part caused by abnormalities of

EFAs which *cannot* be corrected with drugs. Because EFAs are cheap and found in inexpensive oils and vegetables, it would be difficult for drug companies to recover millions spent on advertising new drugs to lower cholesterol. Also, researchers who have spent years "proving" that saturated fat is the culprit do not wish their reputations tarnished or their funds decreased. Government agencies who developed nutritional recommendations which omit the role of EFAs could fear the embarrassment (or even unemployment) which ought to follow a discovery that millions of dollars have been wasted.[6] When I came forward with evidence that EFA abnormalities are quite common, and are a major contributory factor in coronary artery disease and abnormal cholesterol levels, I found that my research was rejected by major public health organizations and my research funds were in great part eliminated by the Federal Government. Fortunately, other scientific groups consider my findings to be highly promising, and continue to call me to lecture and write about them.

Many members of the scientific community have warned me to expect great opposition from groups who have an economic interest in the beliefs surrounding nutrition and heart disease. Hundreds of millions of dollars are spent each year on "proof" that some saturated fats are actually healthy. Additional millions, largely federal and pharmaceutical, are spent pointing the finger at cholesterol as the main culprit in heart disease. In turn, pharmaceutical companies develop and market cholesterol-lowering drugs. Everyone is satisfied with this set of beliefs, including a public which prefers magic pills to the willful self-scrutiny involved in dietary change. I am not a believer in conspiracy theories; corporate leaders of food companies, pharmaceutical companies, and dogmatic researchers did not meet in a dark closet and decide to thwart public revelation of the connection of EFAs to heart disease. But I would not be surprised to find that some individuals or corporations have a lot to gain by delaying my research findings for as long as possible. Nor would I doubt the administration's desire to avoid embarrassment when it is found that the government is squandering hundreds of millions of dollars in useless nutrition and fat research.

The federal government is not supporting enough EFA research

Many well-known scientists believe that the US government prefers to spend money on complex and expensive trials of drugs and invasive procedures rather than safer and more effective nutritional therapies. Medical students and interns spend thousands of hours, entire courses, studying drugs which are often outdated by the time they graduate. Yet they spend only a few hours learning about nutrition. Dr. Irwin H. Rosenberg, MD, Director, USDA Human Nutrition Research Center on Aging at Tufts University, sent me a letter describing nutrition programs, wherein he stated: *"For too long nutrition has been denied its proper role in American medicine. Billions of dollars are spent on the treatment of disease each year, but very little is spent in research on nutrition, which is often the key to the prevention of disease. Few doctors have the time or the inclination to teach those aspects of diet which are essential to their patients' well-being. It's no wonder, then, that misinformation abounds. And many people who are health-conscious end up listening to advice that is unsupported by sound research."*

In fact, as of 1994, there are no official nutritional recommendations or guidelines that tell people that they must eat EFAs. The Food and Drug Administration does not require companies to indicate the amounts of EFAs in their foods, or to even state that the foods contain or omit EFAs. There is no practical way for the consumer to identify foods rich in EFAs and low in *trans* fatty acids.

In 1993 I published a study showing that *trans* fatty acids (**TFAs**) found in hydrogenated and processed oils are associated with abnormal lipid levels and with heart disease. Since then I lectured at the Department of Nutrition, Harvard School of Public Health, Brigham and Women's Hospital (Boston, MA), Boston University Medical Center Hospital, and numerous other medical meetings and centers across the USA. By 1994 major newspapers and TV stations across the country were stating that TFAs were dangerous and a major risk for heart disease. In an editorial in the *American Journal of Public Health,* which was publicized across the country, Drs. Willett and Ascherio (Dept. of Nutrition, Harvard School of Public Health) stated that *"more than 30,000 deaths per year may be due to consumption of partially hydrogenated vegetable fat."* The authors recommend that *"special warning labels should be used on these products* [such as fast foods] *indicating that they were prepared with partially hydrogenated vegetable fat."* This is the same recommendation I have been making to the FDA for more than 10 years. In a related article *"Diet and Health: What should be eat" (Science, 1994;264:532-537),* Dr. Willett comments on the USDA dietary recommendations represented by a "food pyramid" and states: *"Inevitable, such a document represents a mix of well-supported findings, educated guesses, and political compromises with powerful economic interests such as the dairy and meat industries."*

My research indicates that the USDA "food pyramid" recommendations are incorrect because they do not inform people about their need for essential fats. Moreover, the food labels required by the FDA are misleading because they do not require the content of EFAs in foods. ***The most significant nutritional factor in health and disease is having the proper balance of essential fats in your body.***

Despite a keen interest in nutrition, there is very little sound knowledge about the relationship of fat and cardiovascular disease, even among medical personnel. To respond to that interest and to help people to live longer and healthier lives by modifying their eating habits, I decided to write a book presenting the results of my research both to the general public and to medical professionals.

References and Notes

[1] Ironically, this was the same research that the American Heart Association (AHA) had rejected for presentation at their annual meeting in 1993, presumably because it was not considered important for their purposes. I requested an explanation from the AHA and I was unable to obtain a satisfactory explanation.

[2] The Surgeon General's Report on Nutrition and Health. US Department of Health and Human Services, PHS publication No. 88-50210, 1988.

[3] Sinclair, H. Dietary fats and coronary heart disease. Controversy. *Lancet*, 1980; i:414:415.

[4] Ahrens EH. Dietary fats and coronary heart disease: unfinished business. *Lancet*, 1979; ii:1345-48.

[5] Dr. Hugh Sinclair was one of the greatest nutritional researchers in England until his recent death. Sinclair was a direct descendant of King Woldonius of Finland and King Nor of Norway. A brief description of his life is found in an article written by David F. Horrobin, "Hugh Sinclair: A Memoir", Proceedings of the Third International Congress on Essential Fatty Acids and Eicosanoids, American Oil Chemists' Society, Champaign, IL, 1992. The comments that follow are based on that article. Dr. Sinclair did research on EFAs and nutrition. He was honored by the Netherlands, the United Kingdom and the US for "his outstanding accomplishments in relieving the famine" in Holland and parts of Europe after World War II. Dr. Sinclair did pioneering research on ω3 fatty acids. He found that Canadian Eskimos had low incidence of coronary artery **(CAD)** disease because they ate ω3 fatty acids from fish. In 1979 he ate a true

Eskimo diet for about three months to study the effects of fatty acids on atherosclerosis and clotting. In 1956 a famous Nobel laureate removed Dr. Sinclair from his laboratory, took his equipment and made it impossible for him to continue his research. After that, many scientists refused to consider his findings, and for many years his recommendations languished. In 1956, Sinclair wrote a letter to the journal *Lancet*, i:381-383, stating that the great majority of the diseases of Western civilization might be related to abnormalities of EFA metabolism and EFA deficiency. Because EFAs are essential for every cell in the body, a deficiency of EFAs affects every organ. The actual clinical symptoms will depend on the individual genes, the environment, other nutrients and the balance of EFAs. I never met Dr. Sinclair and found out about his work by accident while reading various scientific articles. At that time I sent him some material I had written. Dr. Sinclair wrote me a very nice letter indicating his appreciation for my research. Unfortunately, he died before I had a chance to meet and speak with him in person.

6   For more than 10 years I have been writing to government agencies explaining that EFAs and *trans* fatty acids (**TFAs**) are more important than saturated or monounsaturated fats. I have requested repeatedly that the Food and Drug Administration (**FDA**) require that labels include the amounts of essential, *trans* and *isomer* fatty acids (unusual fatty acids often caused by food processing). I have informed them that information on the amount of calories from saturated fats is practically irrelevant. They have refused to answer. I also wrote to the USDA to explain that their nutritional recommendations are faulty because they omit the key role of EFAs and the potential harmful effects of TFAs and isomers. The USDA, through one of its contractors, refused to take my research into consideration and instead opted for prohibiting me from using USDA funded research and facilities or associating myself with USDA-funded researchers. I was refused funding to prove the importance of EFAs and TFAs in health and disease. I wrote to the USDA to inform them that their "pyramid" was misleading because it encourages people to eat foods low in EFAs and states that oils "provide little else nutritionally" other than calories, when in fact some oils provide EFAs essential to human health. I wrote to the Department of Health and Human Services and the National Institutes of Health to explain that their recommendations to lower saturated fat are misleading because they omit the role of a balance of ω3 and ω6 EFAs. Again, I accomplished nothing. I have spoken with many scientists who done research on EFAs and they have told me similar stories: Their funding was discontinued, their warnings about the needs for EFAs were rejected. It seems as if everybody is happy with the status quo: The government makes ambiguous nutritional recommendations that please everyone, it imposes labels that appease consumers and manufacturers, drug companies can continue to market drugs to lower cholesterol, and expensive treatment for heart disease continues to make thousands of people very rich. By 1994, the winds of change have begun to blow. Several researchers have indicated that TFAs are dangerous to health and may contribute to the deaths of tens of thousands of people. In 1994 I published an article describing the scientific basis for my findings about the role of EFAs in abnormal cholesterol and heart disease, and another explaining why following the USDA pyramid recommendations would cause more heart disease than it could prevent. More articles will follow on the dangers of low fat, low calorie diets, the need for a balance of ω3 and ω6 fatty acids, and the follies of the emphasis on cholesterol and saturated fat.

INTRODUCTION

Nutrition is the key to your good health

This book gives you the information you need to take control of your health. It provides a thorough explanation of how to eat in order to achieve ideal cholesterol levels, lower high blood pressure and prevent the formation of clots that cause heart attacks and stroke. It is my belief that knowledge about nutrition will help you to live a long and healthy life. Modern research has shown that the dietary program recommended here for the purpose of preventing and treating cardiovascular disease will also prevent some forms of cancer. It will also increase overall well being and longevity.

My research has identified some of the most significant nutritional factors in health and disease. The current recommendations of many researchers and public health organizations are that people should eat less saturated fat and less cholesterol, and that they should replace the fat in their diets with carbohydrates. Commercials and news writers state or imply that less fat is better. My research has shown that *the "official" goal of a "zero fat diet" is wrong*. **The relevant factors are total calories from all sources** and the amount of a key type of fat called "**Essential Fatty Acids**" (**EFAs**). I believe that you can eat all types of natural fat as long as you maintain ideal weight, eat a balanced diet and eat enough EFAs. Eating too many carbohydrates is dangerous because the body converts excess amounts of carbohydrates into saturated fatty acids. I proposed that recent government recommendations for a food "pyramid" that encourages people to eat more breads, pasta and cereals is misleading. What matters most is that people eat enough EFAs, in proper proportion to the rest of their diet. Contrary to popular belief, whole grain cereals, breads and pasta are not healthier than high fat foods. High fat natural foods such as nuts, which are high in nutrients and EFAs, may be healthier than low fat breads, pasta and cereal deficient in EFAs.

Many people who seek to maintain their weight on a low calorie, low fat diet are depriving their body of EFAs and are likely to suffer from hormone abnormalities and cardiovascular disease. Young, slim people,

Preface, Introduction, Summary

children and pregnant women are particularly at risk of developing permanent impairments in their mental abilities because their brains are deprived of the EFAs essential for brain function. Deficiencies and abnormalities of EFAs are not immediately fatal. Like high cholesterol and high blood pressure, EFA abnormality is a silent killer that slowly destroys your organs and hits you after middle age. Then, instead of living a full and alert life with full mental abilities, people with EFA abnormalities find they have exhausted the reserves of their bodies, their hearts and kidneys, and impaired the function of their brain cells.

There are many people who want to live longer, lead more productive lives, increase their mental functions and have healthier bodies. A **balance** of the different types of EFAs holds the key to these health improvements. It is not a simple or easy task. It requires learning new facts about nutrition, and often times dramatic change in lifestyle. However, for those who care enough and sincerely want to improve their health, balancing their nutrients, including EFAs, is the best way to go about it.

Cardiovascular disease is the biggest killer of Americans

"More than two of every five Americans dies of cardiovascular disease".[1] Diseases of the heart and cerebrovascular diseases are by far the most frequent cause of death in the USA. Over 50 million people suffer from cardiovascular disease. Over 500,000 people die every year of cardiovascular disease, about twice as many as those who die of cancer, and more than 20 times greater than those who die of AIDS.[2] *Your chances of dying of heart disease or suffering premature handicaps in your life due to hardening of the arteries are far greater than of dying of anything else.* The unfortunate thing is that we help to cause our own deaths; but this means we also can prevent them.

Who dies of heart disease? Reading through newspapers one finds the names of rich and famous people as well as the average folks, all dead at a relatively young age.

- ◆ Senator E. Zorinsky, 58, "died of a heart attack soon after performing in an Omaha Press Club benefit".[3]
- ◆ James F. Fixx, 52, author of two books on running, collapsed and died, apparently of a heart attack, while jogging in Vermont.[4]

- Heinz Nixdorf, 60, founder of the Nixdorf computer company, died of a heart attack in Hanover, Germany, while attending an electronics and computer trade fair. Nixdorf computer 1984 revenues were $1.7B.[5]

- Spaulding, 60, president of the Massachusetts Rehabilitation Hospital in Boston, died in Puerto Rico Friday after suffering a heart attack. [6] (Ironically, his hospital treats people for cardiac rehabilitation and prevention of heart disease.)

- The Dean of a major business school died unexpectedly Monday morning after collapsing in a university office.[7]

- Christina Onassis, shipping heiress and international socialite, dead at 37 of a heart attack.[8]

- Joseph Brown, commander of the frigate USS Constitution, dead at 47 of a heart attack.[9]

- Leo D. Goulet, head of Gerber baby food, dead at 61 of a heart attack while playing golf.[10]

- Giamatti, baseball commissioner, dead of a heart attack at 51.[11]

- Tom Blackaller, three time America's Cup competitor, died at 52 of a heart attack while practicing for a car race.[12]

- Malcolm Forbes, wealthy publisher of business magazines, dead at 70 of a heart attack.[13]

- Tony Conigliaro, famous baseball player, dead at 45 of a heart attack.[14]

- John Candy, actor, dead of a "heart attack at 43, while on location in Mexico".[15]

The list is endless, and it only describes the endpoint of heart disease: death. For each name highlighted in the media, millions more suffer from heart disease and lead handicapped lives. You probably know several people with heart disease. More than 1,000,000 Americans will have a heart attack this year, and about 1/3 of them will die from it. Most adult men over 40 are likely to die prematurely from heart or blood vessel disease caused by eating unhealthful foods. We spend over 20 billion to treat people with heart and kidney disease using surgery, drugs and dialysis, treatments which can never restore the body to its healthy state. Heart disease, and the drugs required to treat it, can weaken the immune defenses of your body, and make you more susceptible to infection and cancer. A weakened heart cannot feed the

Preface, Introduction, Summary

body with life-saving nutrients, destroy toxic chemicals, and fight invaders (i.e., bacteria or cancer cells). Better prevention and nutrition could save billions of dollars spent on heart bypass, angiography, kidney disease and other expensive diagnostic and treatment procedures. The money saved with prevention could help to balance the Medicare budget and provide national health care for everyone, without increasing taxes or placing a burden on employers.

Most heart disease is preventable. Even if you have inherited a predisposition to heart disease you can still prevent it. After all, it's very likely that along with your troublesome genes, you have inherited some damaging dietary habits from your family. A famous cartoonist once said: *"We have seen the enemy and it is us"*. It is up to you to save your life.

You can prevent your heart disease

Why doctors skip nutrition

We are afraid to be told not to eat

A common complaint by patients is: "My doctor never tells me about nutrition. He never tells me what to eat." In fact, most people do not want to hear nutritional advice from their doctor. They do not want to hear about it because they are afraid of what they are going to hear. They are afraid the doctor is going to tell them to EAT LESS. No more doughnuts with the pizza. Beer? Yes, but only on February 29th.

For countless cultural and personal reasons, diet is a very emotional topic. Non-healthful eating is somewhat like smoking: We all know that smoking is bad for us, but some people cannot stop smoking. Do we need a doctor to tell us to stop smoking? Obviously not. So, many doctors no longer tell their patients to stop smoking because if they do, the patients often get upset and find another doctor. We all know the old fable: Kill the messenger of bad news so that the bad news will go away. My own family members have prohibited me from mentioning food, preferring to die rather than face dramatic dietary and lifestyle changes. When they are hospitalized they agree to radical changes, but sometimes it is too late. Unfortunately, when the messenger is ignored, the bad news often arrives in the form of a heart attack or stroke.

Preface, Introduction, Summary

I have seen close friends and family members die because they were ill-advised by friends, relatives and physicians, who told them that one more extra piece of cake could not kill them. It did! I take a dim view of people who visit a sick patient and fill his/her room with cigarette smoke, or of those who insist that people eat excessive amounts of unhealthy food or alcohol at meals and parties under the pretext that "one more will not kill you". We have a responsibility to help the people we care about, or at least not to make it harder for them to make difficult decisions.

Many people prefer to ignore problems, hoping they will just go away. Eating poorly and ignoring the consequences will not improve nor sustain health. If you are reading this book you are the kind of person who is willing to take positive steps to improve your health. Most people want pills, not diet changes. We want to eat any foods we want, and then get a prescription for a magic pill that will make us lose weight and live forever. I wish such a pill existed, but it does not. It cannot exist because you cannot change your body composition overnight. Seeking a magic pill is like seeking the fountain of youth, a cherished fantasy.

We need to pay for prevention

Most doctors want to teach nutrition to their patients. During 1986 and 1987 I helped to prepare exhibits on nutrition and cholesterol-lowering diets for the annual meeting of the Massachusetts Medical Society. I also lecture to physicians on dietary fats and disease prevention. Physicians are very interested in learning about nutrition for themselves and for their patients. Doctors and nutritionists want to eat better to improve their health, and many have followed my advice successfully.

However, presenting nutritional information to patients and treating patients nutritionally is not always easy for reasons that have nothing to do with the validity of the subject. Administrative and economic factors often conflict with optimal medical procedure. For instance, health insurance rarely pays for a nutritional consultation or a visit to a doctor for the purpose of disease prevention rather than treatment. Your insurance is more likely to pay $2,000 for a catheterization, $5,000+ for heart diagnostic tests, and $800 for each day you spend in a hospital, than it is to pay $500 for nutritional tests or $150 for a medical visit to discuss nutrition. It is easy to collect $20,000 for a heart bypass, or $1,500 for medical procedures, but very difficult to collect $150 for a comprehensive nutritional evaluation. The training to provide a comprehensive biochemical nutritional evaluation is often more intensive and complex than the training to become a surgeon. People do not realize the time it takes a nutritionist to review blood test results and consult medical literature, time which is not compensated by the office visit fee.

A blood test for fat analysis that I perform provides a striking example of what can be done in nutritional biochemistry. The test takes more than 10 hrs. over a period of at least one week to calculate the amounts of more than 30 different types of fat in the blood. The test identifies what kinds of fat people have been eating and what kinds of fat they need to eat to correct their conditions. The technology requires the use of many computers and expertise in engineering, physics, chemistry, mathematics and medicine. Several hours are required to interpret each test result. My review of the nutritional abnormalities of the average patient requires more than five hours of time.

Using sophisticated blood tests rarely done by most doctors, expert nutritionists can identify the cause of anemia, or excessive tiredness. They can measure the extent of calcium deficiency, or predict who will die of heart disease. Unfortunately in spite of the value of nutritional studies for the health of the patient, it is difficult to get insurance companies to reimburse patients for nutritional evaluation, or to pay physicians a fair value for time spent analyzing biochemical results, which are frequently more complicated than NMR or CAT scans. Patients, professionals and lay people must work to educate legislatures and insurance companies, so that prevention and nutritional therapy is placed on at least equal footing with heart transplants and kidney dialysis.

Medicine is a complex science.

The human body is an extraordinarily complex machine, with millions of cells and chemical processes. We are made of billions of chemicals operating in a delicate balance that determines life or death. To maintain the optimal balance, the body needs to repair parts that break or wear down, and eliminate surplus material. Each cell is like a small factory. Using enzymes as machines, cells make a wide range of "parts" essential to the body's function and survival. Food provides both the parts for repairs and energy to run the factories. Humans, like other species, have evolved over millions of years to the point where we have unique physical structure, appearance and needs. To satisfy its unique needs, each species requires different "parts", that is, foods or nutrients, and has different "factories", that is, organs and cells which make the needed parts and perform repairs. Although some humans may be "rats", rats are not human. I'm sure you have noticed differences between bees and birds, cats and dogs, and tomatoes and humans. What is an excellent food for a bee or a bird may be a terrible or toxic food for a human.

It is now undisputed that the nutritional needs of different species are quite different. What we feed a tomato plant would not be enough to maintain a human being and vice versa. It is impossible for every species to have all the factories to make everything from scratch, using only air and sunlight. Instead, species, over time, have specialized. The more complex species have factories which produce more complex chemicals. These chemicals provide a higher level of intelligence, but make the species dependent on other species for intermediate chemicals. In this carefully balanced plan of nature, each species depends on others to produce parts or chemicals needed by them. For example, many plants make the vitamins, minerals and Essential Fatty Acids (**EFAs**) which animals need to live, but do not have the factories to make complex EFA derivatives required by the human brain for memory and intelligence.

The task of nutritionists is to identify the optimal diet for humans To decipher our nutritional requirements, scientists depend on two complementary approaches. One approach is a theoretical model of the chemical reactions in the body. Knowing what the body needs and how the chemical factories work, allows us to deduce what the factories of the body need to work efficiently. To test those assumptions, scientists run experiments where people are fed different foods for long periods of time, and determine what foods make people healthier. Unfortunately, it is virtually impossible to run an experiment for years because nobody is willing to eat the same food every day for years. So instead, scientists use the second, "epidemiological" approach. Scientists study groups of people across the world that follow very different diets, and evaluate which group members have the healthiest bodies. Scientists also study the chemical composition of people's bodies to determine how much of each essential nutrient they have. (Examples of essential nutrients are the vitamins, minerals and EFAs). Scientists determine what levels of the essential nutrients are associated with health and what levels are associated with disease. Based on those studies, scientists calculate how much we need to eat of every nutrient.

The objectives of this book

It is my hope that this book will answer most of the questions that people ask about how to improve their health and prevent cardiovascular disease through diet. It will also provide them with the information they need to understand what their doctors say to them, and to ask their doctors pertinent questions about their condition.

I present ideas that are the fruit of work at the frontier of medical research, and not all physicians may be conversant with the full impact of these studies because they are just now being published in medical journals. Readers without scientific background can skip the technical explanations in this book, but they may want to present them to their doctors! These explanations are not necessary for a practical understanding of what to eat and why.

What makes this book different from other books

This book presents the results of my own research. Some of the findings are discussed here for the first time in application to the way people eat. My research is based on humans.

You probably recognize that many scientific studies tell you one thing today, another tomorrow. One researcher says that vitamin E or beta carotene is good for you and prevents cancer. Another finds that it increases cancer or causes more deaths from stroke. It is very difficult, even for scientists, to make sense of the huge amount of data. To compound the problem, most people write about what others write who wrote what others told them. Few have the time to read the original articles. My book is based on my own findings and my experience studying thousands of research subjects and patients. It is based on my personal conversations with leading physicians and researchers around the world, and my reading of original research articles.

My education qualifies me to interpret data. I have a Ph.D. with emphasis on measurement theory and statistics. I have received some of the highest awards from the federal government and participated in most public health committees that deal with health statistics. I have developed methods to evaluate Health Maintenance Organizations (**HMOs**). At one time I was in charge of evaluating HMOs for the federal government, and prepared estimates of costs and benefits to be derived from developing HMOs in the USA, which were submitted to the US Congress as the official estimates for evaluation of health care reform proposals.

In my experience, there are several errors common to many nutritional studies. Researchers do not analyze the actual fatty acid composition of the subjects. Instead, they rely on far less accurate nutritional intake data. Participants in these studies keep journals of their daily food intake. I personally find it nearly impossible to keep track of everything I eat. Similarly, very few subjects can keep accurate records of every food they eat. Even if participants are perfect recorders, the composition of foods depends on many factors and frequently changes without the researcher's knowledge.

In some nutritional research, a few unusual subjects account for most of the results. These extreme points may be due to error in measurement, faulty levels of antioxidants fed to participants, or diets that were not optimized for the body composition of each participant.

Researchers sometimes interpret the data in ways that are not appropriate. Their predictions account for less than 10% of the variability of the data, so that there is 90% not accounted for. Very few researchers publish an explanation of how well their "model" predicts reality, because it will show that their study explains very little about what they intend to explain or predict.

Many studies where people are fed different mixtures of food use less than 100 subjects, and for less than one year. In research, it is humanly impossible to regulate what a person eats for several years. Moreover, there are huge variations in the way people eat. The amount of antioxidants in the food, or the ones taken as supplements, are often not reported to researchers. The actual amounts of EFAs in the foods are rarely known, in part because it costs huge amounts of money to accurately analyze food. Short term studies may produce results which are transient or artifacts of the experimental design. Many researchers are under pressure to find results consistent with their sponsor and reject approaches that are different from what they propose or believe. You may find that a study funded by the dairy industry shows that milk and cheese are wholesome, one funded by the beef industry shows that beef is terrific, and, of course, one by a pharmaceutical company shows that drugs cure disease.

Contents

This book explains the basic concepts of nutrition and diet and the
different types of nutritional components that make up our diets, with
an emphasis on fat. **The type of fat you eat is probably the most
important nutritional factor that determines your health.** Using
this book you will be able to make better food selections and evaluate
the advertising claims made for different food products. You will begin
to realize which claims are justified and which are misleading.

What do you need to know in order to make intelligent choices about
which foods to select and consume? An understanding of the following
aspects of nutrition is crucial.

- **What it means to "eat a balanced diet."** A balanced diet contains
  neither too much nor too little of key nutrients. These key nutrients
  include vitamins, minerals, proteins, carbohydrates, fiber, water,
  and essential fats.

- **How to eat a balance of essential fats and correct metabolic
  fat abnormalities** developed over a lifetime. While a child can get
  all the nutrients he or she needs from a healthy diet, most adults
  need to eat large amounts of EFA supplements in addition to a
  healthy diet to correct for a lifetime of EFA deficiency. Merely
  eating a healthy diet after age 40 is not enough: Heart disease will
  kill long before a healthy diet can cure it. A disease (hardening and
  obstruction of the arteries) that took 40 years to develop must be
  corrected in a few years.

- **Calories and their importance in physical condition.** It is
  useful to understand how the body regulates and controls nutrients
  and calories.

Fortunately, a healthful diet is less costly than an unhealthy diet. And
we can used the money to enjoy life rather than pay a caregiver to push
our wheelchairs.

The fat you eat determines your good health

Our discussion emphasizes fat because it has been shown that the type
of fat we eat is a major determinant of cardiovascular disease, diabetes,
hypertension, and many other diseases that lead to premature aging.
Most of this book explains how to use fats and oils to improve your
health.

Preface, Introduction, Summary

The role of essential fats (EFAs) and fish oils

We humans are made of fat, protein, carbohydrate, vitamins, minerals, water and a few other chemical substances. We get fats in the body not only from the fat in the food we eat, but also from the conversion of excess dietary protein and carbohydrate to stored fat. Proteins and carbohydrates that we eat beyond what our bodies need are converted to a kind of fat called saturated (hard) or monounsaturated fat.

Fats are made of fatty acids. However, the word "fat" is usually used to refer to fatty acids because it is shorter. There is a kind of fat called **polyunsaturated** fat (**PUFAs**), which consists of the essential fatty acids (**EFAs**) linolenic acid (*omega*-3 = ω3) and linoleic acid (*omega*-6 =ω6) and their derivatives. We refer to these fatty acids as "**essential fats.**" Humans cannot make these **EFAs** and must obtain them from their food. EFAs are essential to humans, and most people do not eat enough of them. For these and other reasons, a significant proportion of disease in our society is caused by an imbalance of the types of EFAs that we ought to eat. This book will help you identify and correct EFA abnormalities.

The EFAs are found primarily in vegetables, fish, seeds, and oils. Fish oils and vegetable oils are liquid at room temperature, and usually remain liquid when we eat them. Body structures formed with these polyunsaturated fats are more flexible than the structures formed with hard saturated fats.

We are what we eat

There is a remarkable fact about our food intake and the fat we have in our body. *The kind of fat we store in our body is derived directly from the fat that we eat.* People eating diets high in saturated fat and carbohydrates will accumulate saturated fat in their bodies. People eating mostly polyunsaturated fats will store these essential fats in their bodies. This amazing correlation between food intake and fat storage has enormous consequences for the person who wants to modify his or her diet to prevent or treat cardiovascular disease. Think of it: If you eat hard fat, your arteries will contain hard fat; if you eat soft fat, your arteries are made of soft fat.

The only way to accumulate the essential fats that help prevent heart disease, lower high cholesterol and high blood pressure, and prevent the formation of clots, is to make sure to consume them in your diet.

Eating too many non-EFA calories leads to excess saturated fats in your system. *Decreasing the quantity of saturated fat stored in your body is not only a matter of avoiding saturated fat, as many publications will lead you to believe, but of avoiding unnecessary calories while eating enough essential fats.* A diet high in vegetables and fish leads to the accumulation of essential (soft) fats in your body and better prospects for a future free of cardiovascular disease. Your brain cells will get better nutrients and you will get brighter. (The unfortunate side-effect of this is you will worry more in the face of world problems, environmental disaster and tax time).

About cholesterol

Many physicians and publications speak about the "bad" cholesterol (**LDL**) and the "good" cholesterol (**HDL**). I prefer not to use those terms, because they confuse people and have meaning only as indicators of disease. We do not eat "good" or "bad" cholesterol. We eat cholesterol and fat (saturated, monounsaturated and polyunsaturated fat). Depending on how much cholesterol we eat and the types of fat we eat, our bodies either increase or decrease both good and bad cholesterol. The types of cholesterol in our bodies are primarily determined by the mixture of fats that we eat rather than by the cholesterol that we eat. Eating the proper types of fats helps your body regulate your cholesterol. The mechanisms for this will be explained more extensively later.

No single food is always good or bad: It is the balance that counts

Balanced meals

A general principle of nutrition is that **the body needs a proper balance of all nutrients. Excesses are as bad as deficiencies**. We need a balanced diet of protein, carbohydrate, minerals, vitamins, and fats. Thus, by itself, **no single food is either terribly good or bad. It is the balance of foods that counts**. Eating a balanced diet allows us to eat the foods we like without increasing the risk of getting cardiovascular disease. Eating an unbalanced diet, like imbalances in other areas of life, often leads to disease.

People often ask me: Can I eat bread? Must I stop eating butter? What about steak? Is it dangerous to eat hydrogenated oils? Many foods I like have hydrogenated oils. What can I do about it? If I stop eating hydrogenated fats for a week or a month, will they leave my blood? The answer depends on the other foods they eat and the foods they have been eating for years. A physician can order blood tests that help you to know what kinds of fats and cholesterol you have accumulated during your lifetime. If you have accumulated an excess of the saturated and monounsaturated fat and little essential fat, you need to compensate by eating more EFAs now.

What to eat

Both thin and overweight people need EFAs. In general, in the USA, overweight people have accumulated saturated fat rather than EFAs. Some populations in the world, such as the Eskimos, appear to accumulate essential fats rather than saturated fat because they eat a lot of fish high in essential fats. Their risk of heart disease is correspondingly low. We know that people who have accumulated few essential fats usually have elevated cholesterol and high blood pressure and have a high risk of developing cardiovascular disease.

Your diet should include an appropriate balance of the different types of EFAs found in animal and vegetable foods. Frequently, you will need oil supplements. The balance depends on your lifetime history and accumulated fat and essential fats. Each individual, depending on his particular medical conditions or risk for a particular disease needs a different mixture of EFAs. Some oils will help reduce your high blood pressure. Others prevent clot formation. Some are more effective in lowering the "bad" cholesterol and increasing the "good" cholesterol. Others affect your triglycerides, skin dryness, PMS, etc. We can tell the effects of fats by doing blood tests and evaluating the risk factors present for each person. It is quite different to design a balanced diet for a 2 year old than for a 40 year old man or woman who must correct for 40 years of bad eating.

How to start

I recommend that people follow a careful diet until they bring their risk factors such as elevated levels of cholesterol and high blood pressure to reasonable levels. Then they can resume eating **some** "junk" food as long as they eat foods in proper balance.

This means that a meal high in animal foods should be followed by a period of meals high in vegetable products or fish. Those that cannot

survive without beer, hot dogs and butter may compensate, in part, by
eating selected vegetable oils with their meals.

Start young

To avoid the need for drastic measures we must start with good dietary
habits when we are young. Unfortunately, cardiovascular disease does
not usually hurt immediately after a meal. Because it does not hurt,
people do not associate diet with disease (that is why heart disease is
called the "silent killer"). By the time people get their first heart attack
it may be too late. I often see overweight children whose parents feel
proud that their children are so "robust". But overweight children are
more a symbol of failure to control one's own life than of wealth or good
health.

Taking control of your life

There are very few areas where humans have the power to influence
their own destiny. By changing something so simple as eating habits,
we can change what we are and how we will live. Will we be sickly
people whose lives are darkened by the specter of crippling or fatal
illness, or will we live fully and happily, realizing our potential well into
old age? Are we going to spend most of our lives after 50 moving with
great difficulty because our lungs and heart cannot provide enough
oxygen to our brain, forgetting things because our brain cells are dying
so fast?

It is dizzying to realize how much control we really do have over our
health, and almost frightening to realize how much harm we can do to
ourselves through unwise eating. We must ask ourselves a very
important question: What do we want to be? What is the purpose of a
retirement plan if we will be too decrepit to enjoy our lives? For those
who want to live as long as possible, in full control of their minds and
bodies, this book opens a door to a new lifestyle, with new options and
actions to take that can save lives. Only when we decide to take action
can we reshape ourselves and our lives. The challenges are great, but
what power and freedom we have to meet them! Sadly, it is very easy
to die; it can be very difficult to survive. Patients often feel that living a
healthy life is too much of a burden and they would rather die. But
once life is lost, it does not come back.

How to use this book

The main purpose of this book is to explain how different types of fatty acids affect your health. Each section is organized around one major topic: Nutrition, Diagnostic Tests, Prevention, Treatment, Foods and Diets. Each chapter has a summary and a list of topics at the beginning. You may find it useful to read the summary first, then the chapter, and finally to review the summary again. To assist you with various terms and to place the ideas in context, I have included sections on other aspects of nutrition and health. These sections are simplified and not comprehensive. I have also presented simplified descriptions of many diseases. You should consult other medical books if you require more information.

References and Notes

[1] Source: American Heart Association. Heart and Stroke Facts, Statistical Supplement. Also National Institutes of Health statistics.

[2] Science, News & Comment, Nov. 20, 1987, p.1031. New data clinch heart drug approval.

[3] Zorinsky, age 58. The Boston Globe, March 8, 1987. Front page and p.46.

[4] The Boston Globe picture and statement. July 22, 1984.

[5] The Boston Globe, March 19 1986.

[6] The Boston Globe.

[7] The Boston Globe, Jan 13, 1987.

[8] The Boston Globe, November 20, 1988.

[9] The Boston Globe, July 10, 1987.

[10] The Boston Globe, July 7, 1987.

[11] The Boston Globe, September 12, 1989,

[12] The Boston Globe, Sept. 8, 1989.

[13] The Boston Globe, Feb. 25, 1990.

[14] The Boston Globe Feb. 25, 1990.

[15] The Boston Globe March 5, 1994. As reported, John Candy was a "rotund comedian who starred in 'Uncle Buck and Planes, Trains & Automobiles' ". He was filming a movie when he died of a heart attack. I liked him very much and made me sad to think that his death could have been avoided with an optimal diet.

WHY YOU NEED TO EAT A BALANCE OF DIFFERENT TYPES OF FATTY ACIDS.

BOOK SUMMARY

The 1988 US Surgeon General's report identifies the *type of fat* that people eat as one of the most significant factors in health and disease. Certain types of fats called Essential Fatty Acids (**EFAs**) are critical to good nutrition because humans cannot make them. Just as humans must consume vitamins, they must also get EFAs from food, but in far greater quantities than vitamins. Failure to eat enough EFAs is a cause of hardening of the arteries, abnormal clot formation, coronary heart disease, high cholesterol, and high blood pressure. What should you eat to correct an imbalance of EFAs? That depends on the balance of EFAs in your body. Using the fatty acid profile **EFA-SR,** which measures your EFA status, your physician can determine how to correct an imbalance or deficiency of EFAs.

The diagnosis of EFA abnormalities aids in the prevention and treatment of:

- Cardiovascular disease, stroke, atherosclerosis; poor blood circulation. EFAs reduce, while *trans* and saturated fatty acids increase, the risk of Coronary Artery Disease (**CAD**).

- Hyperlipidemia (abnormal blood fats) and high blood pressure.

- Complications of diabetes, such as eye and kidney problems.

- Complications of pregnancy, including preeclampsia.

- Inflammatory bowel disease; celiac disease; cystic fibrosis; kidney disease.

- Brain and behavior abnormalities in children fed diets low in

EFAs. Such diets include milk & formulas without EFAs.

- Malnutrition; wasting states. The fatty acid test **EFA-SR** aids in appropriate nutritional planning for patients on elemental diets or parenteral (intravenous) alimentation.

EFA deficiency can also exacerbate neurologic abnormalities, Seborrheic dermatitis, coagulation disorders, arthritis, and immune deficiencies. The essential fats known as ω3 (*omega*-3) are critical to proper brain function; those known as ω6 (*omega*-6) soften blood vessels; their balance determines whether you form clots to prevent bleeding or obstruct arteries.

Recent research has found that more than 20% of adults and many children and infants have EFA abnormalities. This deficiency results from insufficient dietary sources of EFAs. Resulting abnormalities are compounded by infant formulas and adult liquid and powder supplements, which do not have enough EFAs, or the correct balance of them. Additionally, mothers with insufficient levels of EFAs may produce EFA deficient milk.

> *Fats are made of three kinds of fatty acids: saturated, monounsaturated and polyunsaturated.*

Popular media has given rise to a common misconception about fats: that is, a fat is exclusively "**saturated**," "**monounsaturated**," or "**polyunsaturated**. All fats are complex mixtures of these fatty acids. Nevertheless, each fat is named after the fatty acid which makes up the majority of its structure. For example, butter is composed primarily of saturated fatty acids (approximately 70%), thus its general classification as a "saturated fat."

The specific amount of each fatty acid within a fat determines whether it is soft or hard. Saturated fatty acids (**SFAs**) are straight molecules. They form foods which are solid at room temperature, such as butter and beef fat. Monounsaturated fatty acids (**MUFAs**) have one "kink" or bend in their molecules. They form foods that are liquid at room temperature, but solid in the refrigerator, such as olive oil. Polyunsaturated fatty acids (**PUFAs**) have 2 or more kinks. They form foods that are liquid even when refrigerated, such as soybean, walnut, canola or flax seed oil. The PUFAs are also known as "**essential fats**" because humans must eat them to survive and cannot make them from

---

other fats. To live healthy lives we must eat PUFAs in significant amounts practically every day.

In general, when we speak of "**fat**", we mean a fat that is solid at room temperature. When we speak of "**oil**", we mean a fat that is liquid at room temperature. Both "fats" and "oils" are made of fatty acids, differing only in their composition. Fats have more saturated fatty acids while oils have more PUFAs.

The kinks in monounsaturated and polyunsaturated oils can be changed from their natural form by cooking, processing or hydrogenation. Hydrogenation is a process that changes liquid oil into a more stable solid which is less likely to turn rancid. This process is commonly used to make margarine and fats used in breads and cookies. Byproducts of this process are *trans* fatty acids (**TFAs**). These fatty acids resemble the straight, saturated molecules which form foods of a solid consistency. TFAs have no known desirable function. They may interfere with normal fatty acid activity, and increase the risk of coronary artery disease. People who eat many hydrogenated oils accumulate TFAs in their blood. With proper diet, they can be eliminated from the blood.

Common Myths

Myth. Eating foods low in cholesterol lowers your blood cholesterol.

The human body makes large amounts of cholesterol. The amount of cholesterol made depends on your overall body chemistry, and particularly the balance of essential fats in your body. Eating cholesterol within the ranges found in most natural foods is probably not an important factor in increasing or decreasing your cholesterol (unless you have some unusual genetic disease).

Myth. Low cholesterol foods are good for you.

Many foods low in cholesterol are high in saturated fat. Many dairy products such as cheese and cream are high in saturated fat. Eating large amounts of saturated fat stimulates your body to make more cholesterol, as a mechanism to counter the effects of excessive saturated fat. Eating large amounts of carbohydrates and sugars has the same effect.

Myth. The way to lose weight is to avoid all fat

The way to lose weight is to eat fewer calories and exercise more. If you substitute calories from fat with more calories from carbohydrate or protein --- as many people do --- you will transform the extra calories into saturated fat. Ironically, you may find yourself gaining weight. Healthy weight loss can be accomplished by replacement of most SFAs, MUFAs, and high caloric processed foods with natural foods low in calories, high in EFAs, and high in fiber. Such foods will fill you up and provide balanced nutrition.

Myth. The less fat you eat the better: Aim for zero fat.

The body needs Essential Fatty Acids (**EFAs**). Eating a zero fat diet will make you deficient in EFAs.

Myth. Some types of EFAs help you lose weight.

Some authors write that some essential fats, such as one called GLA, make people lose weight. Deficiencies of EFAs may trigger the "hunger" mechanism, and correcting EFA abnormalities may produce satiety. However, EFAs are fats and make you gain weight just like any other source of concentrated calories.

Myth. The way to lower your blood's saturated fat is to substitute it with carbohydrates and protein.

All excess calories that you eat from carbohydrates or protein are converted by the body to SFAs and MUFAs. Thus, you may accumulate saturated fat in your body even if you eat a low fat diet. Actually, you may accumulate more saturated fat in your body by eating many calories from low fat foods such as cereals, breads and pasta than by eating equivalent calories from pizza made with oils high in EFAs.

Myth. Monounsaturated fats (MUFAs) prevent heart disease, so we should eat more of them.

Monounsaturated fatty acids (**MUFAs**) are carefully regulated by the body, which can make them from saturated fatty acids (**SFAs**), carbohydrates and protein. The body's store of MUFAs can increase for three reasons: 1) Eating too many MUFAs. 2) Eating calories the body does not require; humans convert some excess saturated fats, carbohydrates, and protein into MUFAs. 3) Eating a diet low in EFAs.

The body makes more MUFAs in response to an EFA deficiency. For that reason, it is highly unlikely that diets high in MUFAs alone will prevent heart disease. Most likely, this myth has arisen because researchers overlooked the fact that in countries with low incidence of heart disease, people eat foods high in EFAs in addition to foods high in MUFAs. MUFAs perhaps do not cause as much an imbalance to the body as saturated fats, but the overriding concern is to eat a proper balance of EFAs.

Myth. Very low fat diets can be used safely by anyone who needs to lose weight.

Very low fat diets cause EFA depletion. Before going on a very low fat diet for a long time (more than one month), you should have a blood test done to determine whether or not you have enough EFAs in your body. If you do not, you need to eat EFA supplements.

Myth. Medium Chain Triglyceride fats do not increase weight.

Medium Chain Triglycerides, recently promoted as a weight loss supplement and source of "quick energy", actually are almost 100% saturated fat. They burn and metabolize like saturated fat. They are an excellent source of calories, like saturated fat, and are very useful for people who need fat for protection against cold or starvation. However, medium chain triglycerides are treated like all other calories in the body. Calories not used for exercise or heat end up being stored as saturated and monounsaturated fat.

Myth. If I eat a few oil capsules with EFAs, I am OK.

Most older adults need the equivalent of 2 or more tablespoons of oil per day. You would need to eat more than 20 small capsules with the proper oil mixture to get enough. If you have a body deficiency of EFAs, you may need to eat even more. Eating the wrong mixture of oil capsules will further disturb any existing imbalances in your body's fatty acid composition.

Myth. If I eat the "healthy diet" recommended by the US Department of Agriculture (USDA) I am preventing heart disease.

The USDA recommends a diet high in carbohydrates and very little fat, claiming that fats and oils "provide calories and little else nutritionally". Unfortunately, most processed foods such as pasta, bread, cereals and rice, placed by the USDA at the base of their pyramid, to be eaten in the largest amounts, have practically zero

EFAs. Moreover, some of the carbohydrates in these foods are converted to saturated fats and upset the balance of EFAs in the body. The USDA's prescribed diet is counterproductive if you replace sources of EFAs with carbohydrates. Being wholesome or organic tells you nothing about the EFA content of foods.

> ### *Myth. All oils are similar, and can be used as adequate EFA supplements.*

Each oil has very different mixtures and quantities of the different types of EFAs. If you start eating healthy foods when you are born, your body automatically adjusts and discards what is not needed. After 10 or more years of bad eating, your body's EFA imbalance makes such regulation difficult. You will need a specially formulated mixture of EFAs unique to your body composition. Different mixtures of EFAs are required for people with different health conditions.

> ### *Myth: Carbohydrates burn fat; so eating carbohydrates helps you lose weight.*

The body needs only about 100 grams per day of carbohydrates to burn fat. Eating more carbohydrates will not help you burn more fat. All calories, whether from carbohydrates or other sources, contribute to your total caloric intake. If you do not use all the calories you eat in one day, you store the excess as non-essential fat in your body.

> ### *Myth: Butter is better than margarine, or margarine is better than butter.*

If you have an optimal body composition of EFAs, small amounts of butter are unlikely to hurt you. Margarine high in PUFAs and low in *trans* fatty acids may be better than butter for eating, although not for cooking. Butter is more stable for cooking at high temperatures.

Types of fatty acids

There are **two Essential Fatty Acids (EFAs), Linolenic and Linoleic acid**. People cannot make either, and therefore must get both EFAs from their diet. People who have not eaten enough EFAs over time become **EFA insufficient**. From the EFAs, humans make many fatty acid derivatives. The polyunsaturated fatty acids (**PUFAs,** also known as **essential fats**) consist of both EFAs plus all of their fatty acid derivatives. PUFAs are divided into two families of fatty acids, each made of one EFA and its derivatives. The *omega-3* (ω3) family derives from Linolenic acid, and the ***omega-6*** (ω6) from Linoleic acid. Scientists named fatty acids using the Greek letter "ω." Included in the fatty acid's name are numbers which refer to the location, type and number of "kinks" or "bends" in its chemical structure.

$$\text{PUFAs = EFA (precursors) + EFA derivatives =}$$
$$= \textit{omega-}3 + \textit{omega-}6 = \omega 3 + \omega 6$$

Grouping the fatty acids into precursors and derivatives enables nutritionists to determine what your body needs. Most people *only* need to eat a proper balance of the precursors, linolenic and linoleic acids. However, some individuals need to eat EFA derivatives because they cannot make enough of them. This inability may occur with old age, disease, or a deficiency of vitamins or minerals. In general, plant foods have only EFAs and no derivatives. EFA derivatives are found in animal fat (mostly ω6 linoleic acid derivatives) and fish fat (mostly ω3 linolenic acid derivatives), and

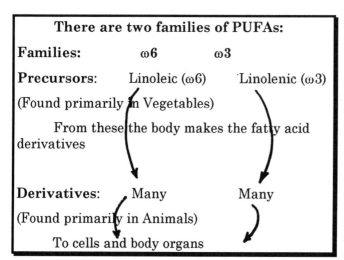

There are two families of PUFAs:

Families: ω6   ω3

Precursors: Linoleic (ω6)   Linolenic (ω3)
(Found primarily in Vegetables)

         From these the body makes the fatty acid
derivatives

Derivatives: Many   Many
(Found primarily in Animals)
    To cells and body organs

some new food and oil supplements. To improve your health you need to learn more about the types of EFAs and their derivatives, and how to work with your nutritionist to eat healthier foods.

Your body is made of food: You are, quite literally, what you eat. If you eat foods high in saturated fat, most of the fat in your body will be solid. Your arteries will become hard, and you will develop high blood pressure. If you eat foods high in EFAs, your arteries will remain soft and the blood is less likely to form clots that obstruct arteries and cause strokes or heart attacks. All cells and organs need EFAs to work well. Balanced hormone production also depends on the amount of EFAs circulating in the blood. When your body is deficient in EFAs, all the organs work poorly and you get progressively more ill.

Preface, Introduction, Summary

It is dangerous to eat too many or too few specific fatty acids.
In contrast to most vitamins, which may be excreted, fatty acids
accumulate in the body. This is why people get fat. Relative excesses
or deficiencies of one fatty acid alter the effects of the others. People
who follow low fat diets may not eat enough EFAs. People who eat too
much fat often eat too much saturated fat. Eating too many ω3
derivatives can impair the blood's clotting function and make you bleed
too easily. Eating too many ω6 derivatives, or too few ω3s, can have the
opposite effect: Your body will make clots too easily, which can cause a
stroke or heart attack by clogging a key artery in your brain or heart.

**A low fat diet, if insufficient in EFAs, increases the risk
of cardiovascular disease.**

Both fatty acid families are involved in the regulation of cholesterol and
triglycerides in the body, and in the formation of many hormones. They
act together and their relative amounts determine which hormones are
produced and how they act in the body. A proper balance is essential to
life. The ω6 has a major role in the texture and appearance of the skin
and the softness of vessels; the ω3 is critical to eye, brain and
neurological function. The higher the ratio of ω3/ω6, the less likely that
a clot will obstruct an artery. If the ratio is high you can bleed easily.

Among abnormalities related to EFAs, the most common is **EFA
insufficiency (EFAI)**. Insufficient levels of EFAs or EFA derivatives
may lead to abnormal vision, hyperlipidemia (high cholesterol or
triglycerides), high blood pressure, abnormal activity of hormones,
reduced cell survival, and impaired wound healing and cell growth.
EFAI is a major factor in cardiovascular disease, kidney disease,
complications caused by diabetes, and probably in neurological diseases
and loss of mental ability. You are likely to have EFAI if you eat very
little fat or calories, or are very thin because you eat very few calories
(as opposed to eating and exercising a lot).

Most people have too much saturated fat in their blood. Even if
sufficient EFAs are present in the body, excessive saturated fat
prevents the blood from carrying enough EFAs to the organs that need
them. This condition is called **Relative EFAI** and it is found in
cardiovascular disease, high blood pressure, and hyperlipidemia. The
fatty acid profile **EFA-SR** can diagnose EFA abnormalities and assist
your health professional in planning an optimal diet for you. This test
reveals which fatty acids you need more or less of. The test shows the

Preface, Introduction, Summary

amounts of major saturated, monounsaturated, EFAs, ω3, ω6, and *trans* fatty acids in the blood. The combined, long term effects of the foods you eat, their processing and freshness, your body's break down and use of food, and exercise make it impossible to predict specific EFA abnormalities. However, people who eat a disproportionate amount of processed foods low in EFAs (such as cereals, breads, pasta), or fruits which are very low in fat and EFAs, have a cumulative dietary history of reduced intake of ω6 and ω3.

Treatment & management

The blood test **EFA-SR** identifies both the problem and the means of correcting it. Optimal nutritional treatment is cheaper and often more effective than medications. Genetic traits, addictive behaviors such as smoking, and preferences such as physical inactivity, are difficult to change. In contrast, the balance of EFAs can be changed by simply eating foods with more EFAs. Your doctor may prescribe oil supplements or oil capsules together with antioxidants such as Vitamin E to match body requirements. The treatment is designed to correct abnormalities identified by the fatty acid profile **EFA-SR** and by the clinical examination of your medical condition. The objective is to eat essential fats in the proportion required to bring your fatty acid profile closer to the one of a healthy person. Fortunately, the diet that works best for cardiovascular disease will often help to prevent other diseases, including cancer. **If you are overweight and are unwilling or unable to lose weight, you still must eat more EFAs to have the proper balance and prevent cardiovascular disease.**

According to your medical condition, weight, and the results of the test **EFA-SR**, your nutritionist determines the optimal mixture of EFAs that you should eat every day. For example, you may need to eat less animal fat or hydrogenated oils, eat more leafy green vegetables, or take one tablespoon of soybean, walnut, or safflower oil per day. Green vegetables and seeds are often high in EFAs. Linoleic acid (ω6) is found in safflower, sunflower, and corn oil. Linolenic acid (ω3) is found in linseed (flax) oil. Soybean, walnut and canola oil have mixtures of linoleic and linolenic acid. Derivatives of linolenic are found in fish oil. Derivatives of linoleic acid are found in Evening Primrose Oil, Borage Oil, some uncommon vegetables, and organs like brain.

Optimal mixtures of EFAs and derivatives may improve cardiovascular disease, hypertension, diabetes & immune status.

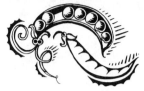

I.1

DIET AND NUTRITION

"The key to nutrition is balance: neither too much nor too little"

Topics: *Your diet. Fat, carbohydrates, proteins, vitamins, minerals, water, fiber. What constitutes a balanced diet. Nutritional status. The body as a machine. Enzymes. What you can do. Natural foods.*

Summary

The foods that you eat make up your diet. Food is composed of nutrients including fat, carbohydrates, proteins, vitamins, minerals, water and fiber. Even though all food contains nutrients, some foods have a better combination of nutrients than others. To remain healthy, we need to eat a balanced diet, which includes all essential nutrients in the appropriate proportions. The nutrients that we eat determine the nutritional status of our bodies. With a healthy nutritional status we can prevent and fight disease. An unbalanced diet leads to poor nutritional status, which contributes to disease. Enzymes are proteins that regulate what chemicals the body produces. Vitamins and minerals adjust the work of enzymes.

You can prevent heart disease

You can prevent heart disease. Even if you have "bad" genes or a history of heart disease in your family, you can still prevent heart disease. And the secret is in the food you eat. Of course, in order to eat, you do not need to know anything about how food works; animals eat and have not studied nutrition. However, animals and plants know instinctively what is good and what is bad for them.

We humans are too intelligent—we have forgotten what is good for us. Influenced by advertising, the food preferences of our family and friends, and by good-tasting artificial foods, we have lost our ability to distinguish healthy foods from unhealthy ones. That is why we need to learn again. Research has demonstrated that very young children in control of their diets naturally choose healthy foods. Liking "junk" foods turns out to be a learned behavior.

This book emphasizes fat because the type of fat we eat is the major determinant of cardiovascular disease, diabetes, hypertension, and many other diseases that occur with aging.

Do you eat to live or do you live to eat?

Eat to live

Many of us need to eat better. Instead of eating to live, we live to eat. Eating has become a national pastime. Early humans ate when they were hungry, in order to survive. They ate in order to have the energy required for daily activities, including hunting and gathering of food. They ate to store up fat to prevent starvation during winter. We no longer chase food; we follow advertisements and chase sales at supermarkets. Today we watch TV. Watching TV rarely requires "energy", except for those without remote control. Yet we eat while we watch. We eat when we meet with friends. We eat when we are alone. We eat at parties. We eat when we are happy and when we are sad. We eat when we have nothing else to do.

Most people eat too much and eat the wrong kind of food

The basic nutrients

The foods that you eat contains **nutrients** that constitute your **diet**. The major types of nutrients (things that we need to eat) are: FAT, CARBOHYDRATES, PROTEIN, VITAMINS, MINERALS, WATER AND FIBER. Calories are the **energy** in food; they are not a nutrient. Most foods contain all these nutrients in different quantities, but some foods have mainly one type of nutrient and very little of other kinds. All foods provide calories. Fat provides about twice as many calories, per weight, as carbohydrates or proteins. Vitamins, minerals, fiber and water do not provide any calories. Even though all food has nutrients, some foods have a better balance of nutrients than other foods.

The nutrients we eat determine the nutritional status of our bodies. With an optimal nutritional status, we can prevent and fight disease. An unbalanced diet leads to an imbalance in our nutritional status, which facilitates disease.

> *The key to disease prevention is to eat a balanced diet and to correct for previous imbalances.*

Nutrition and Diets

The body consists of a multitude of chemical processes. Parts of the body are constantly being destroyed while other parts are being formed. This process of destruction and construction goes on ceaselessly, day and night. It operates on basic building blocks, like the "Leggos" you used as a child. These building blocks are called nutrients. The human body is like a chemical factory where chemicals are made, processed and regulated. Your diet provides the raw materials for these processes: nutrients. Choose them well!

Nutrition vs. diet

Nutrition refers to the overall status of all the chemical processes in the body, such as the digestion and utilization of food, and the raw materials which are used in those processes. The term "diet" refers to the food that we eat on a given day. A healthy diet is one that provides all the essential nutrients that the body requires to remain in good health and to resist disease.

A food or food supplement has "**nutritive value**" when it helps to sustain human life by such processes as promoting growth, replacing loss of essential nutrients, or providing energy.[1]

Nutritional Status

Nutritional status tells us how well your body is. It is the consequence of the utilization of nutrients. Your nutritional status dramatically affects your ability to prevent and fight disease. If your nutritional status is good, you are likely to heal wounds promptly, to fight infection effectively, and often to avoid infection in the first place due to your strong immune system. With good nutritional status, your circulation is excellent, and this helps the body to carry nutrients and disease

fighting elements (such as white cells and antibodies) to those parts of
the body that need them. If your nutritional status is poor, you are less
able to manufacture antibodies and white cells. Your skin and internal
organs become weak, and are less capable of fighting disease or trauma
caused by accidents. A minor bruise could take a long time to heal; a
broken bone or tendon may heal poorly.

*A body with optimal nutrition and nutrients has the
appropriate raw materials to repair itself and to fight
disease and invaders such as viruses and bacteria.
Bad nutrition leads to quick deterioration and
breakdowns.*

What constitutes optimal nutrition?

One of the most difficult issues in nutrition is to determine what
constitutes optimal nutrition. We are bombarded every day with ads
that tells us that certain foods or supplements are perfect for us and we
may die if we do not eat them. Supermarkets and health food stores
surround us with products, each claiming to be better than the other.
Obviously, we need some criteria to decide what is good for us.

One major criterion shapes this book: Humans have been created over
the course of millions of years of evolution. We were designed more
than 50,000 years ago, before supermarkets, cooking, freezers, food
processing and TV were widely available. I think it is wrong to believe
that anyone of us can do better than millions of years of evolution (or,
alternatively, do better than the One who designed us). Therefore, I
propose that we think in terms of the needs of humans that existed
50,000 years ago. When we do that, we find several major factors that
help us make a decision. First, all foods were eaten in their natural
state. Cooking and food processing were not available. All animals and
other species eat food in its natural state. Neither gorillas nor ants nor
trees cook food or purchase ready-to-eat TV meals. This tells us that
natural foods ought to be sufficient, and anything we do to change them
may not necessarily make them better. The key is defining what
combination of natural foods is optimal for humans.

Another fundamental difference was that primitive humans did not
have Cable or satellite TV. With supermarkets closed and refrigerators
unavailable, they were forced to find food almost every day. And food
rarely kept quiet. Sometimes food ran away, sometimes food ran after
early humans. This constant search for food and shelter, while

Diet and Nutrition

avoiding becoming food themselves, required a lot of energy: far more energy and calories than switching TV channels by remote control. We can infer that early men and women probably ate far more calories that we do now. This tells us that humans were designed to eat far more calories than many of us do, and burn excessive calories through hours of active exercise every day. Today, when many of us eat half of the calories consumed by primitive humans, or even less, we need to eat foods which contain nutrients in greater concentration. Additionally, we may need to take specific nutrient supplements. This is one reason why some people need to eat some vitamin and mineral supplements (This does not imply they ought to eat every food supplement on the market). Because many foods are fortified with vitamins and minerals, and because many people take vitamin and mineral supplements, deficiencies of vitamins or minerals are rare in healthy people. However, some people do have deficiencies caused in part by a disease or its treatment. For example, diuretics, drugs used frequently to treat high blood pressure, cause the kidney to produce a lot of urine. When discharged, this urine carries with it minerals. People treated with diuretics often develop deficiencies of potassium, magnesium as well as other deficiencies.

Few Americans are underfed. Most actually eat too much food and too many calories for the amount of exercise and type of work they do. (I am not referring here to professional basketball players or lumberjacks.). Deficiencies of carbohydrates and protein are also very rare, and most people eat plenty of saturated fat. However, a large number of Americans do not eat enough of a type of fat essential to optimal body function, known as **essential fatty acids (EFAs)**. This book is about the role of EFAs in health and disease.

The body as a "machine"

The body has many parts. Some of the parts have specialized functions and we call them "organs" and "glands". Organs have unique tasks to do, while glands make hormones used by other parts of the body. The brain, heart, blood, liver, lungs, kidneys, spleen, skin are organs. The brain thinks and coordinates everything; the heart pumps blood; the blood carries food, oxygen and nutrients; the liver burns or detoxifies the blood; the spleen destroys sick cells; and the skin protects the rest of the body against the environment. The adrenal, ovaries,thyroid and parathyroid glands make special hormones that regulate metabolic rate, calcium, the reproductive cycles and other aspects of the body.

Diet and Nutrition

The pancreas makes insulin and glucagon, which contribute to the regulation of fat and glucose.

The major organs and structural parts of the body are made up of cells. Cells themselves consist of a multitude of small "organelles" and other biochemical components. The organs of a cell, just like the organs of the body as a whole, help to make and repair the components of the cell. Some living organisms, such as bacteria, consist of a single cell: Their whole life cycle machinery is inside that single cell. The cell is surrounded by a membrane which is like the body's skin: It covers the whole cell and protects it from damage. The cell membrane very carefully regulates what goes in and comes out of a cell.

Cells and enzymes

Cell organelles also contain enzymes, a class of biochemical that helps make other chemicals. **Enzymes** are proteins which have a very important function in our bodies: They participate in all chemical reactions. Enzymes, in turn, are highly regulated by vitamins and minerals. If the body requires a certain chemical, it produces more of the enzymes which participate in making that chemical. Then, the blood shuttles the necessary vitamins and minerals to the enzyme, enabling it to function. If too much of a certain chemical is being produced, the vitamins and minerals are eliminated from the enzyme. This causes the enzyme to work less effectively, and ultimately, to be destroyed. Like everything else in the body, enzymes are carefully regulated: Too many or too few enzymes lead to biochemical imbalance, and disease. Excess or inappropriate production of parts always leads to the clogging of our body machine. As always, BALANCE is the key.

How nutrients are used

To maintain the structure of the body we use CARBOHYDRATES, PROTEIN and LIPIDS. These substances are strong and produce a surface or frame which holds all other parts together. FAT is used to make the CELL MEMBRANES adaptable and flexible, not rigid. It also provides the energy (fuel or calories) to keep the machinery of the body working, and provides insulation against the cold and the environment. Like gas in a car, some fat is burned to keep the body running.

What keeps a cell alive

Cells are made of proteins, carbohydrates, fat, vitamins, minerals and water. These substances regulate how the cell works, what the cell produces and how long the cell will live. Some cells seem to live forever, and when they die they are rarely replaced. Scientists have found that many of the cells in the brain, heart, kidney, lung and major organs are rarely replaced when they die. The death of these cells is a major factor in the aging process. It is therefore important to protect these cells! Keeping them alive as long as possible prevents us from getting old before our time. Other types of cells are replaced with younger and stronger cells when they die. These are the cells which typically receive a lot of wear and tear, for example the blood cells and skin cells. The human body has anticipated the need to replace these cells as they die by building the machinery necessary to provide their replacements. For example, many of the bones of the body and the spine have, in their center, a substance called bone marrow. Bone marrow contains cells which manufacture new blood cells.

For all these machines and their parts to work well we need nutrients and calories: **Nutrients provide the components required to manufacture new parts and repair old ones. Calories are the energy that fuels the machinery of the body.**

Good health

The chemical processes of your body are continuously changing and adapting to your needs. When you are in good health, all the chemical processes work together efficiently. The main physical difference between living organisms and a human-made machine is that living organisms self-repair, that is, they acquire the "parts" they need from their food, and use these parts to repair themselves.

Our body is a huge machine that self repairs and makes most of its own parts. Its major parts, such as a leg or a kidney, are composed of cells. Cells are also small factories that use nutrients from food to make parts and produce energy.

Disease

Disease occurs when something in the body does not work well. The causes of disease may be external or internal. Allow me a simplistic

Diet and Nutrition

illustration, the use of a car analogy: An external source of difficulty for automobiles is collision with another vehicle; similarly, human beings may break a limb in an accident or get "hit" by a virus. But internal factors also play a role in causing breakdown or disease. A car will eventually look and run less well due to normal wear and tear. Similarly, the human body often appears to run down due to the normal process of aging. However, some people have 10 year old cars that look new, and others have new cars that look 10 years old, depending on how they treat and maintain their car. The aging process in human bodies also responds to loving care.

How long can you live?

If you treat your body with loving care it will last longer. People often say, "Who cares? Even if I live to be 80 or 90, I will be too senile to enjoy life. I'd rather enjoy life to the fullest (meaning "eat any food and drink a lot") and die at 70 than be careful all my life and wind up as a 90-year old vegetable."

This concept is incorrect. If you are not careful, you may not live to die at 70, but will die at 50 or 40. Moreover, before you die, you may live many handicapped years with hypertension, diabetes, or heart disease. You may be severely restricted in your activities, and have to live with pain and the fear of dying. Moreover, you may become senile sooner than you think. We are all brave when we feel well, but every person I have met who is ill is very fearful of dying. Those who make jokes about living the "good life" are terrified and sorry when hospitalized for their first heart attack, and are willing to do anything to get better.

Remember, some people drive a 1986 auto that looks like it was used for target practice by the army. Others drive a 1927 model that is a joy to drive. Good care makes a difference. **Take good care of your body and it will take care of you.**

Take good care of yourself

You can see now how everything interacts: If your body is healthy, and you eat a healthy diet, then you can sustain the vital manufacturing processes, making the parts you need for replacement or repair. Remember, living organisms not only make the parts they need, but also manufacture the machines that make these parts. A good example of this is the way our bodies produce our skin. The skin is self-generating (it makes itself). Poor nutritional status deprives the skin of

Diet and Nutrition

the correct balance of "parts" for its continued, healthy regeneration. Defective machines produce defective products. Defective skin looks discolored, overdry in some places, overoily in others; because it is working poorly. Healthy skin adapts to your body's needs in a particular environment, and makes you look younger.

The key word in maintaining your body as a smoothly functioning factory is BALANCE.

Balance is the key

Your body is really the sum total of its chemical processes, working together in a state of delicate balance. These processes build new body parts when necessary, produce energy, repair damaged parts of the body and maintain the machinery needed to accomplish all this. All vital functions in this balance are performed using the nutrients obtained from the food you eat. Thus, you can see how important it is to eat a balanced diet: The wrong balance leads to an inefficient and ineffective body machine. When you eat a balanced diet, your body has adequate nutrition and works at its best.

Nutrients, nutrient needs and interrelations

There are different classes or types of nutrients (fat, carbohydrates, protein, water, vitamins, mineral, fiber, others). All nutrients interact, and therefore it is extremely difficult to identify a particular deficiency on the basis of clinical symptoms (i.e., how you feel). Over the years, scientists have attributed certain diseases to specific nutritional deficiencies, and many of these claims have become widely accepted as true. For instance, many people have come to believe that anemia is caused by iron deficiency. In fact, anemia may result from many different causes: It could be due to excessive blood loss, blood destruction (by infection), or insufficient blood production. An inadequate supply of vitamin B12, Folic Acid, or many other vitamins, minerals or fat can also lead to anemia. Again the key is balance: eating the right amount and proportion of the various nutrients that the body requires.

Let's continue our analogy of the human body and mechanical production. Imagine that you have a factory that makes leather shoes. Of course, if you do not have enough leather, you can not make your shoes. But if you fill every tray in the factory with leather you may

Diet and Nutrition

reach a point where the machines stop working because there are no empty trays to put the shoes or get other parts needed to make shoes. Similarly, if you eat too much or too little of a nutrient, you may interfere with the machinery of the body. That is why a nutritional abnormality is difficult to diagnose and treat: you need specialized chemical tests to determine whether you have a deficiency or an excess. You may think you are missing iron, but the cause of the problem may be entirely different. You may have too much iron and too little vitamin B6 or folate. Increasing your iron consumption may increase the imbalance, thus making the cause of the problem even more difficult to pinpoint.

To diagnose a nutritional deficiency or excess you need sophisticated blood and urine tests. Consuming unnecessary supplements can make the problem worse.

Natural foods and natural food extracts

What is natural? The word "natural" is used in many different contexts by different writers. When we speak of a natural food we mean the food in its natural or original form, without significant processing by humans. For example, a "natural" orange is as you find it: on a tree. Extracts from natural products, even if they have nothing added to them, are still "artificial": Orange juice does not grow on trees. Furthermore, some foods contain ingredients that are either not found in nature (that is, chemicals created by humans), or ingredients that are found in nature but not in that particular food. The more a food deviates from its original state, the more artificial it is. All foods contain chemicals that could be toxic if ingested in large quantities. However, one would usually have to eat extraordinarily large quantities of the natural product to get toxic effects. Processed foods, fortified cereals, breads, extracts from food, juices, and food supplements are examples of foods that we eat that are not found in their natural state (have you ever seen a plant that has "bread" as a seed?). Even if the original substance was a natural product, the nutrient concentration of the new product can exceed anything that a person could normally eat. For example, a reasonable person could eat 3 oranges in one day. However, we can use machines to extract key essences from oranges. A person could eat, in one day, the vitamin C found in 500 oranges. This is unnatural. None of our ancestors could eat 500 oranges in one day.

Diet and Nutrition

Extracts may also allow us to get nutrients that we would otherwise miss. However, they also may concentrate undesirable compounds, making it possible to get toxic effects. Moreover, a desirable nutrient may be eliminated during the extraction process. For example, most apple juice, particularly filtered juice, lacks many of the enzymes and fibers of the original apple, which are helpful for digestion. Both potential toxicity and nutrient-elimination are strong reasons to avoid large intakes of artificial products, even if they are extracted from natural products.

Similarly, it is almost impossible to overdose with the vitamins and minerals that you find normally in natural foods. But you can overdose by eating vitamins and minerals in pill form no matter how "natural" they are. However, because we do not exercise enough we are forced to eat a small variety of foods to prevent becoming overweight. As a result, we may not get enough nutrients and we thus need to eat some food supplements.

How to determine what your body needs

The human body is designed to eat a wide range of foods, use what it needs and discard surplus nutrients in urine and feces. As long as we eat natural foods in reasonable amounts, the body can deal with them. The problem occurs when we eat specific nutrients in unnaturally large quantities, because the body was not designed to deal with them.

How can we decide? I follow some simple rules. We were designed to eat natural foods in their natural state. So I try to eat as many natural foods as I can. However, I find that I often "cheat". I cook my meat and vegetables and many other foods because of the danger of bacteria and other infectious agents. I do not exercise as much as I should. I like chocolate and sweets and many other "unnatural" processed foods. Because I do not want to gain weight, I must eat fewer calories than I ought to eat to get enough nutrients from my food. I figure that I eat about half of what I ought to eat. As a man, I should eat about 4,000 to 6,000 calories per day of natural foods if I were to live like my ancestors. But I eat about 2,000 to 3,000 calories, some days even less. Therefore, I must eat an additional half of my vitamins and minerals to supplement my food. One pill with 100% of the RDA (recommended daily dose) of vitamins and minerals, about 3 to 7 times per week, provides me with the nutritional supplementation I need. I figure a little bit extra is needed to compensate for losses in transit, storage, absorption, etc. Perhaps I could eat twice as much. However, I will not

Diet and Nutrition

eat five times as much because there is no way that humans were designed to eat that many vitamins and minerals. The same principles apply to other foods. The amounts of nutrients that the body usually needs to live well are called "**physiological**" **doses**.

There are some exceptions to this rule. People with diseases of the gastrointestinal system that interfere with absorption need to eat higher doses of nutritional supplements. Some diseases respond better when the body eats large doses (called **"pharmacological" doses**) of vitamins, minerals and other supplements. However, other diseases get worse. Feeding extra nutrients to the body may strengthen the immune system in its fight against disease, but it also feeds the cancer cells or bacteria, allowing them to grow faster and better. Too many nutrients may alter the normal physiology of the immune system and the body has to waste resources getting rid of the excessive amounts of nutrients.

I usually get plenty of carbohydrates and protein even with my limited caloric intake. Most Americans are similar in this regard, and therefore we do not need supplements of carbohydrates or protein. Again, the exception is people with specific diseases which require more protein, such as malabsorption, burns, etc.

There are a wide range of other chemicals that the body needs. It is impossible to predict how much is needed for the "average" person. However, eating a wide mixture of natural vegetables and occasional animal protein with little excess fat will provide those nutrients. Animals, being closer to humans than plants, have body compositions similar to ours, and thus can be useful sources of nutrients. Unfortunately, we no longer eat the types of animals that primitive humans ate. The animals that our ancestors ate, the ones which the human body was designed to eat, were lean animals, with a much higher proportion of polyunsaturated fat (essential fats) and far less saturated or non-essential fat. These animals also lacked the toxic human-made chemicals that modern animals carry in their tissues due to 20th century animal farming techniques, water and air pollution.

If you feel that some particular supplement is great for you, and money is no object, you may want to try it. Beware that some supplements that you eat may cause the body to become dependent. Thus, you may have to eat more of it for the rest of your life. If you eat very high doses of vitamins and minerals, your body learns to excrete them and gets accustomed to excreting them in large amounts every day.

Diet and Nutrition

Again, the rules change when you have a disease. Some of the research and recommendations for supplements makes sense. I wish the federal government would spend less money funding drug research and more money evaluating nutritional supplements and their impact on disease. However, this is wishful thinking, because most of the federal research budget is targeted at big bucks diagnostic and treatment procedures and drugs. The money we spend on heart bypass and maintenance of a few terminally ill people would be more than enough to evaluate all food and food supplements, and provide guidelines so that people could live to old age without bypass surgery or kidney transplants.

You can understand why it is very difficult to decide what is a balanced diet. I read many scientific reports and they often provide conflicting or impractical advice. I cannot take a computer to the supermarket and read all the food labels and figure out what I am eating. Instead, I developed the simple rules which I present in this book.

The scientific approach

Birds fly, dogs and elephants do not fly. True? False! Dead birds don't fly; dogs have been known to fly, in airplanes. Although things may not be what they appear to be, there is a body of scientific facts which are believed to be true. In this book we shall deal only with science. Religion and other beliefs, though very important, are not considered. Furthermore, one purpose of this book is to help you live longer. You can help yourself die sooner by smoking, eating too many calories, avoiding a balanced diet, following procedures that have no scientific merit, driving under the influence of alcohol, jumping from airplanes without a parachute, volunteering for an exhibition fight with the world champion, and many other thrilling activities.

The facts I present are based on the scientific approach. The research is based on experiments. One key element makes an experiment scientific: The results must be reproducible when performed by any individual that follows specific instructions. Results that are only obtained by people with the right "karma" or "touch" are religious experiences rather than scientific experiments.

The human body has excellent powers to heal itself. Some people will recover from cancer and other diseases, even without treatment. Thus, practically every treatment can show "proof" that some people got cured. In a scientific experiment, a treatment is considered successful if it cures or improves the health of more people than a comparison treatment (called "placebo"). Furthermore, when the results are repeated by different scientists in another place, the same results must be obtained. Results that only occur when one person runs the test are not considered scientifically reliable.

It is impossible to do every possible experiment. Scientists use mathematical rules to "extrapolate", that is, to make predictions or extend to other situations the results of one experiment. For example, we know that people who jump from 10 story windows are likely to break their legs, even though nobody has done experiments on all windows and all buildings. Good extrapolations or predictions are based on solid scientific principles. However, we often find predictions or extrapolations that incorporate many scientific principles and perhaps one false assumption. Using 99% proper science and 1% fantasy is likely to result in 100% fantasy. For example, humans are made of cells and all cells contain atoms which produce electric and magnetic fields and currents. However, the intensity is very tiny and declines with the square of the distance. After a few feet, the effect of electricity and magnetism of one person is practically zero. Therefore, it makes no sense to say that one person's magnetism in New York is affecting another person's life in London (unless they use the telephone to insult each other).

Every diagnostic and treatment procedure you use, and all activities of your life, must be in balance with your nutritional status. It makes no sense to worry about small contamination in the water or organic foods when you are very likely to die from smoking or risky pleasures such car racing or heavy drinking. Most treatment is aimed to cure a specific disease even though it may cause another problem. If you have an infection or cancer which may kill you within one year, it makes sense to use diagnostic and treatment methods that will kill the bacteria or cancer even if it could cause your death 10 years from now. However, if you do not have an infection or cancer, you do not want to use diagnostic methods that have a very small probability of finding a disease yet may cause you another disease in the future. I personally believe that X-rays, ultrasound and many other diagnostic procedures make significant changes in the body and ought to be used with great caution. In my laboratory we use ultrasound to destroy cells and tissue from test tubes. I would not want ultrasound waves to destroy my cells.

Many publications use invalid extrapolations to explain why some chemicals are good or bad for you. It is impossible for me to argue for or

Diet and Nutrition

against all of them. However, I urge caution and common sense. Think about what makes sense. Think about the way humans were designed thousands of years ago. Think about the principles discussed in this book. And remember that **balance in life and nutrition is the key to a healthier and longer life.**

Limitations of Science

Science is not perfect; it is a system of knowledge based on experiments. Research studies analyze many people, but data acquired is rarely perfect. In a given study, some subjects may not follow the proper instructions. Others subjects may have a disease unknown to the scientists. Some may have unique genes which alter the response being studied.

Some studies are only a few weeks in duration, and the results could be different if they had lasted several years. Animal studies may produce results not applicable to humans. (As someone once said: "some humans may be rats, but rats are not human".) Some food products, by themselves, may not be cancer-causing or atherogenic (produce heart disease). But eating a mixture of many of those products over a long time could produce disease.

When you read studies, ask yourself this question: Have the researchers published data that indicate the validity of their "model"? ("predictive value" or explanation).[2] If the researchers did not publish a measure of the accuracy of their model, or if the model has low predictability, you ought to be suspicious. A model that is not accurate is not good. Many people make predictions about the stock market, but very few make money when the market goes up and down. There are some similarities with science. Upon repetition by another scientist, many studies that had poor predictive models yield different results.

References and

---

[1] This is the definition adopted by the Food and Drug Administration in 1994, Federal Register Rules and Regulations, Jan. 4, 1994, Vol. 59, section on definitions. These definitions will have a drastic impact on the labeling and marketing of edible substances in the US.

[2] The validity of their "model" or "predictive value" or explanation is usually called the R square or predictability of the model. It is quite different from statistical significance that tests whether some result is different from zero. Because everything is different from zero, practically all published research is statistically significant.

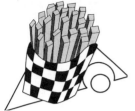

I.2

FAT: SATURATED, MONOUNSATURATED, POLYUNSATURATED (PUFA)

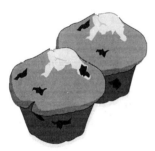

"The type of fat you eat is the type of fat your body stores"

Topics: Fat. Energy. Types of fat. Saturated fat. Monounsaturated Polyunsaturated Essential fat.

Summary

Fat provides energy, insulation against the cold, and determines the flexibility and structure of membranes (the skin of cells). Fat is made of fatty acids. There are several types of fatty acids. Fats composed primarily of saturated fatty acids (**SFAs**), such as butter or animal fat, are hard at room temperature. Fats composed mainly of monounsaturated fatty acids (**MUFAs**) are softer and often liquid at room temperature, such as olive or peanut oil. Fats made of mostly polyunsaturated fatty acids (**PUFAs**) are liquid at room temperature; examples are most vegetable oils. Polyunsaturated fatty acids help to make blood vessels and other body structures, such as the skin, flexible and soft. Most people need to eat fewer SFAs and more PUFAs. Polyunsaturated fatty acids are known as **essential fatty acids** (**EFAs**) because humans cannot live without them and the body cannot manufacture them. We must eat EFAs almost every day, like a vitamin or mineral, but in far greater quantities.

Fat

Fat is found in almost all natural foods. Fat serves as a major source of energy, and helps to make all the major structures in the body. Fat also forms the skins or membranes which protect the body, organs, and cells, and provides the flexibility needed for the skin to do its job. Fat is made of fatty acids. Fat is found in all foods, with each food containing a mixture of fatty acids. The three major types of natural fatty.acids are: saturated (**SFAs**), monounsaturated (**MUFAs**) and polyunsaturated (**PUFAs**). When MUFAs or PUFAs are processed, they form another type of fatty acid called "*trans* fatty acid" (**TFAs**). TFAs are rarely labeled in foods. They do not count as SFAs even though they behave like SFAs. We need to eat a proper mixture of all natural fatty acids while avoiding TFAs.

Lipids, liquid and hard fat

The technical term for substances like fat is "*LIPIDS.*" Lipids are substances that are almost insoluble in water but are soluble in some organic solvents. The lipids include substances such as fats, oils, waxes, phospholipids (such as lecithin) and many other complex substances made by the body and used and needed by all organs in the body for practically every function. Brain, nerves, reproductive organs, liver, and the heart all have different types of lipids uniquely suited for the function of each organ. Most lipids require a specific mixture of fatty acids to achieve optimal function.

When you look at food at room temperature (i.e., about 70 º Fahrenheit or 27 º C), you find both liquid fat, called oils, and solid or hard fat. Liquid fat usually comes from vegetables and hard fat comes from animals. Do not confuse the oils that are liquid fats with mineral oil, motor oil or essential oils. Essential oils are the chemicals that provide fragrances to flowers and perfumes. These oils are not suitable for human consumption.

The body stores fat as energy for times when food is not available. Fat also forms membranes and other body structures, and helps to produce hormones.

Vegetable oils, like most fat in adipose tissue, are made of triglycerides with a mixture of all types of fatty acids. They are usually high in

FAT: SFA, MUFA, PUFA

PUFAs. Since fatty acids are the key constituent of fat, the type of fatty acid in a particular fat determines the type of fat it is.

Saturated fatty acids (SFA)

Saturated fatty acids are usually found in animal foods and make fats hard at room temperature. To simplify, we call a fat rich in saturated fatty acids (SFAs) by the name "saturated fat." These fatty acids are long, straight molecules that are packed very tightly, giving saturated fat its rigid structure. The fat in butter, coconut oil, meat, and cheese is mainly saturated fat. When you eat saturated fat your body accumulates saturated fat, that is, hard fat.

Saturated (hard) fat hardens the arteries

Arteries made with hard fat are hard arteries. Eating saturated fat may lead to hardening of the arteries and heart disease. However, saturated fat is an excellent source of calories and fuel for your body. Certain lines of work, such as that of a lumberjack who cuts trees with an ax eight hours per day, or of an explorer of the North Pole, are very strenuous. People who perform these jobs need to eat saturated fat in order to have sufficient calories for energy. But most people lead an easy life: They are rarely far from a supermarket, they wear clothing and live in heated rooms, and they eat too much, not too little. For them, saturated fat has lost part of its useful function as a source to store extra energy or protect against the *extreme* cold. Instead, *excess* saturated fat has ill effects.

Monounsaturated fatty acids (MUFA)

To simplify, we call a fat rich in Monounsaturated fatty acids (MUFAs) by the name "monounsaturated fat." Monounsaturated fat is usually liquid at room temperature, but it may become hard or mushy (cloudy) when placed in the refrigerator. Olive oil contains large amounts of monounsaturated fat. These fatty acids have one kink or bend in their structure that makes them produce shapes which are more flexible and softer than those produced by saturated fat. When you eat monounsaturated fat you may produce a softer artery than by merely eating saturated fat.[1]

Fats: SFA, MUFA, PUFA

Polyunsaturated fatty acids (PUFA)

To simplify, we call a fat rich in polyunsaturated fatty acids (PUFAs) by the name "polyunsaturated fat." Polyunsaturated fat is liquid at room temperature and remains liquid when you place it in the refrigerator. Most vegetable oils are high in PUFAs.

PUFAs soften arteries

Polyunsaturated fat have many bends or kinks and produce very flexible shapes (such as liquid oils). They form very soft structures that easily adapt to the needs of the body. For example, skin formed with hard fat would be hard, while skin formed with soft fat would be soft and better adapted to the body (and therefore appear to have fewer wrinkles). This, of course, is a simplistic presentation of the scientific issues, but it does explain the difference between soft and hard fat, and how the fat we consume influences the quality of the body parts and organs that our body produces.

Essential (EFAs) vs. non essential fatty acids

Fatty acids (the key components of fat) are classified into two major groups: those that the body can easily make, called Non-Essential Fatty Acids, and those that the body cannot make, called **Essential Fatty Acids (EFAs)**. Since the body cannot make EFAs, we must consume them as part of our diets. This is not true of other types of fat, because the body can easily convert carbohydrates and protein to saturated fatty acids (**SFAs**) and monounsaturated fatty acids (**MUFAs**), but not to polyunsaturated fatty acids (**PUFAs**). In this way, essential fats are similar to vitamins, which we cannot manufacture in our bodies, but must get from external sources. The difference is that *we need EFAs in much much larger quantities than we do vitamins*. We can eat a small pill every day to get all the vitamins and minerals we need. We must eat a lot of food to get all the essential fats we need.

Although saturated fatty acids (SFAs) support important body functions, overconsumption of SFAs leads to cardiovascular disease. On the other hand, polyunsaturated fatty acids (PUFAs) prevent cardiovascular disease, but eating an improper balance of different types of PUFAs is not healthy. Most people eat too many SFAs and not enough PUFAs.

FAT: SFA, MUFA, PUFA

Body fat

The body stores fat to provide energy when food is not available. Fats are usually stored in the body as triglycerides (molecules with 3 fatty acids). Fat is stored everywhere: in your blood vessels, your face, etc. The type of fat stored in your body is determined by the fat and other calories that you eat. Fat which you do not burn for energy is stored for future use. Therefore, if you eat soft fat, you store soft fat; if you eat hard fat, you store hard fat. Moreover, excess food that you eat of any kind--carbohydrate, protein, or saturated fat--is converted to and/or stored as hard saturated fat.

> ### *Enough fat keeps us alive; too much is a burden*

Energy vs. Drive

Let's clarify what we mean by the term, "energy." Energy is *the fuel required for the body to function.* Please do not confuse this definition with the more vague use of "energy" as the desire to do something, drive, enthusiasm, pep, etc. When people feel tired they often think they lack "energy". What they usually mean is that they lack motivation or enthusiasm; they have some sort of problem that makes it difficult for them to work at their best. However, they do not lack energy or "fuel." Rather, an inability of the mind or the body to use energy may be the cause of their problem. Sometimes you may find that your car stalls for lack of fuel even when you have a full tank: It is not lack of fuel, but a problem using the fuel that makes the car stall. Only people starving for weeks in the dessert or the mountains lack energy or fuel. As long as you have fat in your body, the body will use it to provide energy. However, if you lack vitamins or minerals or have another nutritional abnormality, the body will not be able to use the energy effectively. For this reason, getting more "energy" in your life is not a matter of eating an "energy" supplement, but rather following a balanced diet. A balanced diet gives the body the tools it needs to burn energy, both in the form of ingested calories and stored fat.

Besides a lack of vitality, other symptoms often caused by nutritional imbalance are tiredness and muscle pain. This is quite different from not having sufficient fuel. Deficiencies of the minerals potassium, magnesium and manganese cause muscle weakness. People who take pills to urinate, or urinate often, cause their kidneys to excrete these

---

Fats: SFA, MUFA, PUFA

minerals in the urine. Deficiency of carnitine will also cause muscle weakness, although this deficiency is very rare in healthy people. Muscle weakness can also be caused by an imbalance in nutrient proportions. Nutrient interactions make it difficult to correct an imbalance: If you eat too much potassium, for example, you may upset the balance of your other minerals. Furthermore, too much potassium also causes muscle problems and heart abnormalities. Potassium is so potentially lethal that injections of it can be used to kill people.

The message is quite simple: What you feel and what abnormality you may suffer are not always obviously related. You can appreciate why medicine is a challenging mixture of science and art. Tinkering with your body is a risky business.

Other types of fats and lipids

The most common form of fat is a **triglyceride**. Triglycerides are molecules made of three fatty acids hooked to a single base (glycerol). Diglycerides have two fatty acids, and monoglycerides have one fatty acid. Beware that some food labels claim a product has no fats, even though they have diglycerides and monoglycerides. Some labeling requirements do not require that these fats be labeled as "fats." Fortunately, these two types of fat are not dangerous if made from natural foods. In fact, your body makes diglycerides and monoglycerides when it digests triglycerides.

Most of the fat in the body is made of triglycerides. When we speak of being "fat", we mean that we have too many triglycerides in our body. To know if we have too many triglycerides in our body, all we have to do is step on a scale. There is a blood test that measures triglycerides in our blood. When we have too many triglycerides in our blood, we have **hypertriglyceridemia**. High triglycerides in the blood indicate that we have too much fat in our arteries and we have or are at risk for cardiovascular disease.

Another lipid is "**phospholipid**". Phospholipids, such as lecithin, are composed of two fatty acids and the substance choline. We eat phospholipids when we eat cell membranes from leafy vegetables, nuts, soybeans, or animal tissue. Our cells need phospholipids to make cell membranes, but humans can make practically all they need from regular intake of protein, carbohydrates and fatty acids. Although it is possible to measure the amounts of phospholipids in our blood, doctors

FAT: SFA, MUFA, PUFA

rarely measure them because research has not shown how to make good use of this information

Cholesterol-esters are another type of fat made by the body. This fat combines cholesterol and fatty acids. **Cholesterol** is a type of lipid which, when the body has optimal nutritional status, helps to make our blood vessels and cell membranes softer. Cholesterol positions itself between the fatty acids which make up a cell membrane, and makes it more difficult for them to stick together. Cholesterol is also used by the human body to make a wide range of hormones. The body manufactures cholesterol, and carefully regulates its production. As with phospholipids, we do not need to eat cholesterol; the body can make all it requires. Cholesterol imbalances are not caused by simply eating too much cholesterol; we upset the balance of cholesterol by eating an imbalanced mixture of fatty acids. These imbalances cause disease. There is a blood test that measures the amount of cholesterol in our blood. When the amount is high, we have **hypercholesterolemia**. Hypercholesterolemia also may be associated with cardiovascular disease.

References and Notes

[1] The role of monounsaturated fat in health and disease is under research. The human body uses it to regulate some of its chemical processes, as well as to compensate for excessive saturated fat intake. Humans apparently can make all the monounsaturated fat they need. Therefore, we do not need to eat monounsaturated fatty acids. In contrast, polyunsaturated fat is essential, as the body cannot make it. We need to eat EFAs.

Fats: SFA, MUFA, PUFA

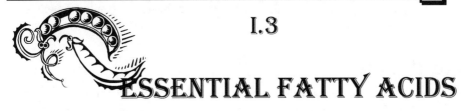

I.3

ESSENTIAL FATTY ACIDS

"The type of fat we eat is the major determining factor in whether we get cardiovascular disease."

Topics: *The essential fats are the omega-3 and omega-6 families. The parents or precursors of essential fats are used to make daughters or derivatives. Animal and fish foods. Eating a mixture of oils. The real culprit in heart disease: not enough essential fats.*

Summary

The essential fats (also known as polyunsaturated fatty acids) are a group of fatty acids that humans cannot make or synthesize. Thus they must be obtained from the diet, in a manner similar to vitamins, but in far greater quantities. There are two families of essential fats, the *omega*-3 (ω3) and *omega*-6 (ω6). The ω3 are made from linolenic acid; the ω6 are made from linoleic acid. Eating both linolenic and linoleic fatty acids allows the body to make all the essential fats it needs. Linolenic and linoleic acids, combined, constitute the Essential Fatty Acids (**EFAs**). They are the precursors (parents) of all the essential fats.

Most people can eat vegetables to obtain all the EFAs they need. Vegetables are high in essential fats; these essential fats are called "parents" or "precursors," and humans can use them to make all the other essential fats (called "daughters" or "derivatives"). We can also obtain the derivatives of the ω3 from fish fat. Some people have lost their ability to derive some essential fats from linoleic and linolenic acids, and therefore need to eat more of the derivatives found in fish, in a few plants and minimally in animal fat. Many people have deficiencies of linolenic (ω3) fatty acids and should eat a mixture of oils including both parents and derivatives. Insufficient intake of essential fats is a more significant cause of heart disease than eating too much saturated fat or cholesterol.

Families of fat

The term "**Polyunsaturated Fatty Acid**," abbreviated PUFA, has been used for many years by health professionals. It also is the general term found in most American diet books and some food labels. Unfortunately, "PUFA" is not a specific enough term. In reality, PUFA refers to a wide range of fatty acids, some of which are artificially made during food processing, and some which are made by the body in response to nutritional deficiencies. In this book we are overlooking these "minor" facts. Instead, we will often refer by the abbreviation, "PUFA" to a group of essential fats that humans need for survival.

Essential fats are grouped in two families, the omega-3 (ω3) and omega-6 (ω3) families (using the Greek letter ω). We call them families because they have many members. Each family member has a different chemical composition and therefore a different medical significance **Each family is headed by one member which we call the Parent or Precursor**. The other members are "**daughters**", or "**derivatives**," meaning that they are derived or produced from their parent.

Essential Fats: The ω3 and ω6 families

Fatty acids form fats like pages form a book, except that fats usually have one to three fatty acids. Even though the appropriate term is fatty acid, we shall often refer to fatty acids as fats in order to simplify the text. The ω3 and the ω6 fatty acids form the families of essential fats. **Linolenic** (ω3) and **Linoleic** (ω6) acid, the parents of each family, are called the **Essential Fatty Acids (EFAs)**. In some old books, and in some publications aimed at the general public, EFAs are called, incorrectly, a vitamin. EFAs are not vitamins; however, they are a vital nutrient which we require in large quantities every day.

The polyunsaturated fats (PUFA) are essential fats. The "**essential fats**" include the fatty acids of both the ω3 and ω6 families. They can refer to either a parent (precursor) or a daughter (derivative). Thus, the words "essential fat" and "PUFA" refer to any ω3 or ω6 fat. The tables in the appendix present the major members of each family of essential fats, and examples of foods containing each type of fatty acid.

Essential Fatty Acids

Precursors and Derivatives

We divide each family into two groups: the precursor and its derivatives. All the **daughters (derivatives)** can be formed from the **parent (precursor)**. *The opposite is not true.* Linoleic and linolenic acid cannot be made from any of their derivatives. In total there are four groups of essential fats: parent and daughter *omega*-3 (ω3), and parent and daughter *omega*-6 (ω6). In general, fat from plants contains the precursors of EFAs while animal fat contains the derivatives.

The derivatives of the **EFAs** (essential fatty acids) can produce physiological changes faster than the parent EFAs found in vegetables. While the human body stores extra EFAs in adipose tissue, stores only small quantities of EFA derivatives. It is more efficient for the body to store EFAs than EFA derivatives for two reasons: first, it can manufacture derivatives, and second, because EFA derivatives are molecules with more bends than EFAs and require more storage space.

The ω3 family

The ω3 family consists of the parent **Linolenic Acid**, found primarily in vegetables, and the daughters found primarily in fish.

Sources of ω3: vegetables and fish

Some authors, when they refer to ω3 fatty acids, mean the derivatives of linolenic acid found in fish products. They confuse daughters with parents. ω3 fatty acids are found in vegetables and they are different from the ω3 fatty acid derivatives found in fish.

The ω3 fatty acid found in vegetables is the parent EFA, linolenic acid. Linolenic acid is found in many seed sprouts, flax seeds (linseed oil),

Family	Parent = Precursor	Daughters = Derivatives
ω3	Linolenic	EPA, DHA and others
ω6	Linoleic	GLA, DGLA, arachidonic
Found in	Vegetables	Animals (ω6), Fish (ω3)

Essential Fatty Acids

soybean and walnut oil, but is not found in safflower, sunflower, olive, or corn oil. Hydrogenation of the oil used in many products like margarine destroys most of the ω3 fat.

Fish and fish oils

Fish and fish oils contain small quantities of linolenic acid and large quantities of the derivatives of linolenic acid. The two most common fatty acids found in fish oil are eicosapentaenoic acid and docosahexaenoic acid (conveniently referred to as **EPA** and **DHA)**. These names are used on the labels of many products currently sold in health food stores and pharmacies.

In my research I have found that the bodies of most people can manufacture the ω3 fats found in fish oils from the EFA linolenic acid obtained from vegetable oils. Because eating fish oils over a long period of time may cause undesirable complications in some people (such as anemia due to internal bleeding in individuals with ulcers and diverticulitis), fish oils should be used with great caution and only for a short period of time until vegetable oils begin to have an effect. In fact, fish is safer than fish oil as part of your long term diet, but fish oils are needed to rapidly prevent clot formation in patients at risk of sudden death due to a clot obstructing an artery.

The ω6 family

The ω6 family consists of the precursor **Linoleic Acid,** found primarily in vegetables, and derivatives mostly formed by humans.

Sources of ω6: vegetables, cattle and poultry

Corn, safflower, sunflower, walnut, sesame, and soybean oils, most leafy vegetables, and seed sprouts contain large quantities of linoleic acid. Derivatives of the ω6 group are found in small quantities in some vegetables and in animal fat. Most animal fat (cattle and poultry) contains small amounts of ω6 derivatives. One such derivative is called arachidonic acid. But animal products contain significantly fewer essential fats than vegetable products. Additionally, animal fat is composed primarily of saturated fat which, as shall be discussed later, interferes with the proper function and use of the EFAs.

Essential Fatty Acids

The role of fat in good health

Most Americans eat a diet high in carbohydrates, saturated fat and partially hydrogenated oils. (Hydrogenated oils are found in foods made with processed fat, such as margarine, breads, crackers, cookies, and pastries.) Most people use corn, olive, safflower or sunflower oils with their salads, and in their cooking. Although these oils provide some linoleic (ω6) fatty acids, they contain few linolenic (ω3) fatty acids. Therefore most people have been eating foods that contain very few ω3 fatty acids. The quickest way to correct for many years of this deficient diet is to eat both members of the ω3 family: precursors and derivatives. A diet which incorporates soybean or walnut oil, supplemented with fish or fish oils, provides both members of the ω3 family. However, it is very important to eat the right balance and most of this book is devoted to this topic.

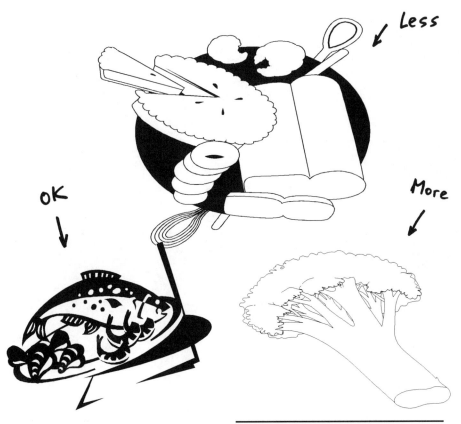

Essential Fatty Acids

People should eat more EFAs

Many nutrition and medical textbooks report that a deficiency of EFAs in adults is extraordinarily rare. Such is also the view of the US Surgeon General who stated that EFA deficiencies are rarely found in the United States[1] (p. 58). Based on the number of cases reported in the medical literature between 1990 and 1993 (other than deficiencies which I reported), the prevailing "wisdom" is that EFA deficiencies affect less than 1 in 100,000 people, or less than 2,000 people in the USA. There are a few researchers who, like myself, think that EFA deficiency is very common. Unfortunately, their findings are not yet taught in medical schools. In my review of medical textbooks, courses and conferences, I have not found a single one which teaches the extent of EFA abnormalities in the USA, let alone how to correct them. My

Type of fat	Family	Major Source	Example
Precursor (parent)	EFA		
Linoleic	ω6	Most vegetable oils, nuts, and seeds. Except tropical oils.	Sunflower (60%) Safflower (60%) Corn , Olive Walnut (50%) Soybean (50%)
Linolenic	ω3	Some vegetable oils, nuts, and seeds.	Linseed (55%) (flax seeds) Walnut(s) (7%) Soybean (7%)
Daughters (derivatives)			
Arachidonic	ω6	Animal fat; future supplements	Liver, organ meats
GLA	ω6	Special oils "Designer fats"	Primrose, Borage Black current oil.
EPA, DHA	ω3	Fish fat = oils	cold water fish, fish oil

Essential Fatty Acids

research indicates that at least 25,000,000 people suffer from significant EFA abnormalities, and the true number is probably much higher. I have found evidence that deficiency of EFAs, both the ω3 and the ω6, are one of the most common deficiencies in the adult population. These deficiencies are likely to be the primary nutritional factor that causes cardiovascular disease, hypertension and the cardiovascular complications of diabetes. Many children also have significant ω3 deficiencies that affect their mental abilities. Therefore it is very important to learn to eat a balanced mixture of ω3 and ω6 fatty acids, starting in childhood.

> ### *Most people need to eat more ω3 and ω6 fatty acids*

The need for precursors and derivatives

Although most Americans eat meat, we know that human beings have no difficulty surviving as vegetarians. Meat is not an essential food for people. However, there are animals, such as those of the cat family, that cannot survive as vegetarians. Our analysis of fatty acids offers an explanation for this difference. Cats and related animals such as the tiger do not appear to have the ability to make derivatives of linoleic and linolenic acid. Therefore these animals must eat meat and fish to survive. However, healthy humans can survive as vegetarians. We have the enzymes which produce all derivatives of the linolenic and linoleic acids. Therefore, eating vegetables and vegetable oils provides us with all the ω3 and ω6 family members that we need. However, as we get old, take drugs, or get ill, the body may not make enough EFA derivatives, and supplements are needed to compensate for this lack.

Some people need fish oils

Some people, due to disease, genetics or a long history of eating diets very low in PUFA, need to eat both EFA precursors and derivatives. Some scientists believe that a large number of people could benefit from eating the ω3 fatty acids found in fish oils, and thus there are corporations manufacturing and marketing fish oil extracts. These extracts contain important linolenic acid (ω3) derivatives EPA and DHA. Other companies are planning to market ω6 EFA derivatives in the near future. The ω6 derivative GLA is already available in primrose and borage oil. [2]

Essential Fatty Acids

My research has shown that most humans do not need to eat fish or animal oils. They can eat the essential fats found in vegetables and some vegetable oils and make all the ω3 and ω6 fatty acids they need, including EPA and DHA. If you are concerned about your ability to manufacture EFA derivatives, due to age, disease, or long term dietary deficiency of EFAs, the best answer is to be tested. The profile **EFA-SR** indicates whether you will benefit from supplementation by derivatives.

Consequences of ω6 deficiency

The signs or symptoms of a particular deficiency depend on the extent of the deficiency, overall nutritional status (i.e., concurrent deficiencies of other vitamins or minerals), individual variability due to disease, age, sex or genetic factors, and environmental variables such as temperature and humidity. The profile **EFA-SR** will usually identify most types of abnormalities.

Studies, mostly in animals, have shown that severe ω6 deficiency is associated with many varying symptoms and disorders. Those occurring upon the skin are most immediately apparent: scaly skin, eczema and Seborrheic dermatitis. Seborrheic dermatitis is frequently seen in infants, and also found in adults behind their ears, on eyebrows, scalp, around the nose and on areas where the skin is folded and is frequently irritated. The skin may exhibit increased water loss, (resulting in dryness) and its healing process may be impaired. Another symptom of ω6 deficiency is abnormal hair loss. ω6 deficiency can also result in disorders of various organs and organ systems, including liver damage, kidney damage, the slow healing of internal injuries, and impaired reproduction (sterility in men, probably because sperm production requires EFAs). Deficiency of ω6 also has a negative effect on the circulatory system. Symptoms in this area include increased blood triglycerides and cholesterol, increased blood pressure, impaired membrane function, hardening of the arteries, artery obstruction, and incorporation of cholesterol and fat in arterial walls. In children, a ω6 deficiency can even result in stunted growth. I have proposed that suboptimal membrane function is a consequence of abnormal EFA metabolism and impairs the immune response, mineral transport, etc. As a result, molecules from inside the cell, such as potassium, magnesium and calcium, leak outside, and those from the plasma outside, such as sodium, leak and accumulate inside.

Consequences of ω3 deficiency

The ω3 deficiencies are associated with neurological impairments such as decreased memory and mental abilities, "strange" or tingling sensations in the nerves, often in the arms and legs, decreased visual acuity (i.e., poor vision), increased tendency to form clots, decreased immune function (decreased ability to resist infections), increased blood triglycerides and cholesterol, impaired membrane function, growth retardation, particularly in infants, young children and pregnant women.

Recently, I spoke with Dr. Simopoulos, who used to chair the Nutrition Coordinating Committee at the National Institutes of Health (USA) from 1978 to 1986 (and is now the President of The Center for Genetics, Nutrition and Health, Washington, D.C.). She sent me many of her articles which summarize results from scientists across the world. It is amazing that so much is known about EFAs worldwide yet so little research is done in the USA. She stated that ω3 fatty acids may decrease cancer mortality, and 0.5 to 1.0 grams of long chain ω3s *"reduce the risk of cardiovascular death in middle aged American men by about 40%"*.[3] For these reasons, I believe that the most important blood test a middle aged men can have is the fatty acid profile **EFA-SR.** If the test reveals that he does not have enough EFAs, he should eat more. Proper diagnosis and treatment could save hundreds of thousands of lives and billions in health care costs. My research is finding similar results with women.[4]

Miscellaneous issues on ω3 and ω6

Egg yolk is a source of PUFAs, particularly in chickens fed foods high in ω3s. Drs. Simopoulos and Salem analyzed the fatty acid composition of chicken egg yolks and found that those fed fish meals or flax had more ω3s. An interesting side note is that Greek eggs were high in ω3s compared with common supermarket eggs. These yolks were also very high in EFA derivatives when compared with Supermarket eggs (which would make them excellent food for infants, see Section IV). The Greek chicken were raised on a farm. The ". . .chickens roam freely and feed on various types of fresh green grass leaves and wild plants including purslane [high in ω3]. . .The chickens also eat insects of all kinds and sometimes eat worms."[5]

Essential Fatty Acids

The tables in the appendix provide you with typical values of most fatty acids in blood for the average person. Practically everybody has fat in their bodies. Except for severely anorexic individuals or those starving in concentration camps or drought regions, everybody has plenty of fat, probably at least 20 pounds. Even those who follow very poor diets have at least one pound of EFAs. For most people, this translates into a range of 25% to 35% of their blood fat in the form of linoleic (ω6) EFA. From this amounts, the body makes EFA derivatives. The body attempts to maintain the levels of EFA derivatives within narrow ranges. Thus, most people have about the same amount of ω6 derivatives, particularly arachidonic acid. This is not true for ω3 derivatives. The amounts of linolenic acid that people eat are very small and some people may not have enough linolenic acid to make ω3 derivatives.

The ratio of **arachidonic acid (AA** = 20:4ω6) to **eicosapentaenoic acid (EPA** = 20:5ω3) is proportional to the ability of the body to form clots. A higher ratio of EPA/AA is associated with decreased clot formation. For most people, increasing the **EPA/AA ratio** requires that they eat more EPA or linolenic acid. Trying to eat less ω6 is counterproductive because most people also have an ω6 deficiency, and even if they eat less ω6 the body would still make AA from the remaining linoleic acid. In fact, if your body level of linoleic acid declines, the body makes more AA in its effort to compensate, and it overshoots! Thus, paradoxically, eating more linoleic acid may decrease the formation of arachidonic acid if you are linoleic acid deficient.

Isomers and *Trans*

In their natural form, saturated, monounsaturated and polyunsaturated fat have specific shapes that create hard or soft structures. The molecules of monounsaturated or polyunsaturated fat have a **kink** or twist (known as a "double Carbon bond") that makes it difficult for them to be knit tightly together. Therefore, they form fluid or soft structures. Saturated fatty acids are straight and can be packed together very tightly. They form hard structures at room temperature, like butter or the fat in beef. It is the unique, kinked shape of polyunsaturated fat which allows it to perform its useful functions in our bodies. Hydrogenation straightens this bend; *trans* **fatty acids** are straight and therefore act like saturated fat.

Cooking changes fat — for the worse

Cooking and processing of unsaturated fat, such as hydrogenation, converts some polyunsaturated fat to saturated, monounsaturated, or to *trans* **fatty acids** (TFAs). Some animals, like cows, have a digestive system that does the same thing to polyunsaturated fat. Thus, you can get some TFAs from beef, not just hydrogenated oils. The TFAs are fats which have a chemical structure between that of a PUFA and that of a saturated fat. They may have undesirable effects, which is a subject of current dispute. High levels of TFAs are associated with coronary heart disease and abnormal cholesterol levels. Some scientists think that at least 30,000 people die each year because of high levels of TFAs (as reported widely in major newspapers and TV stations during the week of May 16, 1994, and reported in the *American Journal of Public Health*). I also suspect that future research will show that many isomer fatty acids are undesirable and may be *indicators* of infectious disease.[6] One thing is certain: TFAs fail to have the desirable effect of essential fats.

Hydrogenated fat contains TFAs

If you read the labels you will find that many processed foods (such as breads and pastries) contain hydrogenated oil. **Hydrogenation** is a process that converts part of the polyunsaturated fat to saturated fatty acids. A side-effect of this hydrogenating process is the production of **TFAs**. Manufacturers hydrogenate polyunsaturated oil to make it more stable, so that it does not smell or taste bad, and so that it has longer shelf life. Hydrogenated oils are then used to prepare processed foods such as bread, cakes, cookies, candies, and shortening. Because most fats are hard at room temperature (that is, they contain a lot of SFAs) they are not hydrogenated. Usually, only oils high in PUFAs are hydrogenated.

Because the government does not require that foods be labeled, it is difficult to find out how many TFAs are in foods. Quite often the label says that a given food contains "partially" hydrogenated oils, to indicate that not all the fatty acids have been hydrogenated. However, there is no way to tell how much of the oil is hydrogenated. Companies use different fats and oils in the same product, often buying whatever is available at the lowest price in the world market. The actual mixture of hydrogenated and non-hydrogenated fatty acids may vary even in the same product of the same brand. Hydrogenated fats are to be avoided. They behave like saturated fats, and contain TFAs.

Without a blood test, it is impossible for you to know how many TFAs you have in your body. Even if you had kept 100% accurate food records for your entire life, you could not know the precise composition of the food you ate or how many of the TFAs were burnt by your body. Your body can burn the TFAs, slowly, but if you eat too many they accumulate. Only a blood test can tell you how many TFAs and other unusual types of fatty acids ("**isomers**") you have in your blood. If the levels are too high, your doctor or nutritionist can place you on a diet that will lower them within one year.

What you need to know

The following factors influence the effects of fats and oils upon your health: the total and proportionate amount that you eat of saturated, monounsaturated and essential fats, *trans* fatty acids and other isomers, the amounts of antioxidants in your diet, your level of exercise, your own metabolism, state of health and body fatty acid composition. In general, small amounts of saturated fatty acids from butter or tropical oils are harmless, particularly if you have adequate levels of essential fats. TFAs are never harmless, but small amounts cause insignificant changes in health status. Isomers, which are other types of fatty acids produced by food processing, may be even more dangerous than TFAs because the body may not be able to eliminate them. We know very little about where the isomers and TFAs accumulate in the body, if they do. Very small amounts of these unusual fatty acids could have an effect out of proportion to their size if they affect some organs, like the heart, more than other organs.

There are several other problems with fat and food processing which have yet to be investigated. Women who eat diets high in TFAs are likely to produce milk high in TFAs.[7] Oil processing produces a wide range of different types of fatty acids that have no known desirable function in humans. Some are called "conjugates" (which some people think may work as antioxidants, but I doubt it). These fatty acids are in very small amounts and can be found in human blood. Whether or not they have any harmful effects is unknown.

Essential Fatty Acids

Popular misconceptions

There are numerous books, articles and brochures written about EFAs. They contain a mixture of useful, misleading and incorrect information. It is practically impossible, even for many experts, to check every fact and thousands of references to foreign articles and authors. I have compiled some of the most common errors so that you can avoid them.

Many books describe ω3 fats and forget to mention the ω6 fats. Others do just the opposite. For example, one well known book for precursors repeats an error found in some nutrition books, which state that there are three essential fatty acids (linoleic, linolenic, and arachidonic), but only linoleic cannot be made by the body. This statement is misleading. Linolenic and linoleic acid are needed by the human body to survive and neither can be made by the body. They are the EFAs. Arachidonic acid is a derivative of linoleic acid. The liver and other organs can make arachidonic acid from linoleic acid and therefore it is not considered essential.[8]

With the recent growth of media publicity surrounding fish oils, many people have heard the term "Omega-3 fatty acids." Many commercials and news reports lead one to believe that ω3 fatty acids are the only important fatty acids, and you can improve your health by merely eating more ω3 fatty acids. This again is a profound mistake. What the human body needs is a proper balance of both ω3 and ω6 fatty acids. Moreover, the ω3 is also found in many vegetable oils, not just fish oils.

Another fallacy is that eating foods low in cholesterol will lower your blood cholesterol substantially. Blood cholesterol levels depend on overall body chemistry, and particularly the balance of fatty acids. Eating cholesterol within the ranges found in most natural foods is probably not an important factor in increasing or decreasing your cholesterol (unless you have some unusual genetic disease).

Another misconception is that the healthiest way to lose weight is to avoid all fat. The way to lose weight is to eat fewer calories, balancing all the necessary elements, and to exercise more. If you substitute your excess calories from fat with calories from carbohydrate or protein --- as many people do --- you will transform the extra calories into saturated fat. Thus, you will still accumulate unwanted body fat. EFA Deficiency will result from eating foods low in EFAs. This condition may increase hunger as the body searches for more EFAs.

Essential Fatty Acids

Carbohydrates burn fat, but eating more carbohydrates will not help you burn more fat. The body needs only a small amount of carbohydrates (about 3 ounces per day) to burn fat. All calories, whether from carbohydrates or other sources, contribute to your total caloric intake. If you do not use all the calories you eat in one day, you store the excess as non-essential fat in your body.

Because the PUFA and TFA composition of foods does not need to be reported in food labels, and manufacturing techniques continuously change the mixture of oils used and the amounts of TFAs produced, estimates of PUFA and TFA intake from dietary records are highly unreliable. Most food labels that list only the amount of SFAs are useless. What you need to know is the amounts of essential fat and TFAs in the food.

Essential Oils vs. Essential Fatty Acids (EFAs)

Oils are related to the word "essence". An "essence" is what characterizes a particular thing. In practice, "essence" refers to the fragrance or flavor that characterizes a food, plant or flower. Chemists extract from plants and foods the chemicals that produce this "essence." These chemicals are called "essential oils". One major application for these oils is in making perfumes. With very rare exceptions, most essential oils should not be eaten in large amounts, although tiny amounts of essential oils are present in many foods, herb's and beverages, and contribute to their flavor or aroma. Essential oils have a chemical structure far closer to petroleum products than fatty acids. Most essential oils are extracted from plants or flowers. While these chemicals, in very small amounts, may not be dangerous to the human body, in large amounts essential oils are likely to be harmful. Eating a little bit of bath oil may not hurt, but eating a lot is not going to make your joints work more smoothly! In fact, some of these oils could act as solvents, meaning they could dissolve membranes and cause severe body damage.

The EFAs are not Vitamin F

EFAs have been referred to as "Vitamin F." There is no vitamin F, but this is only a minor scientific error. Vitamins are essential to life. So are minerals, but we do not call Iron a 'vitamin." Vitamins are small molecules whose primary functions are to regulate chemical reactions, causing them to proceed more quickly or slowly, .and to activate other

Essential Fatty Acids

molecules. The EFAs are components of fats. They have structural, hormonal and regulatory functions. They are not vitamins even though they are essential to life.

Oxidation, EFAs and vitamin E

Vitamin E has multiple roles. One of its roles is to act as an "antioxidant" which protects EFAs and other substances from unnecessary oxidation. Contrary to popular belief, oxidation is not always harmful. **Oxidation** occurs when chemicals are used by the body to generate energy, or when they are transformed into other chemicals. In other words, oxidation occurs all the time. Oxidation occurs when you think, breathe, and clean your body of toxic substances. If you consume too many antioxidants and oxidation cannot occur, you will die. Thus, eating antioxidants when you do not need them is more likely to harm than protect you.

You need **antioxidants** to protect EFAs from *unnecessary* oxidation. Remember, however, antioxidants only protect EFAs; they do not help your body make EFAs. When you are EFA deficient, taking more vitamin E, C, or Selenium is like buying a lot of anti-rust paint for a car you do not have in the first place.

Some brochures state that "Oxidation changes EFAs into destructive compounds called free fatty acids". This is nonsense. **Free fatty acids** are formed by the body as part of its natural chemistry, as an intermediate step in using fats. When a fat is broken down for energy or converted to a hormone, the first step is to free the fatty acids that make up the fat. In this manner, fat can be carried in the blood and transported into cells.

Some authors confuse "free fatty acids" with "free radicals". **Free radicals** are chemicals that oxidize other substances. In the proper amount, they are essential for the body to work (remember, without oxidation, you would die. All of your organs get "fed" through oxidation). However, too many free radicals make your body more susceptible to heart disease and possibly to cancer.

Oxidation changes the molecular structure of fatty acids into useful hormones, or simply into energy. It does not necessarily change them into free fatty acids. Furthermore, changing EFAs into free fatty acids is not "a major factor in the onset of cancer and heart disease" as stated in some brochures. Unnecessary oxidation of fatty acids could create an excess of chemicals called "free radicals" that may damage your cell

Essential Fatty Acids

DNA. This damage can lead to cancer or the accumulation of fat in your arteries. However, eating many antioxidants will not necessarily stop that process.

Some brochures state that refined soybean oil is worthless or that refined oils have no EFAs. This is not true. Refined soybean oil, well prepared, has about the same number of EFAs as other types of soybean oil. Soybean oil has EFAs in one of the best proportions relevant to human health. Refined soybean oil may or may not have enough vitamin E to protect the EFAs from oxidation, and may not have many other substances found in soybeans that could be healthful, but the EFAs are still fairly intact. On the other hand, refined oil is unlikely to contain pesticides. Many pesticides and toxic chemicals dissolve quite well in oil. To make the oil safe for humans, it is necessary to eliminate these pesticides by extraction and refinement. Oils from organic sources may not need this purification process, but it is impossible to tell the levels of pesticides and toxic chemicals in oils or in any other food. There ought to be a law requiring disclosure.

When you open a bottle of refined oil and air enters the bottle, the oil may go bad faster than an oil that has natural antioxidants to protect it from the air (but many refined oils have added natural antioxidants). Thus, it is still possible that unrefined oils are better, but refined oils are probably OK most of the time.

Another popular statement, "EFAs become empty calories when oils are refined," is also wrong. The EFAs are fats, and like all fats, they have calories regardless of source. Whether you get your EFAs from refined or unrefined oils is irrelevant. Both refined and unrefined oils oxidize quickly, or may be destroyed by cooking, temperature, storage, light, and air. What matters is the combination of oil manufacturing, packaging, storage and use.

Some authors indicate that all polyunsaturated oils can be used for frying. I disagree. Highly polyunsaturated oils such as canola, safflower, sunflower, soybean and walnut oil should not be used in cooking at high temperatures for a long period of time (such as in broiling or frying). High temperatures will destroy the structure of the polyunsaturated oils, thus altering their function in the body.

Essential Fatty Acids

Differences with other authors

I disagree with many authors who state the requirements for EFAs as a percent of calories. For example, one author states that "a low-fat diet requires less EFAs, and a high fat diet requires more". My position is different. A diet low in fat requires, proportionately, more calories from EFAs than a diet high in fat because one needs a minimum amount of EFAs which depend on body size. If the individual exercises quite a bit, he can eat a smaller percent of EFAs on a high fat, high calorie diet, and burn the extra fat. However, if the extra fat is accumulated in the body, then he/she needs more EFAs to maintain within desirable limits the ratio of essential to non-essential fats. The objective is to maintain the body ratio of essential to non-essential fats after taking into consideration the mostly non-essential fats burned for energy.

USDA Food Pyramid

In "The **Food Guide Pyramid**", a fancy color brochure prepared and printed by the US Department of Agriculture in August, 1992 (bulletin No. 252), the USDA states: ". . .the small tip of the Pyramid shows fats, oils, and sweets. . . These foods provide calories and little else nutritionally. . . Most people should use them sparingly." I believe this statement is misleading and false. Many oils provide EFAs which are essential to body function. They should not be used sparingly; instead they should be used in sufficient amounts to prevent or correct EFA insufficiency.

I believe that The Food Guide Pyramid is a major nutritional disaster. It contains misrepresentations or omissions of material facts, such as the need for EFAs. It implies that most of your diet should come from carbohydrates (listed at the bottom of the pyramid), which would increase your body's composition of saturated fat.[9] It is an irony of our complex regulatory process that federal employees can provide guidelines which I believe will kill millions of Americans while food companies are prohibited from explaining potential benefits of oil supplements that would save their lives.

Which is better, butter or margarine

Butter consists mostly of SFAs. Depending on the brand, about 60% of the fat in butter is SFAs, the rest being MUFA and a very small amount, often less than 5%, being PUFA. Butter has very few TFAs.[10]

Essential Fatty Acids

Margarine composition varies tremendously from one brand to another and from one week to the next. Generally, the harder the consistency of the margarine, the higher its amount of TFAs and SFAs. Some margarine have less than 10% of fat as TFAs; some have more than 40% of their fat as TFAs. However, as you are reading this, most manufacturers are drastically decreasing the amount of TFAs in margarine in response to recent public outcry. In fact, there are now margarines made without hydrogenation or TFAs, primarily by using "hardening" agents (to solidify the oil, like a gelatin), or by using high pressures and other processes. Most margarines have more EFAs than butter.

How can the consumer evaluate the beneficial effects of EFAs vs. the hazardous effects of TFAs in margarine, and then compare those with the saturated fat in butter? The answer, of course, is that the consumer cannot. Any researcher can design a study comparing butter vs. some brands of margarine and show that butter is better; others can evaluate margarine and obtain opposite results. The body composition of the participants in the study, other components of the diet, amount of exercise and many other factors determine whether margarine or butter is better in regard to improving cholesterol levels, and ultimately reducing risk of heart disease. In Europe they make margarine by mixing saturated with essential fats. These margarines are generally safer because they retain the EFAs and have virtually no TFAs, even though they have more saturated fat.

It is healthiest to avoid both margarine and butter and use raw oils. However, a teaspoon of butter will probably have no bad effects if you are otherwise slim, in good health, and have a good balance of EFAs. A tablespoon of a margarine low in TFAs and high in EFAs can be healthful if the rest of your diet is low in TFAs, but can hurt if you eat too many TFAs from cookies and other foods high in hydrogenated oil. Unfortunately, there is a "catch" here: You cannot tell because practically no foods list the amount of TFAs (and other isomers), and very few list the amounts of EFAs. The government does not require it and therefore food manufacturers can claim whatever they want. Beware of misleading advertising. A whole page ad in The Boston Globe indicated that margarine is better because it is lower in saturated fat. As stated previously, this is irrelevant. What matters it the overall intake of calories vs. calories from EFAs. What matters is what happens in your body, especially your body's proportion of EFAs vs. other types of fat.

Essential Fatty Acids

For cooking at high temperatures, butter may be more stable that some oils or some margarines. Oils change composition at high temperature and may produce undesirable chemicals. For toast, I recommend you use an oil. In any case, butter or margarine will melt when placed on hot toast or a potato. Most of the time it is impossible to tell the difference between the margarine and an oil (except for the salt or flavor added to the margarine). Whenever possible, use an oil in its raw form. Cook with as little oil as possible, but for high temperatures use butter.

For health professionals

Description and Names

Fatty acids are named according to chain length, number of double bonds (**kinks**), and a characteristic end carbon group known as the

---

enzymes/cofactors

PFAi ----------------------------------> DFAi

Precursor Derivatives

i = 3, 6, 7, 9 are the ω3, ω6, ω7 , ω9 families of fatty acids

---

"*omega*" (ω) or "n-" carbon. Example: **18:2ω6** signifies a chain **18** carbons in length, with **2** double carbon bonds, which belongs to the ω**6** or linoleic acid family. The colon (**:**) separates the carbon length from the number of double bonds or kinks.

Saturated fatty acids (**SFAs**) have no double bonds. Palmitic acid (16:0 or 16 carbons, 0 double bonds) and stearic acid (18:0 or 18 carbons, 0 double bonds) are the most abundant SFAs in blood and tissues. Monounsaturated fatty acids (**MUFAs**) have one double bond; polyunsaturated fatty acids (PUFAs) have 2 or more double bonds. The MUFA family, ω9, derives from oleic acid (18:1ω9), and the ω7 derives from palmitoleic acid (18:1ω7).

The major PUFA families are the ω6, derived from linoleic acid (18:2ω6), and the ω3, derived from linolenic acid (18:3ω3). Linoleic and linolenic acids are essential because humans must obtain them from the diet. The derivatives of fatty acids are abbreviated "**DFA**,"

Essential Fatty Acids

("Derivative of Fatty Acid"), and include the family number from which they are derived. The derivatives of linoleic acid are known as DFA6 (including arachidonic acid, 20:4ω6), and the derivatives of linolenic acid as DFA3 (including eicosapentaenoic acid or EPA, 20:5ω3, and docosahexaenoic acid or DHA, 22:6ω3). The most abundant PUFAs are linoleic acid (ω6), arachidonic acid (ω6), and DHA (ω3). Grouping the fatty acids into precursors and derivatives helps to diagnose patterns of deficiency, and thus enables effective treatment with precursors (such as vegetable oil) and/or derivatives (such as fish oil).

The appendix presents several diagrams and tables with the most significant fatty acid metabolic pathways, and the enzymes which activate and participate in these pathways. Additional tables present prevalent levels of fatty acids (25th, 50th, 75th percentiles) and also various fatty acid ratios, both based on results from 200 non-hospitalized adults ages 30-69 (50% men, 50% women) participating in the Framingham Heart Study, and fatty acid composition of common foods.

Biochemical characteristics

- The 4 precursor fatty acids are linolenic (ω3), linoleic (ω6), oleic (ω9), and palmitoleic (ω7), abbreviated **PFAi** (i=3,6,9,7, for the ω3, ω6, ω9 and ω7).

- There are two families of MUFA (monounsaturated fatty acids), the ω7 and ω9. These families are not essential for humans (humans can make them from saturated fatty acids). The body also makes very small amounts of polyunsaturated derivatives of ω9 and ω7. These are not essential derivatives. When the body is EFA deficient, it makes quite a bit more of them. Finding them in large amounts in the blood is an indication that the body is EFA deficient.

- The elongation and desaturation products of the precursor fatty acids are referred to as derivatives, abbreviated DFAi.

- Fatty acids undergo desaturation and elongation in the body using enzymes apparently shared among fatty acid families.

- The affinity for these enzymes follows this order: ω3 > ω6 > ω9 > ω7. (compare the DFAi/PFAi ratios in the appendix).

- PUFA family members are not interchangeable; members of one family ($\omega 6$ or $\omega 3$) cannot be made from the other family.

- Monounsaturated fatty acids can be made from saturated fatty acids. Excess calories from carbohydrates and protein are converted to and stored by the body as MUFAs or SFAs, the specific proportion depending on PUFA levels.

- The conversion of PFAs to DFAs require enzymes which can be inhibited by TFAs, insulin, disease, drugs, and deficiencies of selected vitamins and minerals. However, it is practically impossible to predict enzyme activity. The only solution is to analyze the blood in the manner I described in the journal *Metabolism*.[11]

Relative excesses or deficiencies of one fatty acid alter the metabolism of the others. This property constitutes the basis for treatment of diseases where one wants to avoid accumulation of specific fatty acids.[12] Humans have the elongation and desaturation enzymes required to make derivatives from precursors. However, some individuals have decreased enzyme activity or increased need for EFA derivatives due to age, disease or a deficiency of vitamins or minerals that act as cofactors. These abnormalities can be treated with a diet high in EFA derivatives.

Functions

Fatty acids are critical participants in all cell functions and body systems. PUFAs have at least three main functions: (1) They regulate membrane fluidity and membrane function. (2) They are precursors to **eicosanoids** (prostanglandins, thromboxanes and leukotrienes), with relative eicosanoid production depending on EFA metabolism. (3) They may have enzyme-like activities or be cofactors in enzymes. The availability of EFAs may be the limiting factor in lipid synthesis because glucose, amino acids and other nutrients are rarely deficient in the American diet.

PUFAs = EFAs + EFA derivatives (Precursors + Derivatives)

= (PFA3 + PFA6) + (DFA3 + DFA6)

Omega 3 ($\omega 3$) = PFA3 + DFA3; Omega 6 ($\omega 6$) = PFA6 + DFA6

Essential Fatty Acids

Fatty acids are absorbed through the small intestine and are stored in adipose tissue as SFAs, MUFAs, and EFAs, but only rarely as EFA derivatives. Fatty acids are oxidized for energy or metabolized to other compounds. They are protected from oxidation by vitamins E, C and selenium. Changes in fatty acid metabolism can dramatically impair body function. Platelet aggregation decreases and bleeding time increases in proportion to the ω3/ω6 ratio[13] (specifically, 20:5ω3/20:4ω6).

Hormone precursors

The EFAs are precursors of a group of hormones called "eicosanoids." The **eicosanoids** consist of the prostaglandins, the leukotrienes, the thromboxanes and several other hormones. For historical reasons, these hormones are grouped in different families, according to their precursor. Series 1 derives from DGLA, 20:3ω6; Series 2 derives from arachidonic acid, 20:4ω6, and Series 3 from EPA, 20:5ω3. I suspect that additional hormones will be discovered derived from 20:3ω9, and other fatty acids, but they are produced in very tiny amounts. Although some writers speak about "good" and "bad" prostaglandins, there is no such thing. Each hormone has an important function in the body and we must have the optimal balance for optimal health. Moreover, this is one area where men and women's hormonal balances is quite different. For example, pregnancy, delivery and menstruation are regulated by a balance of these hormones (an issue that rarely affects men directly). Abnormal hormone imbalance contributes to abnormal premenstrual syndrome and abnormalities of pregnancy and delivery.

Fatty Acid abnormalities

Requirements for EFAs are increased in processes characterized by increased cell turnover, such as burns, pregnancy, gastrointestinal disease and inflammation. EFA abnormalities may be caused by genetic disorders, deficiencies or excesses of dietary fatty acids. Severe **EFA deficiency (EFAD)**, found mostly in animals fed EFA deficient diets, causes dermatitis, hair loss, and abnormal cell histology.[14]

Decreased EFAs in blood plasma causes shifts in fatty acid metabolism, leading to increased ratios of Derivatives/ Precursors (**DFAi/PFAi**) and increased ω7 and ω9 MUFA. The trienoic/tetraenoic or **"T/T"** ratio

increases **(Mead acid, 20:3ω9/Arachidonic acid, 20:4ω6)**.
Values above 0.02 are indicative of insufficient EFA levels.[15]

EFA insufficiency (EFAI) is characterized by the same abnormal
biochemical markers as EFAD, but is not a severe enough condition to
produce the overt clinical signs noted in experimental animals made
severely EFAD. EFAI may lead to abnormal eye and neurological
function, hyperlipidemia, hypertension, abnormal eicosanoid activity,
reduced cell survival, and impaired wound healing and cell growth.
EFAI is a significant factor in cardiovascular disease and complications
caused by diabetes. EFAI is diagnosed by low levels of PUFAs or high
levels of markers of EFAD. The figures in the appendix compare levels
of T/T with the ratio of PUFA/NoPUFA (where NoPUFA stands for
fatty acids which are not polyunsaturated, i.e. SFAs and MUFAs).
Levels of T/T > 0.02 or PUFA/NoPUFA < 0.9 are indicative of EFAI.
However, optimal levels of PUFA/NoPUFA are probably around 1.2,
based on subjects with no known disease, desirable lipid profiles and an
excellent health condition (unpublished data).

Low absolute (whole body) levels of the EFAs produce **Absolute EFAD
or Absolute EFAI**, depending on the severity of the abnormality.
Absolute deficiencies are seen in people with gastrointestinal disease
and fat malabsorption, anorexia nervosa, bulimia, diets very low in
PUFA, newborns and premature infants. **Relative EFAI** is
characterized by normal to high plasma concentrations EFAs but low
percents of EFAs (low percent of total fatty acids), elevated biochemical
markers of EFAD, and high concentrations and percents of plasma SFA
or MUFA (see tables in the appendix). Usually, adipose tissue levels of
EFAs are adequate but biochemically inaccessible.[16] This pattern is
found in cardiovascular disease, hypertension and hyperlipidemia.
Paradoxically, we may find increased plasma concentrations of EFAs
because the concentrations of all plasma lipids are increased. In its
attempt to deliver enough EFAs to the cells that need them, the body
releases all types of fatty acids into the blood. However, the proportion
(percent) of EFAs is decreased because there are not enough of them in
proportion to the amounts of SFAs.[17]

Relative vs. Absolute abnormalities are diagnosed using a plot of lipid
or fatty acid concentration (Y-axis) vs. EFA or PUFA % (X-axis) as
illustrated by figures in the appendix.[18] The table below presents an
outline of Absolute vs. Relative EFAI/ EFAD. Absolute deficiencies
require the consumption of large amounts of both EFA families, with a
mixture of ω3/ω6 to be adjusted by periodic blood tests. Relative

Essential Fatty Acids

deficiencies are often due to overweight, caused by excessive consumption of saturated fats. They improve with weight loss. For these patients, small amounts of EFA supplements help optimize the ω3/ω6 balance and prevent undesirable clot formation.

Outline of Absolute vs. Relative EFAI/ EFAD

	Deficiency		Insufficiency	
EFA Status	**Absolute**	**Relative**	**Absolute**	**Relative**
T/T	Very High	Very High	High	High
EFA status indice	Very Low	Very Low	Low	Low
Indicators of EFAD	Very High	Very High	High	High
Fatty Acid or Lipid Concentration	Low/ Normal	Normal/ High	Low/ Normal	Normal/ High
EFA Concentration	Very low	Normal	Low	Normal/ High

There is almost no federally funded research to study the incidence and prevalence of fatty acid and TFA abnormalities. However, we can make some estimates. Abnormal lipid profiles are usually associated with EFA abnormalities, because EFAs are carried by lipoproteins. It is difficult to achieve optimal EFA delivery in the presence of abnormal lipid levels. Depending on where we draw the line, >50% of the adult population has a condition associated with EFA abnormality, such as "undesirable" cholesterol levels, hypertension or atherogenic disease. Many people with "normal" cholesterol levels, such as patients with gastrointestinal malabsorption, have abnormal EFA metabolism.

Based on my research analyzing more than 500 Framingham Heart Study samples and patients, I make the following estimates regarding

Essential Fatty Acids

the non-hospitalized adult population: 5% have widespread substantial or severe EFA abnormalities that ought to be treated immediately; more than 20% have significant widespread EFA abnormalities, frequently ω3 deficiency, that would improve with treatment and thereby reduce future morbidity and mortality.

Hydrogenation and processing significantly eliminate linolenic acid (ω3) from processed foods. The low stability at room temperature of foods high in ω3s, and the government-sponsored recommendation to eat low fat foods, results in food intake patterns very low in ω3s. Until 1994, practically all **infant formulas** had few EFAs, and still today most liquid and powder food supplements for the elderly have no ω3s and few ω6s. Many children lack sufficient EFAs, and consequently are likely to develop mental and behavior problems caused by ω3 deficiencies. Many people over 65 are treated with EFA deficient liquid formulas and foods. A linolenic acid (ω3) deficient diet, combined with a history of low ω3 intake, causes rapid depletion of ω3 body stores. It is not surprising, therefore, that we are finding many elderly individuals with impaired mental abilities. We have found EFA abnormalities in patients with Parkinson's, Huntington's and Alzheimer's Diseases as well as many undefined neurologic-psychiatric abnormalities.

I suspect that many "psychiatric" abnormalities have a biochemical basis in EFAD. Until recently, these views were heresy for which I could be burned. I now have evidence that psychiatric disorders can be caused by EFA abnormalities. Recently, I analyzed two patients with severe fat malabsorption who had non-specified neurologic symptoms. When neurologists found no "organic" disease, one patient had been recommended for long-term psychiatric treatment. The other patient had decreased long term memory and vague mental impairments. In both patients I found severe EFAD, particularly linolenic acid (ω3). Once treated with intravenous lipids, the "psychiatric" disorders disappeared, while memory and mental abilities improved. I suspect that progressive loss in memory and mental abilities caused by abnormal EFA metabolism is a common unrecognized disorder. About 10% of the population has values of DFA3 < 2 % (which I consider abnormally low). Only 6% has DFA3 > 4% which may be desirable levels. The chronic abnormal levels of DFA3s could account for a significant proportion of the prevalence of mental impairments. While we spend billions to find a genetic cause or miracle drugs, we are overlooking the most common reason for mental impairments, a

Essential Fatty Acids

nutritional deficiency of the very long chain PUFAs that are the building blocks for brain function.

Diagnosis of EFA abnormalities aids in the prevention and treatment of:[19]

♦ *Cardiovascular disease[20], stroke, atherosclerosis (hardening and thickening of the arteries), poor blood circulation. EFAs reduce while trans and saturated fatty acids increase the risk of CAD[21];*

♦ *Hyperlipidemia & hypertension;*

♦ *Complications of diabetes, such as eye and kidney problems[22];*

♦ *Complications of pregnancy & preeclampsia due to EFAI;*

♦ *Inflammatory bowel disease; celiac disease; cystic fibrosis;[23]*

♦ *Seborrheic dermatitis;*

♦ *Kidney disease (dialysis patients have EFA deficiencies[24]);*

♦ *Brain and behavior abnormalities in children and infants[25]fed diets low in EFAs. Such diets include milk and formulas without EFAs.[26]*

♦ *Malnutrition; wasting states. Patients on elemental diets or parenteral alimentation often suffer from EFA deficiency.*

Measurements of EFAs in women contribute to better therapeutic intervention on lipid parameters to reduce the risk of hardening of the arteries.[27] Other conditions related to EFA levels include neurologic dysfunction; arthritis, coagulation disorders; abnormal red cells; immune deficiencies and obesity.[28] EFA abnormalities can make people more hungry and also contribute to the complications of obesity.

Treatment & management

In general, the diet that works best for prevention or treatment of cardiovascular disease[29] may also help to prevent other diseases, including cancer.[30] The treatment diet is designed to correct deficiencies identified by the fatty acid profile **EFA-SR**, using foods and oil supplements. Increased dietary intake of PUFA with oil or oil extracts should be accompanied by increased amounts of antioxidants such as Vitamin E and Selenium to match body requirements.

Essential Fatty Acids

The EFA derivatives have a stronger and faster effect than the EFAs, but the body does not store them. Eating EFAs allows the body to regulate and produce the EFA derivatives it needs. This approach is effective in prevention, but it may not correct years of neglect. EFAs are far cheaper and easier to take because they are found in common oils. EFA derivatives of the ω3, found in fish oils, are more expensive, but often are useful in the short term for their prompt decrease of platelet aggregation.

The initial treatment aims to modify baseline EFA levels towards ideal levels, based on each individual's condition. After obtaining fatty acid profiles at baseline, the first step is to treat with a mixture of EFAs such as soybean oil, for 2-6 months (some patients are at such severe risk of forming an undesirable clot that they need immediate ω3 derivatives). After treatment with oils containing EFAs, another blood test to measure fatty acids like the **EFA-SR** is obtained to determine whether the EFA dose should be increased, decreased or changed in its ω3/ω6 ratio, and whether the patient converts EFAs to DFAs.[31] If he/she does not, it may be necessary to treat with EFA derivatives.

Fish and vegetable oils which contain ω3 and ω6 fatty acids help to prevent cardiovascular disease,[32] aid to lower cholesterol and triglycerides and make blood less likely to form clots.[33] They may normalize blood pressure and prevent the complications of diabetes mellitus, improve arthritis and poor blood circulation, and increase the effectiveness of the immune system.

Technical issues on fatty acids

Research has shown that humans apparently only need fatty acids that have an even number of carbon lengths. Bacteria and some plants have fatty acids with an odd number of carbon lengths, i.e., 15. Bacteria also have a wide range of different types of fatty acids that apparently are not needed by humans. Blood testing can detect these unusual fatty acids in blood and their pattern can be used to diagnose a bacterial infection. (Very small amounts are often remnants of food or leftovers from bacteria digested by the intestine, thus not indicative of disease.)

Although the nomenclature used by various authors is not consistent, in general fatty acids of carbon length 4-8 are often called "**Short chain**", those 8-14 are called **Medium chain**, those 14-20 are called Long chain, and those 22 and above are called **Very Long chain** fatty

Essential Fatty Acids

acids. Most SFAs are 16 and 18 carbons long; most MUFAs are also 16 to 20 carbon long; most PUFA are 18 and above carbons long.

The cells, primarily in their membranes, contain a mixture of different types of lipids including triglycerides (3 fatty acids), phospholipids (2 fatty acids and one molecule of choline) and cholesterol-esters (one molecule of cholesterol and one fatty acid). Whether these lipids forms are solid, semi-hard, or liquid at body temperature is fundamental for the function of the cell. A cell must have a precise amount of "fluidity". Too hard and the membrane cannot move things in and out. Too soft and everything becomes "mushy" and leaks in and out. I believe that regulation of cell membrane fluidity is the most important physiological function of the body and all other activities are aimed to maintain cell membrane fluidity within very narrow ranges. Lipids made with saturated fatty acids are solid at body temperature. Lipids made entirely with long chain PUFAs are liquid at body temperature. The body continuously mixes various types of fatty acids to maintain proper membrane fluidity. If we eat too many SFAs and not enough EFAs, the body tries to compensate by making more MUFAs because they are more unsaturated. However, MUFAs cannot effectively perform the function of PUFAs; the body cannot catch up and the cell membranes do not work well. Then, to make the membrane more fluid, the cell incorporates more cholesterol. When there is too much cholesterol and SFAs, they precipitate and form crystals or clumps. These lumps of fat and cholesterol deposit inside the arteries and harden and obstruct them, inciting the platelets to form clots to obstruct the artery. The platelets see this plaque, think that the artery broken, and rush in to protect the body from bleeding to death. Unfortunately, once the cells are full of SFA and cholesterol, losing a little bit of weight will not help clean the arteries. The body uses first the fat in adipose tissue before it reaches down and starts using the accumulated fat in arteries. Weight loss must be significant before arteries begin to clean themselves. Within wide limits, if we eat too much PUFA, the body merely stores it as adipose fat and uses what it needs. It incorporates PUFAs into cellular membranes to maintain membrane fluidity without using too much cholesterol.

The fatty acids in commercial extracts may be prepared from cholesterol esters, ethyl esters, phospholipids and triglycerides. Most supermarket oils are triglycerides. Lecithin is a phospholipid. Most fats in plants are in the form of phospholipids. The lecithin sold in many stores is an extract of the lecithin found in plants. Our chemical analysis of samples of powdered lecithin found that it contains too many strange fatty acids and other chemicals, many whose origin and clinical significance are unknown. Some are known to be undesirable. Triglycerides and phospholipids are the form in which fatty acids are usually found in nature and therefore would be the preferable type of fat. Ethyl esters may be absorbed better than triglycerides, but could have different biochemical effects. We just do not know.

Molecular shape

Research in progress suggests that essential fats are in many different types of foods and have different chemical shapes. The active ingredient in oils, the ω3 or ω6 fatty acid, may be located in one of several molecular positions. We do not know which one is the most active site. Phospholipids contain their essential fats mainly in what is known as position #2 of the lipid molecule. It may be that only essential fats in position #2 have beneficial effects.[34]

Oils have fatty acids in positions # 1, #2 and #3. Among the various oils, the actual quantity of essential fat may not be as important as the amount of essential fat in position #2. This information is not currently available and several years will be required to study the oils and identify where the essential fats are or should be located. Therefore, claims stating that one oil has more essential fats than another are not a sufficient basis for selecting one oil over another. What may be important is that the oil has enough essential fats in position #2. For example, even though safflower oil has more ω6 than corn oil, the amount in position #2 may be about the same. Thus, it may be proven some day that corn oil is as effective as safflower oil. These issues are most important for designing experiments where subjects eat oil supplements. Without consideration for the molecular location of the EFAs, and the actual effect of the diet on fatty acid composition, the results could be misleading.

References and Notes

[1]   The Surgeon General's Report on Nutrition and Health. US Department of Health and Human Services, PHS publication No. 88-50210, 1988.

[2]   Animal fats also contain small amounts of ω6 derivatives.

[3]   Simopoulos AP. Omega-3 fatty acids in health and disease and in growth and development. *Am. J. Clin. Nutr.* 1991; 54: 438-63. Excellent review article.

[4] In 1994 I requested federal funds to study the role of EFAs in cardiovascular disease in men and women using the world-known Framingham Heart Study subjects. With this research we will know how to prevent heart disease, and diagnose and treat abnormalities of EFAs. Of course, this research is likely to show that the emphasis on avoiding saturated fat and cholesterol is misplaced, which could make many government agencies and food corporations unhappy.

[5] Simopoulos AP, Salem N. Egg yolk as a source of long-chain polyunsaturated fatty acids in infant feeding. *Am. J. Clin. Nutr.* 1992; 55:411-4. This paper presents an extensive discussion about the role of egg yolks. I agree that egg yolks could be an excellent source of essential fats. When I was a child we had neighbors who raised chickens. The chickens were also free and ate in ways similar to the Greek chicken. However, our modern high technology for feeding chickens has transformed an excellent egg into a mediocre food.

[6] *Trans* fats have been linked to cardiovascular disease and cancer. This subject is still debated, but almost everyone agrees that *trans* fats are not natural fats for humans, and therefore have no desirable function. These unusual fatty acids may be produced by bacteria or cancer cells and could thus serve as markers of the disease, even if they do not cause it. For that reason, the fatty acid profile **EFA-SR** measures several isomers and odd fatty acids.

[7] This research is likely to be published late in 1994 or 1995.

[8] Small infants may need EFA derivatives from human milk until their organs mature enough to make their own.

[9] If the USDA were a private organization, I believe that the Attorney Generals of most states, and the Food and Drug Administration, would prosecute it for violation of consumer protection laws.

[10] Some researchers still recommend that people eat foods low in saturated fat and ignore the TFAs. I disagree. The process of hydrogenation changes PUFAs into monounsaturated and saturated fatty acids. It is not a well-controlled process. Different companies used different methods and different sources of PUFA oils. A byproduct of hydrogenation is the formation of isomers and TFAs. Most oils are not completely hydrogenated, and are called "partially hydrogenated.". That is, not all PUFAs in them are converted to saturated fat. Some companies convert all the PUFAs into MUFAs and SFAs. Some companies convert some of the PUFAs to MUFAs and SFAs. The amounts are not published. Oils high in PUFA are unstable, but cheap. Because many people prefer a solid product for butter and margarine, and because the public has been told to avoid foods high in SFAs, companies find it practical to start with an oil low in SFAs, and convert the MUFAs and PUFAs to the TFAs. Because TFAs behave as saturated fat, they are more stable and form more solid foods than PUFAs and MUFAs; however, they do not count as SFAs in the label. Thus, using TFAs accomplishes a major purpose: Companies can market a food low in SFAs but with properties similar to SFAs, and the consumer, ignorant of these differences will buy it. Because food labels do not require a list of the amount of TFAs, companies can hide the amount of TFAs in their foods and claim that their foods are low in SFAs.

It is possible to combine an oil high in PUFA with one high in SFAs, such as a topical oil, to make a margarine that contains PUFAs, no TFAs, and is also solid. However, many consumers have been told that topical oils are dangerous. Furthermore, topical oils count as SFAs, while TFAs do not count. So companies feel: why fight the perfect system? They can cheaply produce foods low in SFAs, which consumers will prefer because the food label says they are low in SFAs.

Research is funded by companies to prove that their products are safe and effective. Government committees approve the use of food labels that do not require a list of TFAs or EFAs. Instead, they require listing cholesterol and SFAs. Drug companies can make drugs to lower cholesterol made by the body. Everybody is happy. The consumer is told to buy foods low in SFAs and cholesterol and therefore people feel that they are eating healthy foods. There are many more aspects of this story. I cannot explain all the political and economic reasons for nutritional recommendations. They are a better subject for a Congressional inquiry.

There are several alternative methods to solidify an oil and make margarine. One product mixes water and some oil. However, because it is low in fat, it cannot be used for cooking, only as a spread. One such product is Smart Beat. Another company uses high pressure to "solidify" the oil. The consistency is similar to whipped butter. One such product is Spectrum Spread. Other companies used a process called "interesterification". The idea is to mix a fat high in saturated fat, such as a tropical oil with an oil high in PUFA. The molecular exchange creates fats with a different mixture of fatty acids which are somewhere between a solid and a liquid. There is no hydrogenation and no formation of TFAs or unusual isomers. Most likely, the body will digest these new fats and use them as it as SFAs and PUFAs. If you eat enough PUFAs, the small amounts of the SFAs is not dangerous. Obviously, the purpose here is to create a texture similar to margarine or butter (otherwise, you might as well eat the oil). **Note**: All names are subject to change because I have combined information from various technical journals. Many of the names are registered or trademarked and are included here only to assist you to identify them.

[11] Siguel EN, Maclure M. Relative enzyme activity of unsaturated fatty acid metabolic pathways in humans, *Metabolism*, 1987;36:664-9.

[12] This approach was popularized in the movie "Lorenzo's oil," although the treatment described may lead to EFA abnormalities.

[13] Anderson PA, Sprecher HW. Omega-3 Fatty Acids in Nutrition and Health. *Dietetic Currents*, Vol. 14-No. 2, 1987.

[14] Rivers JPW, Frankel TL. Essential fatty acid deficiency. *Br Med Bull* 37(1):59-64, 1981.

[15] Siguel, et al. Criteria for EFA Deficiency in Plasma. *Clin Chem* 33:1869-1873, 1987.

[16] Siguel EN. Nutrient Charts: Essential Fatty Acids. *Nutr. Support Service.* 8:24, Sept., 1988.

[17] There are two types of concentrations of fatty acids, one within lipoproteins, which we refer to as relative concentration or percents of fatty acids, and the other within whole plasma. My research found that the body compensates for EFA insufficiency (absolute or relative) in several ways: (a) by increasing the rate of conversion of precursors to derivatives, thereby maintaining fairly constant the sum of percents of EFA derivatives within lipoproteins, and (b) by increasing the production of MUFAs. Our recommended treatment to correct for EFA insufficiency depends on whether it is absolute or relative. Absolute requires greatly increased intake of both ω3 and ω6. Relative requires weight loss to reduce levels of SFA and MUFA, and perhaps increases or ω3 or ω6 to correct an EFA imbalance or EFA insufficiency. The goal is the same: to achieve the fatty acid profile of a healthy person.

[18] Siguel, EN. Method And Apparatus for Diagnosis of Fatty Acid or Lipid Abnormalities. *US Patent* No. 5075101.

Essential Fatty Acids

[19] Siguel EN, Schaefer EJ. Aging and Nutritional Requirements of Essential Fatty Acids. In: Beare J, ed. *Dietary Fats*, Champaign, Il. Am. Oil Chemists Society, Chapter 13. (1989).

[20] Miettinen TA, et al. Fatty-acid composition of serum lipids predicts myocardial infarction. *British Med. J* 1982, 285:993-6.

[21] Siguel EN, Lerman RH. Fatty acid patterns in patients with Angiographically documented coronary artery disease. In Press, *Metabolism* , 8/94.

[22] Horrobin DF. EFAs and the complications of diabetes mellitus. *Wiener Klinische Wochenschrift*, 1989; 101:289-93.

[23] Lepage G et al. Direct transesterification of plasma fatty acids for the diagnosis of essential fatty acid deficiency in cystic fibrosis. *J. Lipid Research*, 1989; 30:1483-1490.

[24] Dasgupta A, Kenny MA, Ahmad S. Abnormal fatty acid profile in chronic hemodialysis patients: possible deficiency of EFAs. *Clinical Physiol & Biochem*, 1990; 8:238-43.

[25] Simmer EJL, Gibson RA. EFA deficiency in parenterally fed preterm infants. *J.Paediatr Child Health*, 1993; 29:51-55.

[26] Abstracts at Am.Oil Chem. Society Annual Meeting, Journal *INFORM*,Vol. 4 (3/1993).

[27] Darioli R, Mailie M, Jacotot. Valeurs standard des acides gras esterifies du serum chez la femme adulte en bonne sante. *Ann.Nutr.Metab* 1987;31:282-291.

[28] Rossner S, Walldisu G, Bjorvell H. Fatty acid composition in serum lipids and adipose tissue in severe obesity before and after six weeks of weight loss. *Int. J of Obesity* 1989; 13:603-612. (Conclusion of this article: obese patients have low EFAs).

[29] Schaefer EJ, Rees DG, Siguel EN. Nutrition, Lipoproteins, and Atherosclerosis. *Clin Nutrition*, 5:99-111, 1986.

[30] Siguel EN. Cancerostatic effect of vegetable diets. *Nutrition & Cancer*, 983;4:285-9.

[31] Siguel, EN et al. Monitoring the Optimal Infusion of Intravenous Lipids: Detection of Essential Fatty Acid Deficiency. *Arch. Path. and Lab. Med.* 110: 792-797, 1986.

[32] Meydani SN, Siguel EN, Shapiro AC, Blumberg JB. Fish consumption and mortality from coronary heart disease. *New Engl. J Medicine*, 313:822, 1985.

[33] Warren SE, Siguel EN, Gervino E, Salzman, EW, Smith, M, Silverman, KJ, Pasternak, RC. Effects of cod liver oil on plasma lipids, eicosanoids, platelet aggregation, and exercise in stable angina pectoris. *J. Applied Cardiology*, 3(4):227-236, 1988.

[34] In the future we may find that a diet with essential fats in the position #2 of the triglyceride or phospholipid molecule may be better than a diet with large amounts of essential fats in positions #1 or #3 because the EFAs are used more effectively by the body.

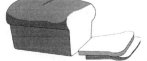

I.4

CARBOHYDRATES AND PROTEIN

"The structure of life"

Topics: *Carbohydrates. Complex carbohydrates. Proteins. Excess protein and carbohydrate is converted to fat.*

Summary

Carbohydrates provide building blocks for the body and transform fat into energy. The body stores very small amounts of carbohydrates, enough for one day's work. Therefore we need to eat a minimum of two to three ounces of carbohydrate every day. More is not harmful, but the extra carbohydrates not burnt as energy are converted to fat and stored as fat. It is best to eat the complex natural carbohydrates found in whole grain cereals, vegetables and fruits. They contain many vitamins, minerals, and essential fatty acids, as well as large helpings of fiber. Simple carbohydrates, such as sugar, fructose and syrups, do not contain the nutrients found in complex carbohydrates. Therefore they should be avoided.

Proteins provide the structure that supports the body, very much like the beams that support a house. Most hormones and all enzymes are proteins. They regulate all the chemical reactions in the body and help to manufacture all the parts that the body needs. They are the machinery of the body. We need to eat protein every day to repair wear and tear on the body. Excellent protein is found in egg whites, tofu, animal tissue and many legumes, grains and vegetables. It is not found in fruit. Extra protein is converted to fat and/or burnt for energy and the residue is excreted by the kidneys. Humans need about 0.8 grams of protein per kg. of ideal weight. For a 70 kg man (about 154 pounds) it is 56 grams, for a 55 kg woman (about 121 pounds) is it 44 grams (approximately the amount in 7 large size egg whites).

However, different types of protein have different amino acid composition. One needs a balanced mixture of amino acids every day.

Carbohydrates

We need a minimum of 3 ounces per day

Carbohydrates provide building blocks for the body. They also help to transform fat into energy. We need very little, about 3 or 4 ounces (100 grams) each day to burn the fat we use in one day. *Although carbohydrates are needed by the body to burn fat, this does not mean that by eating more carbohydrates you will burn more fat.* Only a very small amount of carbohydrates are required to burn all the fat you use in one day. Most people eat too much carbohydrate. All the excess carbohydrate that you eat is stored as hard saturated fat, thus making you gain weight.

Extra carbohydrate is stored as fat; it does not burn fat

Contrary to popular belief, eating more carbohydrates will not burn more body fat. The amount of fat that you burn for energy depends on what you do: The body is very efficient and only burns the fuel it needs. A very active person will burn more fat than a sedentary person, independent of how many carbohydrates he or she eats.

Eating complex carbohydrates is better than eating fat for the following reasons: You can eat more than twice as much carbohydrate as fat (by weight) and obtain the same number of calories. Furthermore, foods with complex carbohydrates contain fiber, vitamins, minerals and essential fats, which are all important ingredients in a balanced diet. Because natural foods rich in carbohydrates contain lots of fiber, you can eat in vegetables many times the weight of one cup of ice cream, cheese or other fat rich foods. Complex carbohydrates fill you up and also provides essential nutrients which makes your body feel "full".

Simple carbohydrates do not contain nutrients

Simple carbohydrates are small molecules. Complex carbohydrates have large chemical structures. Sugar is a simple carbohydrate. Most *natural* whole grain cereals, grains and breads contain complex carbohydrates. Refined products often have simpler carbohydrates. Buying natural rather than processed foods is one way to obtain

Carbohydrates and Protein

complex carbohydrates and avoid simple carbohydrates. Notice
that the term "natural" here does not refer to how the food is grown, but
to how it is processed. Extracts from foods labeled" organic" or
"natural" may also be refined and consist of simple carbohydrates.
They may also have had their vitamins, minerals and fiber removed, or
consist of simple foods that the body digests too quickly and converts to
fat.

Sugar and fructose

Many people think that carbohydrates are different from sugar. In fact,
they are quite similar. Sugar, technically called sucrose, consists of two
building blocks: glucose and fructose All carbohydrates are converted
to glucose (one of the two ingredients of sugar) and can also be made
from glucose. Simple carbohydrates may be absorbed by the intestine
faster than complex carbohydrates.

Fructose usually tastes sweeter than glucose. It is often found in
syrups. This is important to remember because many products, to
prevent being labeled as having too much sugar, use fructose instead.
However, fructose allows you to use less calories to obtain the same
sweetening effect as glucose.

Sugar and fructose are natural products

Sugar, glucose and fructose are "natural" products, extracted from
plants and fruits. Therefore, a product may be labeled as "all natural"
and still contain sugar or fructose. We do not know whether sugar is a
dangerous product. What we know leads us to believe that too much
sugar, like too much of any product, is dangerous. But small amounts
of sugar or fructose, in the context of a healthy and balanced diet, may
be quite acceptable. Most of us do eat too much sugar in the form of
cookies, ice cream, pastries, etc. The danger of excessive sugar
consumption lies in the capacity of sugar to fill us up and thus prevent
us from eating other foods necessary for a balanced diet. Excessive
sugar and carbohydrate consumption often leads to the consumption of
too many calories, making us overweight. And finally, it can put a
strain on the pancreas, eventually leading to blood sugar disorders.

Complex carbohydrates contain many nutrients

Complex carbohydrates are composed of many glucose molecules. In a
sense they are like groups of sugar attached to each other. The complex

Carbohydrates and Protein

carbohydrates found in natural foods have vitamins, minerals, and other nutrients attached to the carbohydrate.

Eat more complex carbohydrates

Almost all nutritionists agree that you should eat fewer simple carbohydrates and more complex carbohydrates. You will then get more nutrients, vitamins, minerals, fiber, and essential fats. You will also gain less weight because you will tend to eat more food containing fewer calories. This recommendation is the same as suggesting that people should eat more natural, unrefined foods and vegetables. Vegetables are high in nutrients, which consist not only of vitamins and minerals, but also of many other chemicals that prevent disease. They also have a high ratio of EFAs to other fatty acids.

Proteins

Proteins are an essential nutrient. They provide the structure which supports the body, very much like the beams that support a house. Most **hormones and enzymes are proteins**. Thus, proteins also play a key role in the functioning of our bodies. They regulate the chemical reactions in the body and help to manufacture the parts that the body needs. They are the machinery of the body.

Proteins are formed from amino acids

But what are proteins? Chemically, proteins are long structures, shaped like chains, with links of different shapes. They are formed from simpler compounds called amino acids, of which there are about 20 different kinds. Amino acids make up proteins like beads form a necklace. About 10 of the 20 amino acids that our bodies need to build proteins are called **"essential amino acids"**. The word "essential" here is used in the same way that it is in the term "essential fatty acids". It labels those amino acids that the human body cannot manufacture by itself, but must obtain from external sources. The other amino acids can be produced from the essential amino acids found in food or from other bodily compounds. A protein may contain thousands of these amino acids, and the specific amino acids in the chain determine the function of the protein.

*Proteins are essential to repair our body and
make enzymes. They provide structure and regulate
production of other substances. We need to eat a small
amount of a balanced mixture of proteins every day to
repair the body's broken parts*

We need to eat 2-4 ounces of protein every day

The body stores only very small amounts of amino acids, and therefore it is possible to have nutritional imbalances due to insufficient amounts of selected amino acids in the diet. We know very little about acquired diseases due to chronic nutritional imbalances in the mixtures of amino acids, although we have discovered many genetic diseases which produce abnormal mixtures of amino acids.[1] A relative deficiency or excess in one amino acid may produce a multitude of effects. For example, it can affect the rate of production of all proteins that contain that amino acid. Or it can affect the way other substances work and produce catastrophic effects which appear impossible to trace due to multiple organ involvement. Think of it: You are building a complex bridge and suddenly do not have a certain type of screw. You continue to build the bridge, but in many places you can not fasten it properly because you do not have the right screw. Many dangerous things can happen when the bridge is finally used.

It is possible to measure the mixture of amino acids in blood or urine, but it is rarely done in routine clinical evaluations because we know little about how to interpret the results. In addition, the test, when properly done, is expensive. There are a wide range of protein and amino acid supplements in the market. Whether or not you need any of them could theoretically be determined by your doctor and some complex biochemical tests on your blood.

We need to eat a proper mixture of amino acids

The type of protein we need to eat has a certain mixture of amino acids. Scientific research has determined how much we need of each type of amino acid. This has led to the establishment of general guidelines. Egg whites and animal protein have a wide range of amino acids which are fairly balanced, so that if you eat animal protein you usually will get the amino acids you need. Plant protein has fewer amino acids, but a daily variety of vegetables, grains and legumes may provide all the amino acids you need.

Carbohydrates and Protein

A balanced mixture of vegetables contains all the amino acids

Eating the wrong amino acid mixture is quite likely to make your body inefficient and eventually make you sick. Everyday we need to eat a certain amount of protein, about 40 to 100 grams or 2 to 4 ounces per day. As a rule of thumb, each ounce of fish, fowl or meat provides 6-7 grams of protein. I the only protein is from such animal sources, one would need to eat at least 6 ounces daily. If caloric needs are met on a whole foods vegetarian diet, adequate protein intake is usually assured. The intestine breaks protein down into small parts (amino acids) that can be absorbed. The body uses those parts to make other proteins. If we do not eat enough protein the body slowly begins to digest less important parts of itself, such as muscle, to protect more important parts like the brain and the heart. If we eat too much protein, the excess needs to be excreted by the body and we increase the work of the kidney. Some scientists feel that eating too much protein leads to excessive wear and tear on our organs, particularly the kidney and perhaps the liver.

For health professionals

Peptides

Scientists used to believe that all protein in the diet was broken into amino acids and the amino acids were then absorbed by the intestine. However there is experimental evidence that small peptides, which are several amino acids linked together, may be absorbed intact. These peptides may resemble hormones. They may also produce allergic responses.

Some people, because of disease or diet or genetic differences, have weaknesses inside the lining of the intestine. Through these weakened walls, which appear to have very tiny holes, large proteins can enter the body. The body detects these "foreign" proteins and thinks they are part of an invading virus or bacteria and attacks them. In the process of attacking them, it produces antibodies and other attacking agents. In the midst of all this "friendly fire", there are some "friendly" casualties. In its zeal to attack the invading proteins, the body may err and destroy parts of itself. Most often, the damage is very tiny and unseen. But sometimes the body "bombs" or attacks the wrong place or attacks it too much and causes severe harm. We know these disorders

Carbohydrates and Protein

as "autoimmune diseases", meaning that the body's defense mechanisms attack itself and causes harm.

Therefore, the nature of dietary protein could influence the type of disease we get because it determines both the availability of amino acids and changes in the concentration of hormones. Future research may explain these issues. In the meantime, avoid having only a single source of protein,[2] and avoid products that consist of unusual protein extracts.[3] Like all extracts, they may be extracted from a natural product, but the extract itself is artificial and may cause an amino acid imbalance.

Eating the proper mixture of fatty acids may help prevent the development of this and other immune disorders. Intestinal cells with the optimal mixture of fatty acids make it harder for foreign matter and protein to pass through them. These undesirable leaks create an immune response which many scientists think is a cause of auto-immune disorders (where the body attacks itself). Furthermore, the white cells and other parts of the immune system work more effectively when your body has the right mixture of EFAs.

References and

[1] Before you think you have one of these genetic diseases, you should know that most genetic disorders of protein or amino acid metabolism are extremely rare and most of these individuals die during their early childhood.

[2] Natural protein is found in egg white, meat, poultry, fish, milk, legumes, grains, vegetables and many other foods.

[3] Some artificial sweeteners are made with a few amino acids. Eating too much of a few specific amino acids may create a biochemical imbalance of those amino acids and affect the function of the body.

Carbohydrates and Protein

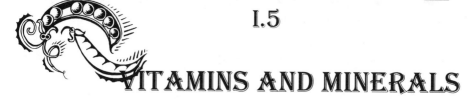

I.5

VITAMINS AND MINERALS

"It is the little things that make life different"

Topics: *Eat a balanced amount of vitamins and minerals Who needs extra vitamins and minerals. The most common deficiencies.*

Summary

Eat a balanced amount of vitamins and minerals for the proper function of the chemical reactions in our body. The best way to eat vitamins and minerals is from a mixture of natural foods. In case of suspected deficiencies one should have a blood and urine test to identify the specific deficiency and then take supplements until the deficiency is corrected. People losing weight, those eating small amounts of food (because they do not exercise) or those with specific diseases often need multivitamin supplements. Common deficiencies are vitamin B_{12}, folic acid, C, iron, and calcium.

What are vitamins and minerals

There are about 12 vitamins and 10 minerals that scientists believe to be necessary, each found in varying amounts in most foods. Vitamins are relatively small molecules made from many different elements. Minerals are very tiny molecules that represent basic elements in nature. Minerals cannot be destroyed (except in atomic reactions), but they can be deactivated by combining them with other chemicals.

Vitamins and minerals have related functions: They help to hold structures together, like a type of glue. They also participate in chemical reactions, helping to regulate and control the speed of the reaction. For example, in cold weather, the body needs to produce more heat. In warm weather, the body needs to evaporate more water.

Vitamins and minerals help to coordinate these reactions and ensure that they work properly. Vitamins wear out and need to be replaced. Minerals are lost by the body (in feces, urine, evaporation) and also need replacement.

After many years of research, scientists have determined which vitamins and minerals we need and in what quantities.

> *Every day we need a very small amount of vitamins and minerals to replace those used. Too much or too little over a long time is usually harmful.*

In order to be effective, vitamins and minerals must exist in certain relative proportions. Too much or too little shifts the chemical reactions in the wrong way. The key is balance, the common theme in nutrition and life. The best solution is to eat a mixture of many natural foods and let the body do the balancing, by conserving what is needed and discarding excesses.

Most people may be eating the wrong mixtures of vitamins and minerals

Almost every book on nutrition has a table of vitamins and minerals. Almost every day some magazine or newspaper tells you the wonderful effects of vitamins and minerals.

So, the more the better? Unfortunately, not. In fact, some people may be eating too many vitamins and minerals while others may not be eating enough. So what can you do? There are two approaches: The scientific one and the practical one. I will first provide the scientific guidelines and then explain the practical guidelines.

Scientific guidelines

The **RDA**. The RDA or required daily allowance has been created by the government. It is the quantity of each vitamin and mineral you must eat every day. The guidelines are very rough, and you can eat as much as 50% more or less or skip days or weeks without any bad effects. Most food labels include the RDA for each vitamin and mineral and how much the food contains.

Vitamins and Minerals

What foods have vitamins

Knowing the vitamin composition of foods which the government now requires on most food labels, after many blood tests, and armed with a computer where you type in every food you eat after carefully weighing it, you can determine how much you have eaten of each vitamin and mineral. Then you can determine from tables which ones you ate too much or too little of. You could then look in other tables and find which foods to eat to compensate for these discrepancies. However, if you do not have a computer, access to a huge laboratory, thousands of dollars to pay for blood tests or the patience of Job, you are in trouble . . . and may have to follow my practical guidelines.

Effects of deficiencies

Because each vitamin and mineral most likely participates in thousands of physiological processes, each one affects practically all organs of your body. You can read a few hundred books to understand what effects are caused by what combinations of deficiencies of vitamins and minerals. You can read articles every month about the benefits and dangers of vitamins and minerals. Unfortunately, we do not know precisely (and it may be impossible to know) what effects are caused by mild deficiencies, the ones most likely for you to have. Severe deficiencies of a single vitamin or mineral are extremely rare in the USA and in most parts of the world. Combined mild deficiencies produce effects which are impossible to detect without sophisticated instruments. But you can still read tables on the effects of vitamins and minerals and use them as a conversation topic to impress your friends or to worry over needlessly (in case you have nothing else to worry about).

Practical guidelines

The truth is that the relationship between vitamin or mineral deficiency and disease is too complex. Studies done years ago on animals or starving people are not applicable to our society.

Even if you knew precisely what you have eaten, it is very difficult to calculate how much of each vitamin and mineral a person eats each day. To complicate matters, only portions of the vitamins and minerals eaten are absorbed! It is very difficult to know whether you need greater or lesser quantities of vitamins or minerals because it is very difficult to evaluate whether you have a deficiency or excess. Many of

Vitamins and Minerals

the effects of mild deficiencies or excesses could take 10 years before they lead to sickness or disease.

Sophisticated blood and urine tests can evaluate a vitamin or mineral deficiency or excess sometimes, but not all the time. Excesses are usually easier to diagnose, but mild deficiencies are extremely difficult to diagnose. However, people can live without such knowledge. Even physicians eat food without knowing whether or not they have vitamin or mineral deficiencies. I do not know a single physician who specializes in nutrition and has access to the most sophisticated computers and test instruments who keeps track of how much he eats each day of each vitamin or mineral, or who has blood tests done every year. It is just too difficult.

Eat a balanced meal and do not worry

So, what can you do? Easy. Do not complicate your life. Eat a balanced meal (as indicated in this book) and you will not need to worry. Use supplements only in special cases.

When to use supplements

- When you are losing weight and drastically reduce your food intake.

- If you exercise rarely and eat very low calorie foods to maintain your weight.

- If you eat a very imbalanced diet, with more than 50% of your calories coming from processed rather than natural foods.

- If you have a specific deficiency due to disease, pregnancy or some other condition identified by your physician.

- If you take a drug that makes you lose vitamins or minerals. For example, many diuretics (pills taken to lose liquid in patients with high blood pressure or cardiovascular disease) make you lose potassium and magnesium. You need periodic blood tests to determine how much supplement to take.

- If you have a disease that causes malabsorption, such as Inflammatory Bowel Disease or Cystic Fibrosis. Under these circumstances you may need large doses of supplemental vitamins and minerals, often larger than the doses you can buy without a prescription.

Vitamins and Minerals

Otherwise, by eating vitamins or minerals without any need for them you could cause more harm than good. Your body chemistry is altered by the improper balance of nutrients. Your body energy is spent eliminating the unnecessary vitamins and minerals; this may produce waste and stress your liver, kidney and other organs.

Do we need fortified foods?

The best way to eat vitamins and minerals is as part of the regular foods you eat. Use fortified foods if they replace vitamins or minerals eliminated by processing, not if they add vitamins or minerals. In general, a product that advertises itself as having 100% of most vitamins or minerals should be avoided. Together with other foods you eat, you would probably be eating too many of those vitamins and minerals. There are some exceptions. For example, most women do not eat enough calcium and calcium fortified foods may be helpful.

Vitamins

Vitamins are classified in two groups: water and fat soluble.

Water soluble vitamins dissolve in water. These include:

> *B complex: B1 (thiamin), B2 (Riboflavin), Niacin, B6 (Pyridoxine), Pantothenic acid, Folic acid, B12 (Cobalamin), and C.*

Fat soluble vitamins do not dissolve in water, but do dissolve in fat. These include:

> *A, D, E, and K*

Minerals

Calcium, Phosphorus, Sodium, Potassium, Magnesium, Chloride, Sulfur, Iron, Iodine, Zinc, Chromium, Copper, and Manganese are commonly listed as the minerals we require.

100,000 people, or less than 2,000 people in the USA. There are a few researchers who, like myself, think that EFA deficiency is very common. Unfortunately, their findings are not yet taught in medical schools. In my review of medical textbooks, courses and conferences, I have not found a single one which teaches the extent of EFA abnormalities in the USA, let alone how to correct them. My research indicates that at least 25,000,000 people suffer from significant EFA abnormalities, and the true number is probably much higher. I have found evidence that deficiency of EFAs, both the ω3 and the ω6, are one of the most common deficiencies in the adult population. These deficiencies are likely to be the primary nutritional factor that causes cardiovascular disease, hypertension and the cardiovascular complications of diabetes. Many children also have significant ω3 deficiencies that affect their mental abilities. Therefore it is very important to learn to eat a balanced mixture of ω3 and ω6 fatty acids, starting in childhood.

Most likely deficiencies

Vitamins

- B_{12} if you eat very little animal meat.

- C if you do not eat enough raw vegetables and fruits.

- D if you do not get enough sun (quite common in the USA), however many products such as milk are D fortified.

- A if you do not eat enough vegetables.

- E if you eat refined oils: If you eat oil supplements as indicated in this book you need to eat more Vitamin E, approximately 60 to 150 units (called International Units, IU) per day.

Minerals

- **Calcium**: Unless you eat plenty of green vegetables and dairy products, you should take approximately 500 mg per day as a calcium supplement.

- **Iron**: One multivitamin pill usually has 18 mg of iron. One or two such pills each week will give you all the iron you need *if*

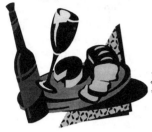

I.6

FIBER, WATER AND OTHER NUTRIENTS

"Keep things flowing and soft"

Topics: *Fiber. Water. How much you need. How to tell.*

Summary

Fiber does not contain calories and may not be essential. However, fiber helps our bodies to function better; it may prevent diseases such as heart disease and cancer, and it fills us up. Natural foods high in fiber contain a wide range of other substances that prevent heart disease and cancer. Water is essential to life. There is a simple test to tell whether you need to drink more water.

Whole foods

When we eat whole natural foods we eat a wide range of substances. Besides the well known nutrients, such as vitamins, minerals, carbohydrates and proteins, whole foods contain thousands of other substances whose effects are barely understood today. Some substances, known as "phytochemicals", make it more difficult for cancerous cells to grow. Others, like fiber, bind to toxic substances or excessive cholesterol and excrete them from the body. Nobody knows what is the ideal mixture of these substances and nobody will ever know, because there are thousands of them and it will be impossible for you or me (even with the best computers and nutrition knowledge), to keep track of how much we eat of each substance every day. Therefore, the best advice is to eat a variety of fresh wholesome foods in their natural state, preferably foods in season.

Fiber or roughage

There are basically two types of fiber. One is the **crude fiber** found in foods in their natural state, and often removed by most food processing techniques. The other is **dietary or soluble fiber**, included with most foods. Fiber tables are often confusing because they mix both types. There are many different kinds of dietary fiber. Scientists currently think that there are about five major kinds, but research is at a preliminary stage. People can live many years without fiber, but modern research suggests that eating fiber may help people to live longer Right now, we do not know which types we really need and how much of each one, so it is difficult to provide accurate guidance. Again, the best advice is to eat a variety of natural foods.

Some fibers prevent constipation; others lower cholesterol

Most fiber is a kind of carbohydrate that the body cannot digest and absorb. Because the body does not absorb it, it is also referred to as "roughage." Two kinds of fiber are the cellulose and hemicellulose that constitute the structural framework of plants. They add bulk to the diet, and make you feel less hungry. They help to carry other nutrients. This fiber also helps to regulate the frequency and amount of feces that we produce. It works like a natural laxative and prevents constipation and diverticulitis. Other types of fiber, such as pectin and gums, may attach to cholesterol and bile byproducts in the intestine, and reduce the cholesterol that we have in the blood. This type of fiber may help people with diarrhea and inflammatory bowel disease, and those with high cholesterol.

Too much fiber can interfere with mineral absorption

Fiber may prevent some undesirable substances from being absorbed by the body, but may also prevent some beneficial substances from being absorbed. Eating a balanced mixture of natural foods allows the body to regulate what the body needs.[1]

Most people need to eat more fiber

We do not know how much of each fiber we need to consume. But what we do know is that most Americans eat too many processed foods

Fiber, Water, Nutrients

without fiber. Cakes, pastries, beer, pizza and cookies are examples of refined products that contain little fiber. If you eat a balanced mixture of foods in their natural state, such as vegetables, cereals, grains and fruits, you will get all the fiber that you need without having to worry about different types of fiber.

Some people think that they can eat a diet of refined foods (i.e., pizza and beer) and then correct their imbalance by eating supplements of minerals, vitamins and fiber. To use a car analogy, this is like ruining your car by driving it with dirty oil and crashing it against walls and other cars, then adding a rust inhibitor to protect the engine: It may make you feel better, but it does not correct the larger abuses.

If you have been eating a diet low in fiber and want to increase your intake of fiber, you may wish to change your food habits slowly, allowing time for your body to adapt to the new diet. Otherwise you may find a drastic change in your bowel habits.

Water

Water is an essential nutrient. As a matter of fact, although the human body appears to be solid, about 70% of it is water.

Water helps the body to get rid of unnecessary nutrients and other waste. If you do not drink enough water, you make it difficult for the body to get rid of chemicals it no longer needs. The kidney filters the blood and excretes the dangerous chemicals it finds in the blood. If you drink slightly more water than needed you merely have slightly more urine, which is often healthy. So, if you are thirsty, drink water. However, drinking far too much water would make you lose important minerals in your urine and you could become deficient.

How to tell whether you need more water

If your urine is deep yellow, you are probably not drinking enough water. You should have light yellow, almost clear urine. However, if it is too clear and transparent it could mean you have too much water in your diet.

The amount of urine you produce is also significant in determining whether you drink a sufficient amount of water. You should urinate at least 1 liter (1.2 quarts) of water every day, preferably 1 to 1 ½ liters per day. The optimal amount depends on your health and can be determined in consultation with your physician.

Fiber, Water, Nutrients

Miscellaneous

Lecithin and choline

Lecithin is a type of phospholipid. Phospholipids contain two molecules of fatty acids. In contrast, triglycerides, which is the type of fat found in fats and oils, consist of three fatty acid molecules. Phospholipids are made by humans from choline or a few other compounds, and fatty acids found in fats and oils. Phospholipids are key components of the membranes of cells. One of the fatty acids in a phospholipid is usually an EFA. Most people can make choline from other things we eat, but people with malabsorption due to gastrointestinal disease may need extra choline. Lecithin is not very stable, and there are wide ranges in manufacturing practices among those who make or sell lecithin. The active ingredient in lecithin that prevents cardiovascular disease is the EFA, which you can also obtain from vegetable oils. Eating foods rich in membranes, such as leafy vegetables, seeds or lean (low fat) animal muscle, is the best way to incorporate lecithin into your diet.

Phytochemicals

Phytochemicals are chemicals found in edible plants. They protect the plants from disease and have many effects yet to be discovered. They appear to inhibit cancer growth in humans. Each plant or fruit has different types of phytochemicals in different amounts. You will hear that one is found effective against one type of cancer, another against a different type. Your best strategy is to eat a wide mixture of natural fruits and vegetables which have these chemicals in the right mixture for humans. Research is proving that there are many natural chemicals in whole foods which have important roles in human health in a way similar to vitamins. Most likely, the chemical composition of a plant is unique to each climate and season. We cannot keep track of thousands of desirable chemicals or nutrients that we eat every day. Thus, *the best solution is to eat a balanced variety of natural foods.*

References and notes

[1.] Many companies market extra fiber to add to foods. Try to eat a balanced mixture. Too much of one type, such as wheat bran, may not be desirable. Fiber bars, to be used as snacks, may curb your appetite, but natural food fiber is more desirable.

Fiber, Water, Nutrients

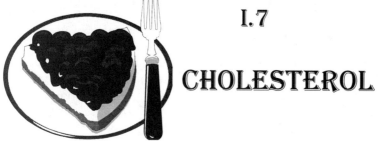

I.7

CHOLESTEROL

"Cholesterol is essential to human life, but not to the human diet."

Topics: *What cholesterol is and why it's important. Eating fewer calories and cholesterol. Why fat is important. Vegetables contain little cholesterol.*

Summary

To prevent cardiovascular disease and some types of cancer you should eat fewer calories and less cholesterol. The most important factor is the type of fat you eat. Eating a proper mixture of essential fats and few total calories lowers the amount of saturated fat and cholesterol in your body. Vegetables contain no cholesterol, and also furnish you with essential fats which lower your cholesterol. Eating more vegetables, vegetable oils and fish oils, while simultaneously cutting down on hard fat and total calories, is the best nutritional strategy to decrease your cholesterol.

Introduction

The US Surgeon General's report[1] identifies the ***type of fat*** that people eat as one of the most significant factors in health and disease. Most people eat plenty of carbohydrates and protein, and they usually get enough vitamins and minerals, too. Any occasional deficiency in this area can be corrected by the appropriate vitamin or mineral pill. When the body contains excessive amounts of vitamins, minerals, or many other substances, they are usually destroyed by the liver or excreted by the kidneys. The situation is quite different with fat. The fat we eat is stored as fat in our body.

There are many different types of fats, and we can have fat imbalances in the presence or absence of excessive fat. Both very thin and very overweight people can have fatty acid imbalances, as well as people who are in between. The body needs an optimal mixture of essential fats and only you can provide them by proper eating.

> **_Balance in fat intake is the most important nutritional factor in health and disease_**

Cholesterol

Cholesterol is a special type of fat found primarily in animal foods. It is important because it helps to form membranes and hormones that the body needs. **Humans do not need to eat cholesterol: Our bodies can fabricate it from other foods we eat**. In fact, most of the cholesterol in the body is made by the body. Therefore, unless you eat outrageous amounts of cholesterol, your consumption of cholesterol does not have a major effect on your blood cholesterol levels.

Most people eat too many calories which are converted to hard saturated fat

Eating the wrong kinds of fat for many years stores the wrong kind of fat in the body. It is not possible to correct those errors by merely taking another pill. It takes years to correct for years of improper eating. We accumulate too much saturated fat in our bodies not only from eating too much saturated fat, but from eating too many calories of any type. To compensate for excessive amounts of saturated fat in the body, the body makes more cholesterol. The reason for this is that cholesterol, in reasonable amounts, has a "softening" effect on blood vessels made hard by too much saturated fat. In technical terms, cholesterol makes cell membranes more fluid by inserting itself between SFAs in the membrane. Unfortunately, when we eat too many calories we accumulate too much saturated fat, and in its attempt to correct one wrong (too much hard saturated fat), the body overproduces cholesterol. This excess cholesterol then accumulates in the vessels and forms hard crystals which obstruct the arteries. Because most Americans have been eating too much fat and the wrong kinds of fat for years, they have accumulated excessive and unhealthy saturated fat in

Cholesterol

their bodies and thus have too much cholesterol deposited in their arteries.

We need to eat more vegetable and fish oils

We need to eliminate excess saturated fat from our arteries, and replace it with polyunsaturated fat. You can see that the problem is far more difficult than merely taking iron to correct for iron deficiency. A change in eating habits is required. How big a change depends on what your previous diet was like. If you already have cardiovascular disease you need a drastic change to achieve a drastic improvement. A small change would benefit your body by slowing the progression of the disease, but that may not be enough. Instead of dying within 10 years, you may live 12. If you are over 40 you cannot afford to wait 20 years to correct for the bad eating habits of the previous 40. We must follow a balanced diet, of course. But the diet needs to be supplemented with a mixture of essential fats (oils) tailored to your own individual needs and body composition.

We need cholesterol. Only in combination with excess saturated fat in the body does it become dangerous.

Cholesterol serves to keep the membranes of cells fluid, and also helps to make many hormones that the body needs. Cholesterol, by itself, is very important to humans. It is only "bad" when we accumulate too much of it and the body cannot eliminate it. Many scientists like myself believe that cholesterol is not the problem. Cholesterol, by itself, is not dangerous. What is dangerous is the combination *in the body* of excessive saturated fat and cholesterol. Many authors mistakenly assume that this dangerous combination in the body comes from the diet, and recommend that people eat less saturated fat and cholesterol. Such a recommendation is incorrect. Remember that excessive calories from all sources get converted to saturated fat. The way to reduce saturated fat and cholesterol in the body is to have the proper balance of essential fats, as well as to eat the appropriate number of calories. This combination will turn off the body factories that make saturated fat and cholesterol.

> *The proper balance of essential fats and calories turns off the body factories that make cholesterol*

Cholesterol

Cholesterol + saturated fat spells danger

The real health hazard is eating too many calories and not enough polyunsaturated fat. It is not necessary to consume cholesterol in one's diet: The body makes all you need. If you eat too much cholesterol but a healthy balance of fatty acids, the body usually stops making it and excretes the excess. However, if you do not have enough essential fats and you accumulate saturated fats, the body keeps on making cholesterol in an attempt to maintain the fluidity of membranes. Eating polyunsaturated fat helps to stop this excessive production of cholesterol.

When you eat too many calories which get converted to saturated fat, the body thinks that it needs more cholesterol and it makes more cholesterol.[2] For that reason it is ideal to be slim, eat fewer calories, and eat more polyunsaturated fat to help the body eliminate unnecessary cholesterol.

An exception for active people

Thin people who are very active rarely need to worry about saturated fat: they burn the fat and other foods for energy. Consider two persons who eat the same types of food, **Mr. Thin** and **Mr. Fat**. Suppose Mr Thin eats more food (of the same kind) than Mr Fat but exercises more. Mr Thin will then eat more saturated and more essential fat than Mr Fat. But Mr Thin will burn the saturated fat because he exercises more and therefore burns more calories. His body will contain more essential fat and less saturated fat than Mr Fat. The consequence is that Mr Thin will have less cholesterol and he is less likely to have a heart attack.

> *People who exercise less need to eat less total calories and proportionately more calories from essential fats.*

It is the type of fat and total calories you eat that matters, not just cholesterol or saturated fat

It is important to eat less cholesterol. But it is even more important to eat fewer total calories. You may have heard that egg yolks contain large amounts of cholesterol and therefore they are to be avoided. It is true that egg yolks contain quite a bit of cholesterol. However, if you eat a healthy diet high in essential fats (polyunsaturated fats), you may

Cholesterol

be able to eat a few egg yolks each week without a corresponding increase in your cholesterol. In fact, dairy products high in saturated fat (like many cheeses) may be more dangerous than egg yolks. And egg yolk also contains many PUFAs, which is a desirable quality.

Animal fat is high in cholesterol and low in PUFA

The most important thing you can do to reduce your cholesterol is to eat less of the fat found in animal foods and eat more polyunsaturated fats found in vegetables. Because vegetables contain practically no cholesterol, and quite a bit of fiber (fiber has zero calories), you will find that a reduction of fat from animal foods reduces the amount of saturated fat, total calories, and cholesterol that you eat.

> *Eat more vegetables and you will eat more essential fats and less cholesterol. This is one of the best ways to reduce your total cholesterol*

Why lower cholesterol

All scientific studies have found that people with elevated cholesterol in their blood are more likely to have a heart attack. In fact, recent studies suggest that people with elevated cholesterol suffer from all types of cardiovascular disease, and are also more likely to get colon and rectal cancer. For that reason the federal government and all health associations recommend that you have your cholesterol checked frequently and, if elevated, you take steps to reduce it.

"Good" vs. "Bad" cholesterol

I do not like the terms "good" vs. "bad" cholesterol. There is just one type of cholesterol. Depending on where it goes and how it is used by the body, cholesterol may be good or bad. When people do not have the appropriate balance of fatty acids, the body must compensate in any way it can. One way is to increase the production of cholesterol. Cholesterol helps the cells compensate for their lack of EFAs and maintains the cell membranes' fluidity. Without cholesterol, the membranes would become hard and vessels would be as hard as butter. Instead of emphasizing the alleged "good" or "bad" cholesterol, we must emphasize the good or healthy distribution of fatty acids in our body.

Cholesterol

High cholesterol and high blood pressure are not diseases: They are indicators of health status

High total cholesterol and high blood pressure indicate that the body is not healthy. They are useful diagnostic and monitoring tools because they are inexpensive, and they tell us how the body works. When you listen to the noises made by your car, you can sometimes tell that certain noises indicate problems. The objective of fixing your car is not to eliminate the noise (which could be corrected by wearing earplugs), but to correct the problem that causes the noise.

We do not want to just lower cholesterol or blood pressure. We want to correct the disease that causes elevated cholesterol or high blood pressure. This is one of the reasons why I believe that we should rarely use drugs to treat high cholesterol or high blood pressure. The drugs rarely treat the problem that causes high blood pressure or high cholesterol. They merely lower cholesterol or high blood pressure. Drugs treat the symptom, not the disease. Because we are what we eat, changing what we eat can make our bodies healthier.[3]

References and notes

[1] The Surgeon General's Report on Nutrition and Health. US Department of Health and Human Services, PHS publication No. 88-50210 (1988).

[2] The reason for this proposition is highly technical. Cells require a flexible ("fluid") membrane to function properly. Polyunsaturated fat and cholesterol help to maintain the membrane fluidity. Saturated fat makes the membrane hard. When the membrane has too much saturated fat, the cell makes more cholesterol to compensate for the excessive saturated fat. Of course, it would be better for the cell to have more polyunsaturated fat. But the cell cannot make it: Polyunsaturated or essential fat can only be obtained from the foods you eat. If you do not eat enough essential fats, the cells do not get enough. Therefore, your cells resort to the best alternative available to them: They make more cholesterol to compensate for the lack of EFAs and try to keep their membranes fluid. Cells also make more monounsaturated fat to compensate for the lack of PUFA.

[3] Of course, it is also important to have the right attitude, to exercise, and to minimize the effect of environmental pollution.

Cholesterol

I.8

NORMAL AND ABNORMAL CHOLESTEROL LEVELS

"You want to be healthy, not average"

Topics: *"Normal" means average. Normal or average cholesterol levels. Healthy cholesterol levels. Why cholesterol is important. When to treat.*

Summary

In medicine the word "normal" means average. When your physician says that you have a cholesterol level below normal he means below average. Because most "normal" or average values are around 240 (in mg/dl, the way concentrations are measured), many people have been told that if they have a cholesterol level below 240 they are "normal". Unfortunately, being average in this country means that you are likely to die of cardiovascular disease. For this reason, a government panel has recommended that people aim for a cholesterol level below 200. You can live longer and prevent cardiovascular disease by reducing your cholesterol to healthy rather than average levels. At the very least, you should try to bring it below 200, but the ideal value is closer to 150 than 200.

Normal means average in medicine

"**Normal levels**" for a blood test are the range of values used to determine where a particular person fits relative to the population (see Part II). Normal levels for any blood test are derived from the average for the population. If the "average" person in the population is healthy, then you are compared to that "healthy" person. But if the average person is not healthy, then you may be called "normal" even though you may not be healthy.

For example, the average cholesterol in the USA for people 40 to 50 years old is about 250 mg/dl. You need not be concerned with the units because most laboratories measure cholesterol in similar terms (however, the USA is changing to international units --- used in Europe --- and some laboratories now report in both the old and the new units). Thus, if your cholesterol is below 250 you may be called "normal" and if it is above 250 you are called abnormal. But most people between 40 and 50 are not in very good health. They usually have "average" to severe cardiovascular disease. If the average income in the USA were $18,000/year, would you be happy to be average?

You want a healthy, not average, cholesterol level

You should not be happy when your physician tells you that your cholesterol is the same as the average person. Ideally, your cholesterol would be the same as that of the average "healthy" person. For that reason we need to know the average cholesterol of a healthy population.

How normal levels are calculated

For many years physicians have been using normal or reference levels derived from different sources. Some hospitals take the average of all their patients and call that "normal". Others take the average of all the patients that are not hospitalized (the ones seen in their clinics) and call that "normal". Sometimes a random sample of people are used to establish normal values.

Because of the different populations used to establish normal values, some laboratories have a normal range of 150 to 350 mg/dl while others have a normal range of 150 to 250 mg/dl. To get those numbers laboratories compute the average of a group of people, then find the range which includes 90% of this population. 5% of the population will fall above and 5% below that range. Using this approach, the older "normal" levels for cholesterol were about 250 mg/dl. In my experience I still find physicians who use the older reference values.

There are two things wrong with this approach when it is used with cholesterol. Since most people in the USA have cardiovascular disease and elevated cholesterol when compared to people in other parts of the world, you find that the "normal" range is quite high. A person with a

---

Normal and Abnormal Cholesterol Levels

cholesterol level of 140 mg/dl may be labeled "abnormal" when in fact he is quite healthy, and someone with a value of 220 mg/dl may be labeled "normal" when in fact he has a high risk of dying of heart disease or stroke. So being "normal" in the United States is not necessarily something to strive for.

Recently revised normal levels are below 200, but still aren't low enough

To correct for those problems the National Institutes of Health established committees to reevaluate recommended levels of cholesterol. The government committee had to make a very difficult decision. They were afraid that if they prepared complicated guidelines, physicians and patients would not follow them. Moreover, if the normal cholesterol level were too low, too many people would be labeled "sick", which would scare the public. Therefore, I believe that the committee determined that a cholesterol level below 200 mg/dl is adequate, and over 200 is not acceptable. Because this decision would require that more than 10,000,000 people get treatment, thereby overwhelming medical facilities and increasing insurance costs, the committee created guidelines (reproduced elsewhere). Fortunately for pharmaceutical companies, most people do not care enough about their lives to change their diets, and people with abnormally high cholesterol are content with taking a few pills, cutting salt in their diet, and from time to time eating less saturated fat and cholesterol. However, this is simply not enough, and in fact is practically useless to prevent heart disease.

Initially the guidelines indicated that it was OK for cholesterol to increase with age. Later, general guidelines applicable to everybody were established. Some researchers think that older people should not aim for a state of health as good as a young person, and therefore they should not attempt to prevent premature death. Others, like myself, believe that older people have a right to attempt to be in the best possible health, and they ought to be provided guidelines to aim for the best possible health. If they do not want to follow them, that is their right. There is no known physiological reason why older people should have a higher cholesterol. The fact that cholesterol increases with age indicates that people deteriorate as they get older, and does not suggest that it is healthier to have a higher cholesterol. Recently researchers have begun to use a group of people believed to be in very good health as the yardstick for setting "normal" values. Thus, we may eventually

Normal and Abnormal Cholesterol Levels

see a revision indicating that "healthy" total cholesterol levels
for all people, young and old, should be between 100 and 150 mg/dl.

Healthy levels are under 150 mg/dl for all ages

What is healthy? If you had a choice, what would be the **ideal level**? If
we look at the cholesterol levels of populations that have very little
heart disease we find that a value between 100 and 150 mg/dl is
reasonable. Heart disease is almost never found in people with
cholesterol below 150 mg/dl. In fact, very healthy people have been
found to have values below 110 mg/dl, but it requires a very strict diet.
The diets proposed in later chapters will help you bring your cholesterol
below 150 mg/dl without much effort.

Most of the healthy men and women we have tested have values below
140 mg/dl. It is not unreasonable to have a value of 120 mg/dl,
assuming that you are otherwise healthy. On the other hand, a value of
180 mg/dl is not bad. Research indicates that your risk of heart disease
increases when your cholesterol is much higher than 150 mg/dl.[1]

Use the ratio cholesterol/ HDL cholesterol

So far we have been talking about total cholesterol. This single value
could be misleading. Some people have high total cholesterol and high
total HDL. The HDL refers to cholesterol found in a type of particle
called High Density Lipoproteins that carry fat in the blood(see Part II).
Having high HDL is usually good.

To evaluate the risk for heart disease we need to consider both the total
cholesterol and the HDL cholesterol, using the **Cholesterol/HDL
cholesterol ratio**. (See Part II for other ratios). Instead of talking
about cholesterol, it is better to talk about the Cholesterol/HDL ratio.
You want to have low cholesterol but also want a high HDL. What
seems to be important is to keep the Cholesterol/HDL ratio below 3,
preferably close to 2. Around 3-4 you have an average risk of heart
disease, that is, you are likely to die of heart disease.

When your Total Cholesterol/HDL ratio is above 5, your risk is much
higher than the average person. That is, you have a very high
probability of a heart attack. Remember that most people in America
die of cardiovascular disease. Therefore, to be average means to
prematurely die of cardiovascular disease. If you are worst than
average, then you are almost certain to die soon of cardiovascular
disease, or develop severe impairments that will make it far more

Normal and Abnormal Cholesterol Levels

difficult for you to enjoy life. You will have shortness of breath, difficulties walking, will feel tired most of the time, and start to lose brain cells because the heart cannot pump blood with oxygen and food all the way up your head. Soon you will start forgetting things, which unfortunately helps you forget about the need to take care of your life. Soon, life takes care of you.

You want to be healthy, not average

The graph below shows the distribution of cholesterol in the US population (percent of the population with specific cholesterol values).

References and notes

[1] There are exceptions to this recommendation. There are people that have high total cholesterol and high HDL cholesterol and appear to have reduced incidence of heart disease. There are a large number of chemical reactions modulated by enzymes which are controlled by genes. These genetic differences produce people with high cholesterol and low incidence of heart disease, and people with low cholesterol and high incidence of heart disease. However, practically all benefit from seeking an optimal balance of EFAs in their blood. In this book we do not seek to reduce cholesterol as the end point. Rather, we seek to balance EFAs in the body and reduce cholesterol as a consequence of such balance.

Cholesterol Distribution in the U.S. Population (Males/Females Combined, NHANES II 1976-80),[2] and Potential Changes in the Distribution

Figure 2

Population distribution of serum cholesterol values. The borderline-high and high cutoff levels are shown as dotted lines to indicate the proportions of the population above or below 200 or 240 mg/dL (5.17 or 6.21 mmol/L).

Ages 20-74

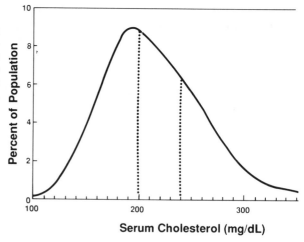

Serum Cholesterol (mg/dL)

Normal and Abnormal Cholesterol Levels

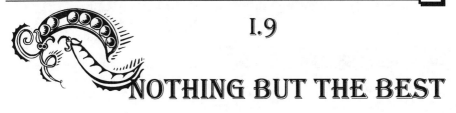

I.9

NOTHING BUT THE BEST

"Help your body regulate itself"

Topics: A balanced diet. Eat a mixture of all types of foods in their natural state. Do not make one food the basis of your diet. Eat more vegetables, fruits, grains, and cereals and less animal fat. Extracts from natural foods are not "natural". Fads, quackery and rip-offs

Summary

The key to a healthy body is a balanced diet. You should eat a mixture of all types of foods in their natural state and not make one food the basis of your diet. Eat far more vegetables, seeds, and fruits, and less animal fat. Eat more foods in their natural state, that is, raw foods, and eat fewer cooked foods or processed foods. Avoid refined products, or concentrated extracts. Extracts from natural foods are not "natural", even if they come from natural foods. Do not overeat, but exercise so that you can eat enough food with all the needed nutrients without gaining weight. Processed foods are not necessarily dangerous; we may never know whether they are or not. When in doubt, think this way: Nature probably knows best; hence opt for natural foods.

When buying food keep in mind these general guidelines. Nature knows what is best for your body. What is best for a bee or an elephant is not what is best for a 35 year old human. A product that may kill cancer cells may also kill healthy cells. If you have cancer, you may want to take the risk in the same way that you may remove a breast or prostate or leg with cancer. But why kill yourself otherwise?

Calories

Calories are not nutrients. **Calories** are a unit of measurement of energy, just as we have units of energy that measure how much energy in a gallon of gas or oil. You need calories to make the body work and to keep it warm. The following table describes how many calories are in each type of nutrient. Try to memorize this table.

Nutrient	Calories/gram
Fat	9
Carbohydrate	4
Protein	4
Vitamin	0
Mineral	0
Water, Fiber	0

All nutrients contain some calories. However, in practice, we eat so few vitamins and minerals that we can say they contain no calories. All the calories we eat are found in fat carbohydrates, and protein.

Carbohydrates and protein contain approximately equal amounts of calories. In 100 grams of either protein or carbohydrate we find 400 calories. Fat, on the other hand, is a more efficient source of calories. . In 100 grams of fat we have 900 calories, more than double the calories in protein or carbohydrate. Many of us do not need all those calories, but starving people do need them and fat is the way to get the most. However, for the average American, who is not starving, eating fat makes you gain weight twice as fast as eating the same amount of protein and carbohydrate.

Most foods that are high in fat are low in water and fiber (butter, cheese, cookies), while foods high in carbohydrates (vegetables and fruits) are high in water and fiber. Therefore you can eat far more of the latter, and still be consuming fewer calories.

> *Fat is the greatest source of calories. Most of us eat too many calories.*

Excess protein or carbohydrate equals excess fat

Every day you need a small amount of protein and carbohydrate to rebuild cells and make the body function properly. Any amount in excess is converted to fat and stored as fat. All the fat in your body that is not burnt as calories or used for other functions is stored as saturated or monounsaturated fat. You can become overweight from eating too much protein, carbohydrate or fat. But fat makes you overweight faster because it has more calories per unit of weight.

Nothing but the Best

RDA = Recommended Daily Allowance

Scientists have established a recommended daily allowance for each nutrient except EFAs. You can find these allowances on food labels. The **US RDA** stands for "United States Recommended Daily Allowances".[1] Most products you buy in the supermarket tell you what the US RDA is and how much of a particular nutrient is contained in that food. For example, a can of vegetable soup may say that it contains 25% of the recommended daily allowance for vitamin C. If you do not get the full allowance in one day there is really no cause for concern; the RDA is a VERY ROUGH estimate of a person's need for a particular vitamin or mineral. The important thing is to consume quantities of nutrients close to the amounts suggested by the RDA so that over a period of time your average daily consumption of each nutrient is approximately the RDA.

If you eat a little bit more or a little bit less you are unlikely to get in trouble. Your body can excrete the excess or draw from its stores if you do not eat enough. However, if you rarely eat calcium or iron or another vitamin or mineral over long periods of time you will develop a deficiency of that nutrient. If you consistently eat more than the RDA every day, you may develop toxic effects.

Regulation and equilibrium

The human body is a wonderful machine that can accept widely different ranges of food and adapt to them. However, it is possible to harm that machine by feeding it too much or too little of any particular nutrient. The body can regulate itself within narrow limits of environmental conditions, food, exercise and mental status. Excessive amounts of one nutrient produce ineffective utilization of the other nutrients

For example, if there is too much heat in the environment, the body cannot cope with it; if there is too much cold the body cannot produce enough heat to keep itself warm. Similarly with foods: Too much or too little may damage the body because it exceeds its ability to self-regulate. We are very fortunate that our bodies will store nutrients so that we do not have to eat every day and can, within limits, compensate for not always eating a balanced diet. But we must not abuse our bodies. The best way to assure that we eat balanced meals is to use foods in their natural state.

Nothing but the Best

Proper nutrition allows your body to self-regulate for a healthy life

The body self regulates

If the body finds that we have too much of a certain substance, it simple burns it (metabolizes it, usually in the liver) and/or throws it out in the urine or feces. If it does not have enough, it tries to absorb as much as it can or substitutes it with something similar. As long as you eat natural foods, you are very unlikely to develop excesses of any particular nutrient because the body can get rid of its excesses. But if you eat processed foods, you may be eating far too much of some nutrient.

If you eat too little of a nutrient in a given day, your body adapts by using its reserves. However, if you deprive your body of a critical nutrient for a long period of time, you may slowly empty its reserves and damage your body.

These principles apply to fatty acid metabolism but with an important twist: Humans do not secrete excessive fat; instead we accumulate it. When humans were designed, supermarkets were not available and food was scarce. Therefore, the ability to store excessive food was important for survival. Bodies which could not store extra calories would not survive a tough winter and these genes were eliminated through evolution.

Exceptions: When you are sick

Although our body can adjust to the food we eat, sometimes we need to eat to adjust to our body's needs. An accident, an infection, aging and heart disease are examples of situations when we must change our diet to help our body cope with new problems. As we get older our body loses its ability to regulate itself with maximum efficiency and we must be more careful with the foods we eat.

Corrections for a lifetime of poor eating habits

You may need to eat food extracts or supplements such as oils, vitamins and minerals to correct for past dietary errors or for genetic abnormalities. I am not implying that every person ought to eat every food, vitamin or mineral supplement. However, there are over

10,000,000 people in America who should take supplements to correct for existing disease or past nutritional imbalances. There are more than 3,000,000 people who have a severe disease or genetic abnormality that will cause premature death unless drastic steps are taken. These people will benefit from large doses of supplements and essential fats even though the same amounts would be dangerous for another person.

Many people have been eating the wrong foods since they were children. Most kids in the USA eat cookies, pastries and foods rich in saturated and partially hydrogenated fat as part of their school meals. In fact, my experience indicates that most of the school lunch programs contribute to heart disease later in life. Many government-sponsored food supplements for women, infants and children are EFA deficient and high in calories and saturated fat. In order to assure compliant eating by kids, public schools feed them highly processed foods. Even the alleged "healthy" or "wholesome" foods are often hazardous. Many of these foods are highly processed and have been deprived of all EFAs and many natural nutrients. One redeeming feature of "healthy" low calorie foods may be that they encourage children to eat fewer calories, an important issue because far too many children are overweight. Many good parents have been taught by custom to keep their children overweight in case food becomes scarce. This was important to prevent starvation in World War I and II, but is now very dangerous in America, where starvation is rare but obesity is common.

Parents who encourage their children to eat healthy meals have a hard time fighting the system: Most kids learn to like processed foods better than natural foods.[2] By the time a child becomes an adult, he or she probably has poor nutritional status, reflecting 20 years of bad eating. This may sound blunt, but where health is concerned the truth is the best medicine, no matter how hard it is to hear. Once we know where we stand, we can act. We can begin to rebuild our health.

Change your diet slowly to allow your body to adapt

A balanced diet: key to a healthy body

You should eat a mixture of all types of foods in their natural state and not make one food the basis of your diet. Eat more vegetables, fruits, grains, and cereals and less animal fat. Eat more foods in their natural state, that is, raw foods and eat fewer cooked foods or processed foods.

Nothing but the Best

Avoid refined products, or concentrated extracts. Extracts from natural foods are not "natural." They are an artificial product even if they are labeled as natural. Do not overeat, but exercise so that you can eat enough food and get all the needed nutrients without gaining weight. Processed foods are not necessarily dangerous; we may never know whether they are or not. But when in doubt, think this way: Nature probably knows best. Hence opt for natural foods.

References and notes

1 There is another meaning of the term RDA which is used by the National Academy of Sciences and stands for Recommended Dietary Allowances. Both allowances are quite similar, but only the US RDA is required on food labels. If this sounds confusing, write to your Congressman and ask him to cut down unnecessary government red tape and create more uniform standards.

2 It is rare to find a child who will prefer a carrot or even an apple to a chocolate chip cookie or a hot-dog.

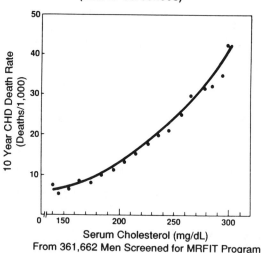

Figure 1
Relationship Between Serum Cholesterol Level and CHD Death Rate
(MRFIT Screenees)

Serum Cholesterol (mg/dL)
From 361,662 Men Screened for MRFIT Program

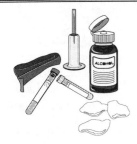

II.1

BLOOD TESTS

"The proper test will help your doctor to determine which foods to curtail and which supplements to take."

Topics: *Diagnostic tests. How to diagnose good health and disease. Blood and urine tests.*

Summary

Research has shown that certain medical test results are associated with good health and others with disease. Evaluating tests is difficult and requires highly advanced technical expertise. The same test may give different results at different times, because people's physiology change, and unavoidable minor laboratory errors do occur. Dietary changes may also influence results. Moreover, different laboratories use different instruments and methods, producing different results. Therefore, one single value is not important. What is important is the trend. Like the stock market: A single cholesterol value may go up or down, but the trend is most important. It is desirable to obtain "baseline" values when you are healthy, so that a doctor may compare them to later results and detect early signs of disease.

Why you need to know about tests

Although your doctor will order tests for you and give you instructions, if the test is not properly done you are the one who suffers. Sooner or later most of us, or a close family member, need to have blood tests done. Learning the basics of how to provide the right blood sample saves you time and assures that the test results are meaningful. Good test results provide the foundation for better treatment.

The use of tests

This chapter contains technical information for those who want to learn about tests. It contains material that may be difficult or technical for some people. Our purpose is to describe many of the common and not so common blood tests. Understanding tests will help you to obtain more reliable test results and better communicate with your physician.

Tests are done to identify and diagnose a specific disease, measure the severity of the disease and help to select the appropriate treatment. Almost all tests have possible side effects. Although one test may have a mild effect, the cumulative results of many tests are dangerous. During my medical residency in laboratory medicine, part of my job entailed reviewing test results at two major hospital centers. On ill patients so many blood tests were performed that often a patient became more anemic and required a blood transfusion because of all the tests. I recommended that venipuncture (blood drawing) be done using the smallest possible tube, and that blood tests be ordered only when they were essential. Quite frequently, doctors and nurses were not aware of the large amount of blood being drawn. Today most hospitals have shifted to small tube sizes, but drawing too much blood still remains a common problem.

Therefore, before a test, prudent physician should ask themselves: Will the result help to treat the patient? Some tests provide diagnostic information which does not change treatment. They are useful for research purposes, to confirm a diagnosis, to prevent a lawsuit, or to monitor the effects of treatment. From the patient's perspective, it is important to find out what the health provider plans to do with the test results. He/she should tell you something like this:

"If the test results are in ____ range, we will do "A"; if they are in ____ range, we will do "B".

If he/she does not give you such guidelines, ask for them. Knowing what to expect reduces stress and will prepare you for the future.

I disagree with a common practice of informing patients only when test results are abnormal. I believe people should receive copies of all their test results, normal or abnormal. I know that I am very worried when I suspect a health problem, and I want to know the results, positive or negative. Receiving test results minimizes two possible errors: the tests are lost or the health provider has forgotten to inform the patient about them. My recommendation is for patients to always insist that a

Blood Tests

copy of their test results be sent to their home. Most test results are available within 15 days. Call if you do not receive them after 15 days.

Some tests help to convince a patient that he/she needs to change his/her lifestyle. People rarely get motivated to lose weight until their doctors tell them that they have a high cholesterol value or high blood pressure.

No one can have all tests done

During their examination, doctors asks patients: "what tests has your other doctor ordered." And often the patient responds: "ALL". "My doctor ordered all the tests". This is a typical statement I hear and it conveys a common misconception about medical testing: that is, that one actually can be tested for every possible disorder or disease. Unfortunately, some people think that the doctor is liable if he fails to diagnose every conceivable disorder because he failed to order the "right" test.[1] It is easy to know the right tests after one knows the diagnosis!

No doctor ever orders all meaningful and useful tests. There are well over 10,000 tests commercially available, and over 100,000 at research laboratories in various stages of commercial development. Soon there will be millions. You could easily spend $1,000,000 just to do useful and meaningful blood tests. You barely have a gallon of blood, sufficient for a few hundred tests at most. If you had all those tests done you may find out how well or sick you are. But that would be irrelevant: You would die because you would no longer have any blood left. Most physicians agree that the most blood you should have drawn during a period of 4 weeks is 250 ml (about 8 ounces), and only if it is essential. One small tube is about 10 ml or about ½ ounce. I personally think that you should not have more than 50 ml (about 3 tablespoons) drawn every 4 months unless you have a complicated disease.[2]

Blood tests: general indications

Always provide fasting blood (blood after not eating for 12-14 hours). The best blood is obtained as follows. For several days before the blood test you should eat your usual meals, without eating too much of one thing or another. The day before the blood test you should have your usual breakfast and lunch. Your dinner should be very low in fat

Blood Tests

and calories. You should **finish your meal around 6-8 PM**. For the next 12, preferably 14 hours, until the next morning when you have your blood drawn, you should eat nothing, except for drinking water. That is, if you finished eating by 7 PM, you should have your blood drawn about 9 AM. You should not be thirsty: this could concentrate your blood. Likewise, your blood should not be dilute, so do not drink water 2 hours before the blood test. Your blood should be drawn between 12 and 15 hours after you finished your last meal.

Example: have a light dinner and finish at 6:30 PM. Drink water if thirsty until bedtime. In the morning drink water when you get up, before 6:30 AM. Now you are ready to go to the laboratory between 8 AM and 9 AM. Some people think that because they have to fast before their blood is drawn, they need to eat more food to compensate. So they eat a big dinner. This is a mistake.

Arrive at least 15 minutes early. Arrive early at the laboratory and sit and wait for a while. This will calm you down and calm your system. For example, if your blood pressure is to be measured, it is better to be sitting for at least 15 minutes before your blood pressure is taken. Similarly, try to be seated for at least 15 minutes before your blood is drawn. If you must move to another office, get up sssloowly and move ssloowly. That way you will not alter your system. Drastic changes in your body alter the hormones and your blood tests may be slightly altered.

References and Notes

[1] This also explains a major flaw is most health insurance reform proposals. Many people believe that we can afford to treat everyone with every diagnostic and treatment procedure that would improve their health. People from all over the world call me and ask me to help them and state that "money is not a problem"; "I will pay whatever it takes", they say, to cure their cancer, heart disease, etc. I tell these people that I ask for a $1,000,000 deposit to start to review the medical literature (over 100,000 articles). For approximately $10,000,000,000 we can reproduce most organs. The fact is that if we spend money on all the diagnostic and treatment procedures that will likely help each person, we would need more money than is available in the world. In practice, doctors do the diagnosis and treatment procedures that they know or remember within the time available for seeing one patient. This also explains why a lawyer can usually find a test that the doctor failed to do. There is usually a test that could diagnose or help to prevent or treat the disease. We learn about it after the person dies, but often we could not tell before

[2] Blood has key nutrients, including trace minerals, and cells with "memory" of past events, such as infections and the ability to fight them. Some people may find it hard to replace the lost blood. We may never know.

Blood Tests

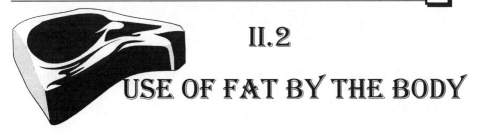

II.2

USE OF FAT BY THE BODY

"Fat leads to Fat"

Topics*: Fat. Lipoproteins. HDL. LDL. Risk of heart disease. Ratio of HDL/Cholesterol.*

Summary

Fat is carried in the blood inside tiny particles called lipoproteins. Blood is made up mostly of water, and since fat does not mix with water, it must be transported in these lipoproteins. There are several types of lipoproteins of different sizes which carry cholesterol, other fat and vitamins. One of these particles is named HDL (often referred to by the media as "good cholesterol"). People who have a lot of HDL are less likely to get heart disease than people with a small amount. Physicians measure the total cholesterol in the blood and the cholesterol inside HDL and compute a risk of heart disease by dividing Cholesterol/HDL cholesterol. Based on your Cholesterol/HDL cholesterol ratio, a physician can tell whether you have a high or low risk of getting a heart attack.

Lipoproteins are blood vehicles that carry fat

Blood has two major constituents: **cells** (red and white and platelets) and plasma. **Red cells** carry oxygen to organs, **white cells** defend the body against foreign invaders like viruses and bacteria, while **platelets** form clots to stop bleeding. The **plasma** is the liquid part of the blood and it consists mainly of water mixed with nutrients and other chemicals.

Cholesterol and other fats and lipids are carried in the blood, inside vesicles (**particles**) called **lipoproteins**. These particles resemble small spheres. They contain the fats and vitamins that do not mix well with water. If you put oil in water you will see that it forms unequal "clumps" and mostly moves to the surface. Ideally, the body would like to have nutrients equally distributed in the blood, so that they can reach even the smallest vessels. If the fats and vitamins traveled freely in the blood, they would clump as oil does in water and many parts of the body would not receive enough nutrients. The body's solution is to encapsulate the fat and vitamins inside lipoproteins. These lipoproteins are made of fat and protein. They dissolve easily in water because the outside of the ball dissolves in water. In this way, the body carries lipoproteins well mixed with the blood. Cells and organs feed from these lipoproteins and dissolve them to obtain the nutrients inside. Inside the lipoproteins we find all kinds of fats (SFAs, MUFA, and PUFAs) as well as non-water soluble vitamins A, D, E & K. These vitamins do not dissolve well in the water which constitutes the plasma.

The body needs a specific amount of each type of lipoprotein and each lipoprotein has to have a proper balance of ingredients. If we have too many, we have **hyperlipoproteinemia**; too little and we have **hypolipoproteinemia**. If the balance is not correct, or if the lipoproteins are abnormal in composition, we have **dyslipoproteinemia**.

Substances inside lipoproteins

Lipoproteins are like small balls. The outside of the ball consists of proteins, cholesterol and phospholipids that are soluble in water and blood. Inside the ball are molecules which are not soluble in water; being inside a water-soluble coating is their way of traveling in the bloodstream. Molecules which are carried inside lipoproteins include: triglycerides (fats that contain 3 fatty acids), cholesterol-esters (a mixture of one molecule of cholesterol and one fatty acid), vitamins and a few other substances.

Scientists have found that they can group the different types of lipoproteins into several major types. Lipoproteins are named (or grouped) according to their densities, i.e. how heavy they are. The three main types of lipoproteins are called HDL, LDL, and VLDL. **HDL** means High Density Lipoprotein. **LDL** means Low Density Lipoprotein. **VLDL** means Very Low Density. Each particle carries a

Use of Fat: tests

mixture of fats, but specializes in the transportation of a specific type of fat.

It is very difficult and expensive to count the number of lipoprotein particles in a blood sample. Instead, laboratories separate the particles using a technique called "centrifugation" that separates the particles according to how heavy they are. It is the same as leaving the blood standing, and allowing the heavy particles sink to the bottom. To measure HDL and LDL, scientists measure the cholesterol contained in the HDL and LDL types of particles from a given individual's blood. It is an indirect way of counting the particles. Because these particles carry cholesterol, measuring the cholesterol is easier than counting the number of particles of each type.[1] When doctors speak of HDL, they actually mean the amount of cholesterol in HDL. If you have a lot of cholesterol inside HDL, doctors assume that you have a lot of HDL and say you have "high HDL." If you have a lot of cholesterol inside LDL, doctors say you have a "high LDL."

From these test results physicians compute several ratios:

◆ Total Cholesterol/ HDL cholesterol (the cholesterol in HDL)

◆ HDL/ LDL (the cholesterol in LDL)

◆ Total Cholesterol/ Total Triglycerides

After many years of research, doctors have prepared tables that tell them which levels and ranges of various cholesterol ratios are associated with good health or disease.

Cholesterol is merely an indicator of your health

Having more cholesterol inside HDL is "good"; having more cholesterol outside HDL is "bad"

Increased HDL particles suggest low risk

Scientists have found that if you have many HDL and few LDL particles, your risk of heart disease is low. Research has shown that by measuring these fats one can estimate the relative risk of cardiovascular disease and determine the appropriate therapy. Physicians use tables that indicate whether a person has a high or low

Use of Fat: tests

risk for heart disease, according to their cholesterol and triglyceride ratios.

You may wonder why is HDL "good" and LDL "bad". Studies have shown that people with high HDL have less incidence of heart disease and those with high LDL have a higher incidence of heart disease. The truth about how HDL and LDL work is not known. My research suggests that people who have a good ratio of EFAs to saturated fatty acids have many HDL particles that carry away unnecessary fat and cholesterol. People who eat too much saturated fat require many LDL particles to carry the excess fat and cholesterol. Because there is so much fat in these people's blood, some fat and cholesterol become attached to their arteries, and eventually cause the arteries to harden. Furthermore, your body attempts to compensate for excessive amounts of hard saturated fat by making more cholesterol, which softens the hardening effects caused by saturated fat. Having relatively high HDL compared to total cholesterol or LDL tells you that you have relatively high amounts of EFAs compared to other fatty acids. If you have too many saturated or monounsaturated fatty acids in your body, you need many LDL particles to carry them.

Common misconceptions

Over the years, some writers have referred to HDL as "good" cholesterol and LDL as "bad" cholesterol. Actually, all cholesterol is the same. The difference lies in where it is. When we say that you have a lot of HDL, we mean that the cholesterol in HDL is high. This indicates that you have many HDL particles. A high HDL cholesterol also suggests that you are less likely to have heart disease. Therefore, your objective is not to "eat good cholesterol and avoid bad cholesterol". *Your objective is to modify the fat composition of your body so that you your body makes less total cholesterol, and more of your cholesterol is in the right places.* One way to move towards these objectives is to eat to correct imbalances of fatty acids, and to get one's blood tested for fatty acid imbalance.

Cardiovascular disease and hardening of the arteries

If your total cholesterol is high and your HDL cholesterol is low, then your LDL is usually high, your arteries are hard and you are more likely to form clots than healthy people. This means that your risks of

Use of Fat: tests

getting a heart attack or a stroke are much higher than the risks of a person who has low total cholesterol and high HDL.

However, remember that cholesterol is merely an indicator of your health. We use cholesterol because we have not been able to easily measure the types of fat in your body until now. But we must be careful not to overemphasize cholesterol and overlook *the major culprit in cardiovascular disease: Insufficient levels of EFAs*.

It is now possible to actually measure the specific mixtures of fats in your blood using a test called the **EFA-SR**. Doctors may order this test which can replace traditional measures of cholesterol. This test is more expensive than a cholesterol test because it measures over 30 different kinds of fatty acids in your body, and shows precisely what deficiencies or excesses you have. The results go to the root of the problem, and also point the way to a nutritional solution. The test EFA-SR is like a multidimensional x-ray or CAT scan of your fat. The results of many measurements are plotted using sophisticated computers to obtain diagrams that diagnose your fatty acid status.

References and Notes

[1] For research purposes, doctors also measure the amount of triglycerides, phospholipids and other substances. But it would be far too expensive to do this for every patient.

Use of Fat: tests

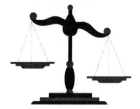

II.3

TESTS FOR

CARDIOVASCULAR

DISEASE

"Measure the risk of developing heart disease"

Topics: *Common blood tests for cardiovascular disease. The ratio of HDL (the cholesterol in HDL) to Total Cholesterol. The Bleeding Time (a small cut in your arm). The Fatty acid profile **EFA-SR**.*

Summary

The most common and useful blood tests for cardiovascular disease measure characteristics of the blood and the way fats are carried in the blood. Other tests measure the tendency of the body to form clots. The most useful tests are the ratio of Total Cholesterol or **LDL** (the cholesterol in LDL) to **HDL** (the cholesterol in HDL) and a fatty acid profile. The Bleeding Time (a small cut in your arm) helps to determine whether you have a tendency to form clots (hypercoagulation). A new test, which analyzes fatty acids is the **EFA-SR** (Essential Fatty Acid Status Report). The **EFA-SR** measures how much of each type of fat including *trans* fatty acids, is in your body, and tells you how much you need to eat of each type of essential fat to achieve the proper balance.

Cholesterol tests

High cholesterol is a sign, not a disease

Cholesterol tests, like many other blood tests, are used to evaluate the likelihood that you will develop heart disease. High cholesterol is not a disease; it is merely a warning sign that you may have or may develop cardiovascular disease. Because the human body makes cholesterol, cholesterol is not an essential nutrient.

Having a value too high usually means that your body makes too much cholesterol rather than the common misconception that you are eating too much of it.

In contrast, having too much of an essential nutrient, like zinc, usually means that you have eaten too much of it, or your body is destroying itself and releasing too much zinc into the blood.

Total Cholesterol.

Total cholesterol measures the total cholesterol in your blood. When physicians speak about cholesterol, they refer to total cholesterol. Most people have between 180 and 260 mg/dl for cholesterol (mg/dl are units like ounces). There is continuous discussion about "ideal" cholesterol levels. By agreement of a government committee, it was decided that cholesterol greater than 200 mg/dl would be considered abnormal. This was done, in part, to avoid causing panic in the US population where millions have high cholesterol, and also to avoid flooding the emergency room with patients afraid of dying from high cholesterol.[1] However, many scientists consider an ideal total cholesterol to be between 100 and 150 mg/dl, with about half of it in HDL.

Doctors use a variety of test results to evaluate the risk for cardiovascular disease. If you have high cholesterol, but most of that cholesterol is in particles called HDL, then you are not at high risk for cardiovascular disease. Remember, HDL are particles that carry cholesterol and other fat in the blood.[2] Cholesterol is very important to the body and therefore you need to have cholesterol. However, you want to have neither too little nor too much.

HDL Cholesterol

The laboratory measures the cholesterol in the HDL particles found in plasma (the liquid part of the blood). Having a high HDL is usually a good sign. Most people have between 40 and 60 mg/dl. This is an indirect way of counting the HDL particles. You want the number to be greater than 60, or about 50% of your total cholesterol.

Cardiovascular disease tests

LDL cholesterol.

It is difficult to count LDL particles. Instead, most laboratories compute the number of particles from other things that the laboratory measures. You do not need to worry about how it is calculated, but you want it to be below the recommended levels (see appendix). It is often healthier to have it lower than government-established guidelines *if* you bring it lower with proper diet and exercise (this suggestion does not apply to lowering it with drugs). One of the formulas used to calculate LDL is:

LDL = Total Cholesterol - HDL(Cholesterol) - Triglycerides/5

VLDL Cholesterol.

This is another particle that carries cholesterol. It is desirable to have a low VLDL, like 20. Direct measurements of VLDL are rarely done for clinical purposes; instead it is used for research. VLDL is often calculated from Triglycerides as follows:

VLDL = Triglycerides / 5

Total Cholesterol divided by HDL cholesterol

To evaluate health status physicians divide Total Cholesterol by the cholesterol found in HDL particles:

Total Cholesterol / HDL Cholesterol

A good ratio is below 3; ratios between 3 and 5 are "average" and ratios above 5 indicate a significantly higher (than average!) risk of heart disease.

Examples:

"**Good**": LDL = 150 (T.Chol.) - 60 (HDL) - 60 (Trig)/5 = 78

T. Chol / HDL (Chol) = 150 / 60 = 2.5

"**Bad**" : LDL = 260 (T. Chol.)- 55 (HDL) - 120 (Trig)/5 = 181

T. Chol / HDL (Chol) = 250 / 55 = 4.0

Cardiovascular disease tests

Values of Total/HDL Cholesterol for various percents of the population

	5%	10%	25%	50%	75%	90%	95%
Males	3.00	3.30	4.00	4.90	6.00	7.30	8.00
Females	2.60	3.00	3.50	4.30	5.20	6.50	7.30

The risk of Coronary Artery Disease vs. Total Cholesterol/HDL

There are numerous studies on the relationship of Total/ HDL cholesterol. Just to provide a general idea of what other people's test results look like, I prepared this table based in part on data published in the Journal *Circulation*[3] and based on the Framingham Heart Study.[4] Because these values vary from time to time, they are to be used only as rough guidelines.

This table means that 10% of the males have Total/HDL cholesterol below 3.30, and 10% have it above 7.30. About 10% of women have Total/HDL cholesterol below 3.00 and 10% have it above 6.50 (or, equivalently, 90% of women have values below 6.40). Do you get it? Do you know how your values compare with this group of people? Are you in the bottom 10% (best) or top 10% (worst)? Because so many adults have heart disease in America, if you are above the 50% mark in this test compared to this people (above average), chances are quite high that you will have heart disease.

Triglycerides

Triglycerides is the technical name for things we call fat. For example, oils and the fat in meat are composed of triglycerides. Triglycerides are the main carriers of fatty acids from adipose tissue to other parts of the body. They consist of three fatty acids. Cholesterol is a different type of "lipid" or substance that does not dissolve in water. Cholesterol is smaller than triglycerides.

Researchers are evaluating the meaning of the triglyceride blood test. One reason for inconsistencies of results is that people do not follow the specific instructions about fasting that we described before. If you eat before a blood test, your triglycerides go up. But if you follow the rules

Cardiovascular disease tests

given before for preparing yourself for a blood test, triglycerides provide important clinical information that your doctor can use to better plan your diet. Most people have values of triglycerides between 60 and 200 mg/dl, the lower the better. However, a value too low indicates starvation or the fact that the body is unable to utilize fat.

Coagulation tests (tests for clots)

These tests measure whether your blood forms clots normally, too easily or too slowly. A clot formed too easily is one which forms when there is no need for a clot. For example, inside an artery that is not broken.

Bleeding Time

The test for bleeding time is designed to see how long it takes for your blood to clot. It is a simple procedure. The technician makes a tiny cut in your arm with a special razor blade. He then measures how long it takes before the blood clots. The cut heals and it is difficult to see. It rarely hurts because the cut is superficial. The average person has a bleeding time between 3 and 8 minutes, depending on the technique used, the type of razor blade, etc. Ideally, you should have a value between 6 and 10 minutes, higher for people at risk of heart disease. Too short a time indicates that your blood coagulates too rapidly, suggesting that you may be prone to form clots inside your arteries. Too long a time means that your blood does not clot quickly enough and you may be prone to bleeding.

A long bleeding time may help people with hardening of the arteries.

If you are quite healthy the results are not very important unless you have values that are very different from the average person. But if you have hardening and partial obstruction of your arteries, you want to have a bleeding time between 8 and 12 minutes to prevent clotting. With this goal you are trying to balance benefits and risks. It is rare to bleed excessively, but it is common for a clot to obstruct a partially closed, hardened artery.

A very long bleeding time can give you anemia

On the other hand, if you have an ulcer or similar internal bleeding problem, a shorter bleeding time is desirable. Otherwise you could lose too much blood internally and become anemic. This sometimes happens

Cardiovascular disease tests

to people who take aspirin, because aspirin inhibits clot formation. This is one reason why aspirin may prevent some heart disease deaths. Bleeding is also a contributory factor in the type of strokes where a vessel in the brain bleeds. A second kind of stroke occurs when a clot obstructs a brain vessel.

Because aspirin and other antiinflammatory drugs may increase your bleeding time, you should stop taking these drugs for at least 10 days before you have your bleeding time done. The same warning applies to the Platelet Aggregation test (below).

Platelet Aggregation

Platelets are the cells in the blood that form clots. This test measures how well your platelets form a clot ("aggregate"). The test requires that blood be collected in a special tube and later be timed for platelet aggregation. It is related to the test for bleeding time. To measure the tendency to form clots which obstruct arteries I prefer the bleeding time test because it is easier to do and easier to interpret. Other physicians prefer to measure platelet aggregation. Any good laboratory can do excellent studies of platelet aggregation and bleeding time. Either test is adequate. Newer and better technology has significantly improved our ability to study clot formation. The proper test results helps to determine whether you have a tendency to form clots too easily. If you do, ω3 fats will help you prevent clot formation.

Apoproteins

This test is the new fad in blood studies. Apoproteins are a special type of protein that helps to regulate the way fats are transported in the blood. Studies have shown that the quantity of each type of apoprotein that people have in the blood is related to the probability that they will have a heart attack. It therefore helps to tell how sick you are.

My main criticism is that the results of this test tell you what may be wrong with you but do not tell you how to correct it. There are many apoproteins and different tests to measure them. Knowing the level of each apoprotein does not help to plan a better diet. You cannot eat more to correct excesses or deficiencies of apoproteins. All apoproteins in food, like all proteins, are digested and destroyed by the stomach.

Measuring apoproteins may be useful for a small segment of the population, including people with severe lipoprotein genetic disorders

Cardiovascular disease tests

(about 5% of the population) but it is primarily used in research. My clinical experience suggests that the fatty acid profile, sometimes supplemented by the total cholesterol, triglycerides and HDL cholesterol, provides the information that your doctor needs to plan your diet.

The fatty acid profile **EFA-SR**

There are many different ways to analyze the blood and count how many fatty acids are there. The analysis of fatty acids is called a "**Fatty Acid Profile**". One type of fatty acid profile is presented in this book, the **EFA-SR**, which is a report on your Essential Fatty Acid Status. The profile **EFA-SR** measures the most common different kinds of fatty acids in your body. This test indicates, directly, if you have too many SFAs and not enough essential fats in your body. It provides detailed information which can be interpreted by your doctor to plan a diet with emphasis on what foods you should eat (or avoid) to correct your specific fat abnormalities.

Both hospitals and laboratories can send blood for analysis. The test requires about 0.5 ml of plasma (less than 1/2 a teaspoon) using a purple top tube. The smallest tube is sufficient. Further instructions are attached in the appendix. Because the test can be used to analyze different types of fat in the body, we explain some of the different applications later in this book.

The analysis of fat in your blood helps to explain how your body uses your fat. It also provides information regarding your past dietary history. Your doctor may order an analysis of the fat in your blood cells (which reflect the status of your cells) or the fat in your blood **plasma** which reflects overall body status. Plasma fatty acid analysis is the most common form of the test. More specialized analysis in specific cells, such as white cells, helps to identify disorders that contribute to diseases such as asthma, diabetes mellitus or immune deficiencies.

Assessing the risk of coronary artery disease (CAD)

Your physician uses test results to estimate the chances that you will get a heart attack or a stroke. He has a reference table of normal or average values that he uses as a reference point. If your numbers fall

Cardiovascular disease tests

in the normal range, he considers you "healthy". If they lie outside the normal range, he considers you as probably not "healthy" or at risk of having CAD. In practice, some tests results are within the normal range even when a person has CAD, and others are outside even when the person is healthy. The physician compares all the results and makes an overall judgment of whether you have low, average or high risk of heart disease or premature death.

The best tests for risk assessment are: the fatty acid profile, Total Cholesterol, HDL Cholesterol, Total Triglycerides and Bleeding Time. A physician may order more than one test. However, more tests do not necessarily provide more information. Research has shown that many test results duplicate the findings of other tests or cannot be translated into specific recommendations for improved health. In a study published in the *New England Journal of Medicine*, researchers found that the ratio of total cholesterol to HDL cholesterol was very useful to predict the risk of myocardial infarction (heart attack). However, the measurement of different types of HDL (there are at least three different types), or the measurement of different types of apoproteins A-I, A-II and B (the proteins that make the spheres called lipoproteins) did not add additional information beyond the information provided by total/HDL cholesterol.[5]

Another newly popular test measures a special type of lipoprotein called **Lp(a).** Some researchers believed that this unusual lipoprotein was a marker of risk of heart disease. I personally discourage the use of markers of disease such as Lp(a). Even if we find that some people have abnormal Lp(a) levels, there is little we can do about it. Because Lp(a) is made by the body, it is impossible for people to eat more or less Lp(a). Instead, they will have to rely on drugs that alter Lp(a) levels or presumed relationships between nutrition and Lp(a). I see Lp(a) testing as another boom for the drug industry. Every time a marker of a disease is found which can be altered by drugs, drug companies have the opportunity to profit from selling drugs that improve that marker (whether or not they improve the disease is often impossible to prove). Dr. Ridker and coworkers found that there was little association between lipoprotein (a) and risk of myocardial infarction. The results of their study "do not support using lipoprotein (a) measurement to screen middle-aged Caucasian men for increased risk of myocardial infarction".[6]

Remember that most diagnostic tests describe the physical disease, not the underlying cause. Nutritional tests are the exception. They

Cardiovascular disease tests

identify a specific deficiency or excess that causes a disease and tell you how to change your diet. The fatty acid profile directly measures your nutritional status, and therefore helps to plan your meals and oil supplements. This test also measures the *trans* fatty acids, the fats you find in hydrogenated and processed fat.[7] All other cholesterol, apoprotein and blood clotting tests are indirect measures of your health or nutritional status. They do not specifically tell you what you must eat or avoid to improve your health.

References and Notes

[1] I had professional friends who insisted in seeing me *immediately* because their cholesterol test results were elevated.

[2] The previous chapter describes the use of fat by the body and the different particles that carry fat, such as HDL and LDL.

[3] Castelli WP, Abbott RD, McNamara PM. Summary estimates of cholesterol used to predict Coronary Heart Disease. *Circulation*, 1983; 67:730:734. You should see this journal for complete information.

[4] The Framingham Heart Study studies about 4,000 people from the city of Framingham, Mass. These people are followed every year to evaluate whether or not they get heart disease. The study is funded by the National Institutes of Health. Some of the data on fatty acids presented in the appendix are also based, in part, on the analyses of subjects that participate in the Framingham Heart Study.

[5] Stampfer MJ, Sacks FM, Salvini S, Willett WC, Hennekens CH. A prospective study of cholesterol, apolipoproteins, and the risk of myocardial infarction. *New Eng. J. Medicine*, 1991; 325:373-81. Also cited in Willett WC. Diet and Health: What should we eat. *Science*, 1994; 264:532-537.

[6] Ridker PM, Hennekens CH, Stampfer MJ. A prospective study of lipoprotein(a) and the risk of myocardial infarction. *JAMA*, 1993; 270:2195-2199.

[7] **Analytical methods**. Lipids extracted from samples are hydrolyzed. The fatty acids are converted to fatty acid methyl esters and separated with high resolution Capillary Gas Liquid Chromatography using long columns, preferably 100 m. Peaks are identified by comparison with known standards. Using computers, peak areas, ratios, concentrations, and percentages of individual compounds and groups of selected compounds are calculated. Each peak is individually reviewed to verify that it is properly integrated and identified using patented methods These methods were used to analyze fatty acids in the Framingham Heart Study, one of the longest running and best known studies of heart disease. These methods were reviewed by several committees of the National Institutes of Health who described them as "state-of-the-art GLC methodology." Separation of TFAs from cis fatty acids requires sophisticated technology because there are more than 20 different types of TFAs and isomers (fatty acids with structure different from the one that the body needs) produced by hydrogenation, food processing and bacteria.

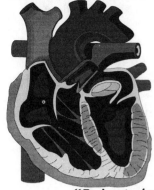

III.1

CARDIOVASCULAR DISEASE

"Bad arteries account for most deaths in the USA"

Topics: *Cardiovascular disease. Thick arteries. High blood pressure (hypertension). Stroke. Brain damage. Clots. Warning signs.*

Summary

In acquired cardiovascular disease, that is, disease that is not genetic or due to infection or accident, the arteries are thick, hard and narrow. This forces the heart to work harder to pump blood. Even so, less blood reaches the cells in your body and some cells die. Hard arteries increase resistance to blood flow and lead to high blood pressure because the heart pumps harder. Excessive blood pressure can rupture a vessel inside the brain and produce brain damage. Most people with cardiovascular disease also have a tendency to form clots that obstruct the arteries. This occurs because the platelets which form clots are "sticky" and the arteries are narrow. These clots lead to heart attack or stroke.

Aspects of cardiovascular disease

Blood consists of **plasma** (liquid part), **red cells** (carry oxygen), **white cells** (form the immune defense) and **platelets** (form clots to protect against bleeding and close holes in vessels). Cardiovascular disease manifests itself in many forms, but all forms of the disease share the same elements:

- Thickening and hardening of the arteries (**arteriosclerosis**).

- Obstruction or partial obstruction of the arteries with fat deposits called plaque (**atherosclerosis**).

- **Clot formation** inside an artery, usually the final event that leads to a stroke or a heart attack (myocardial infarct). If the obstructed artery is small, it leads to small tissue destruction. You may not feel it, but if it continues it has a cumulative effect and leads to malfunction of the heart and/or decreased brain function.

- **High blood pressure**, which can rupture an artery. Lowering the blood pressure with drugs means that the pressure is not high enough to reach all parts of the body and slowly some parts of the kidneys, brain and heart die.

Atherosclerosis, arteriosclerosis and thrombosis

Most people have a combination of arteriosclerosis (thickening and hardening of the arteries) and atherosclerosis (obstruction or partial obstruction of the arteries with fat deposits called plaque). The result is that the *arteries are hard and narrow*. This combination makes it difficult for the blood to circulate efficiently and reach all the cells. Remember that blood carries nutrients and oxygen to the cells. Without sufficient blood, cells die and organs age prematurely. Furthermore, the heart has to work harder to pump blood through the hard and narrow arteries. The arteries of the body start at the heart. When they start, they are very big and broad. As we move away from the heart, the arteries divide into smaller arteries to reach even the tiniest parts of the body. Like the water supply in your city, the heart has to pump very hard to get blood to all parts of your body. If you live in an old apartment high in the city you may notice that when many people use water, the water pressure decreases. If pipes are old and rusty and have accumulated deposits of junk, water cannot flow easily. Similarly, if you try to use a very old water hose to water your plants, you may not get as much water pressure as you get from a new, flexible hose, which can stretch to adapt to accommodate more water flow.

Your arteries behave in the same way. The parts of the body that are at the end of the system of arteries do not get enough blood if the arteries are hard and partially obstructed. To compensate for this obstruction and lack of flexibility, the heart pumps harder. This causes an increase in your blood pressure. Because the pressure is higher, the chances increase that a small and tiny vessel in the brain or heart will break. The chances are greatest for hard vessels that are brittle and

Cardiovascular Disease

weak, because of the accumulation of junk (usually saturated fat and cholesterol) within them.

When a vessel such as an artery breaks, you have internal bleeding. If there is a lot of bleeding, you are in trouble. Fortunately, most of the time the vessel that breaks is a tiny one in an organ such as the kidney, the skin or the outer part of the heart. In those cases the blood just leaks into the body cavity where there is plenty of room for it. Eventually, the body forms a "clot" that heals the vessel and you have almost no damage, except for an internal "bruise" that heals after a few weeks. However, when the bleeding occurs in the brain, there is no place for the blood to go because the skull is rigid. Even a small amount of bleeding can cause enough internal pressure to destroy part of the brain.

A "**thrombus**" is the technical name for a clot in a blood vessel, or in the heart itself. A thrombus is caused by the coagulation of the blood (in technical terms, the aggregation of platelets). The main purpose of clotting is to close ruptured vessels, but sometimes the body is confused by the junk (plaque) inside an artery. The body thinks that it is broken, and tries to "close" it. By mistake, instead of fixing the outside of a broken vessel, if fixes the inside and it closes a good vessel. Sometimes the thrombus stays in one place for a long time; other times it starts in one place, such as a leg, and moves to another place. When the thrombus obstructs a major artery, all parts of the body that receive oxygen and food from that artery start to die. Key organs like the brain and the heart may die within minutes.

Often, an individual's body slowly develops atherosclerosis and arteriosclerosis. As the arteries get narrow, the body compensates by making many more arteries around it. In this situation, even if the main artery is obstructed, the collateral arteries continue to feed the organ. Interestingly, a person who slowly develops heart disease is in part protected from "sudden" death due to obstruction of a major artery. By contrast, a person who has relatively healthy arteries and suddenly develops a clot that obstructs an artery in the heart may die because there are no "collateral" or supplemental arteries to replace the obstructed one.

The disease "**thrombosis**" is the formation or presence of one thrombus, or many thrombi. Platelets move inside the blood vessels like cars on a highway. When the vessel is narrow and there are many platelets, they hit each other and often form small groups or tiny clots.

Cardiovascular Disease

Often these tiny clots disintegrate without any effect on the body. But all too frequently, the platelets become excessively adhesive or "sticky" and we have too many small clots running around. These small clots stick to each other and soon we have larger clots or thrombi (the plural of thrombus).

Ideally, we want the body to form a clot when we have a puncture in a vessel so that we do not suffer internal bleeding. We particularly require this mechanism in the brain, where a tiny bleed would let blood inside the skull. Because the skull is very rigid and there is no room for the leaking blood, the blood presses against the brain and destroys it. This is the reason why a "hematoma" (*bruise* or blood accumulation due to a bump or similar accident) is quite dangerous in the brain. The same hematoma in an arm or leg causes no harm except a purple spot that disappears after a few weeks.

If the platelets do their job, a small puncture of a vessel is promptly plugged. However, if the platelets become overactive and aggregate more than they need to, they form clots and begin to obstruct arteries. If they obstruct a small artery, they cause "minor damage," such as slight destruction of your heart or brain, which you may not feel at first. But over a period of years, this small damage becomes cumulative and causes abnormal function. For example, many small damaged parts of the heart cause improper pumping or rhythm of the heart, which we call arrhythmia.

When the clot is small and obstructs a minor artery, you may not feel any pain or consequence for many years. Many organs do not have "nerves" inside. Thus, even repeated minor damage causes no pain. The same thing happens in your skin: A small cut may not cause any pain, but you can see it. However, the skin recovers, while cuts and bruises inside your organs may cause permanent damage. Sometimes a small clot obstructing a brain vessel causes you a **headache** because there is not enough oxygen reaching a part of the brain. Other times it may cause you heart pain, what we call **angina**.

When the clot is large and obstructs a major artery, you have a **stroke** or **heart attack**. The effect is immediate and within a few minutes it can cause paralysis or death. People who have atherosclerosis or arteriosclerosis have vessels that have reduced diameter. They also have areas where there are partial "obstructions" to the flow of blood caused by big chunks of fat and cholesterol. When this happens, even a small clot can cause a major obstruction. Thus, the combination of

Cardiovascular Disease

abnormal platelet aggregation and partial obstruction of the arteries due to atherosclerosis is deadly.

If your arteries are very narrow, you are faced with a difficult choice. Should you take drugs to "thin" your blood and make your platelets less likely to form clots (these are called anticoagulants, and aspirin is one of these drugs), and risk the possibility of bleeding? Or should you do nothing? The answer varies from one doctor to another and from one person to another. Because each person's metabolism changes from week to week, due to cost and practicality it is impossible to do blood tests every week to decide how many aspirins to take, etc. Instead, doctors often "play it by ear." If the patient has evidence of severe obstruction in his vessels, the doctor recommends an anticoagulant because the risk of dying from an obstruction is greater than the risk of dying from bleeding. Many doctors believe that an aspirin a few times per week is justified because few people die from bleeding and many die from arterial obstructions. Aspirin may prevent a heart attack or stroke because it makes your platelets less "sticky."

I think this is a very dangerous treatment. There is a better and safer alternative: Improve the balance of your essential fats so that they make your platelets work better and adjust to your system. You can change the balance of your ω3 and ω6 fatty acids. Using optimal mixtures of essential fats you can make your platelets less "sticky" and less likely to form clots, without impairing their ability to plug a hole to prevent bleeding.

Heart Disease

The combination of increased stress on the heart and decreased blood available to all cells, including heart cells, leads to heart disease. Chest pain or angina is a common symptom of heart disease. Chest pain occurs when the heart cells do not receive sufficient oxygen and other nutrients. Stress, like exercise, increases your metabolism and increases the demand for oxygen, forcing the heart to work harder.

People with **poor blood circulation** may also have pain in other parts of the body, particularly the legs and hands. These parts of the body are located at a distance from the heart and are the ones most likely to suffer from insufficient oxygen and nutrients. When there is insufficient blood and oxygen, the body "aches". When you get very cold

Cardiovascular Disease

hands or feet and not enough oxygen, your feet or hands may hurt. When the brain does not get enough oxygen, you get headaches.

To increase its ability to pump blood, the heart works harder. If the heart has to work harder all the time, it increases in size. An enlarged heart requires more oxygen and nutrients and is therefore more vulnerable to poor circulation and damage. Thus, the vicious cycle of disease leading to more disease is continued.

We often speak of a "weakened" heart. In reality, we are talking about a heart that is not strong enough to comply with the high demands imposed on it by the body. You may have a perfectly healthy heart, but your body has become so large that your heart can no longer feed the entire body. Most people, as they get older, get bigger while the heart gets smaller (because tiny parts of it die with age). The solution to this serious health problem is to decrease our body size and soften the vessels to improve blood circulation.

The cells of the heart, like the cells of most other body organs except for the skin, do not reproduce once the individual reaches adulthood. In fact, the function of most organs (such as the heart and kidney) decreases with age. Therefore, as we get older, we ought to have smaller bodies to match our less capable heart and kidneys. **Cardiac insufficiency** occurs when the heart cannot meet the demands of the body and pump enough blood and oxygen. **Kidney insufficiency** occurs when the kidney cannot meet the demands of the body to clean the blood and throw away waste. The result is that toxic waste accumulates in the blood and interferes with other nutrients and harms the body. The only effective solution is to decrease the size of the body, that is, be thinner.

Heart attack or myocardial infarction

What people call a "heart attack", which is a relatively sudden injury to the heart, may occur in many different ways. Over many years, due to continuous periods of insufficient oxygen, parts of the heart die. When the damage is slight, you may not feel anything. When it is more significant but not yet deadly, you may feel pain, sometimes called "angina". This lack of oxygen occurs when the heart is working near its limit and can barely cope with the body demands. Then almost any additional activity or exertion will push it over its limit and parts of the heart, brain or kidney will fail to get enough blood.[1]

Cardiovascular Disease

When the damage to the heart is large enough for you to feel the pain and be at risk of dying immediately, we call it a heart attack. Sometimes a heart attack is merely the cumulative result of many tiny "myocardial infarctions". The word "myocardial" means heart muscle. The word "infarct" means an area of tissue that is dead because it did not receive enough oxygen and nutrients.

Besides having an infarct caused by cumulative small losses of tissue, you can have a clot that obstructs a large artery and causes the death of a large chunk of tissue. This is probably the most common cause of **sudden death** or a heart attack. Several things may trigger the formation of clots (which can also cause a stroke). Usually you are already in a state where the blood clots easily ("**hypercoagulable state**").[2] Eating a meal very large in saturated fat makes it easier for the body to form clots. Thus, some people have heart attacks shortly after a large meal. In the morning, after sleeping for many hours, the platelets appear to be more "sticky" (or sleepy) and the blood moves more slowly, giving them more time to stick to each other. Researchers have found that many heart attacks occur shortly after people get up in the morning. Sudden stress or exercise usually triggers the other type of heart attack, where the heart must work beyond its limits and, being unable to feed itself, causes its own death.

Hypertension

When arteries are hard and/or narrow, the heart has to pump harder to move blood through the body. The combination of stronger pumping action by the heart and hardened, narrow arteries produce elevated blood pressure. The phenomenon is quite similar to what happens to a water hose. An older, harder hose requires stronger water pressure for the water to circulate, and is more likely to burst due to the increased water pressure.

The body reacts in predictable ways and has a reason for its actions. Quite frequently, high blood pressure is caused intentionally by the body in its attempt to pump or send enough oxygen and food to parts of the body served by narrow and partially obstructed vessels. But the attempt to correct one problem may cause other problems.

High blood pressure is dangerous because the high pressure inside the arteries may rupture a vessel and produce internal bleeding. It may also contribute to hardening of the arteries and associated damages to all the organs. When blood pressure is too high, the danger of a vessel

Cardiovascular Disease

bursting is very high. When balancing the danger of a burst vessel versus the danger of not pumping enough blood or oxygen to the parts of the body that need it, doctors usually find it better to decrease the immediate risk of a broken vessel. Doctors treat hypertension with drugs to decrease the blood pressure because it can kill people rather quickly. However, when we reduce high blood pressure with drugs, we often reduce the ability of the heart to supply all the vessels and parts of the body begin to die, particularly the brain. This process takes many years before we see any effect, but after 10 to 20 years it has caused significant harm to your body. A 40 year old man who has severe hypertension and takes drugs to reduce his blood pressure may find that by the time he is 60, he has lost a significant portion of his kidneys, heart and brain.[3]

Stroke

There are *two different types of stroke: blood obstruction or blood leak.* In the former, a clot forms in the brain, obstructing an artery and leading to the death of cells in some part of the brain. Depending on what part of the body was controlled by the dead cells, a person may lose the function of an arm, a leg, or memory. In the second type of stroke, a vessel breaks and spills blood inside the brain. This blood creates pressure which damages and kills brain cells, leading to loss of brain function such as paralysis of an arm. The treatment for each kind of stroke differs from the other. Both are risky because trying to treat or prevent one type makes you more likely to get the other. If you take drugs to "**thin**" your blood, you are more likely to bleed; if you eat foods to prevent bleeding (saturated fats), you are more likely to form clots. Keeping the optimal balance is difficult and requires advanced testing and technology, and I believe it is practically impossible by artificial means such as drugs. Instead, we can keep optimal clot balance through optimal nutrition, including a balance of essential fats.

There are cases where doctors can actually determine which type of stroke the patient is in danger of having. For example, some high blood pressure sufferers have a tendency to bleed and their blood vessels are hard, brittle, and thin. They may not have enough platelets (due to disease or drugs). These people will usually suffer the type of stroke where a blood vessel bursts and spills blood into the brain.

People whose high blood pressure is primarily due to thickening of the arteries, that is a narrowing of the passage through which the blood

---

Cardiovascular Disease

flows, usually have sticky platelets. They also have more of them than the average healthy person. They are more likely to have a stroke consisting of a clot that blocks the normal flow of blood.

Your age, current and past health status, and many other factors alter the number of platelets and their ability to adhere (stick) to each other. An infection may sometimes cause the platelets to become more sticky. Thus, whether you have one type of stroke or another depends on your body status, and also on some triggering event, such as an infection, stress or a small bump in the head, that may cause obstruction or bleeding.

Treatment with oils will vary in each case, especially since oils rich in ω3 fatty acids can increase the tendency to bleed and therefore can be dangerous for patients who bleed easily, but would be quite helpful for patients whose blood clots too readily. In general, one must eat quite a lot of fatty acids to have significant effects. Before starting a program of EFA supplements, your doctor should analyze your blood for EFAs and determine whether or not you need more ω3s and how much you ought to take. Taking a "blind" dose of fatty acid supplements without a blood test is like playing Russian roulette with your life. If you take too little oils, it will probably have an insignificant effect; if you take too much, it can cause internal bleeding, and the permanent damage which results from stroke.

Diabetes

Diabetes Mellitus is a disease caused by the inability of the body to properly use glucose in the blood. Glucose is the main chemical ingredient in sugar and carbohydrates. One form of the disease is due to a diseased Pancreas which cannot produce enough insulin. People with this disease most often require insulin injections and have "Insulin Dependent Diabetes" or "Juvenile Onset Diabetes" (because the disease often starts in childhood).

Another type of the disease, called Adult Onset Diabetes, is due to a general inability of the body to utilize glucose efficiently. This disease often starts when a person is in his or her late 40's, and gets progressively worse as people get older. It is associated with arteriosclerosis and hypertension. Adult onset diabetes is also associated with increased need for insulin, but patients can often

Cardiovascular Disease

manage with oral drugs that lower the high glucose in the blood. One of the most common causes of adult onset diabetes is being overweight.

Diabetes alters the metabolism of fat in your body. It makes it more difficult for the body to make derivatives of the EFAs. It also makes it more difficult for the body to receive enough EFAs. It contributes to the process of having your body produce abnormal levels of cholesterol and triglycerides. It contributes to the hardening and thickening of your arteries, and partial obstruction of arteries. One frequent consequence is that small vessels in the eye work poorly and in part obstruct your vision.

In diabetes, the kidneys and heart do not receive enough oxygen and slowly die. Kidney disease is a common consequence of diabetes. It is incurable, because it is caused by the slow and irreversible death of the kidney. A similar problem occurs with the brain and the heart. Partial obstruction of the vessels of the legs cause pain and make it difficult for the blood to feed them and fight infections. A minor infection in a toe can cause a diabetic person to lose a foot because the body cannot send enough blood to fight the infection. Losing a part of a leg to "gangrene" or an infection is a common problem for diabetic people. Most of the complications of diabetes are due to arteriosclerosis and atherosclerosis. Both are preventable by eating a proper balance of essential fats.

Combined Effects

Elevated cholesterol and triglycerides (types of fat in the blood) lead to deposition of fat in the arteries, which harden and obstruct the arteries. The reduced blood flow (poor circulation) is insufficient to feed all the cells and some cells die for lack of oxygen or nutrients. Diabetes makes things even worse because it deprives the cells of the glucose needed for energy. The result is that the body begins to age prematurely. All organs deteriorate and cannot accomplish their function. This means that the kidney, liver, brain, etc., work progressively less efficiently as we get older. The liver can barely keep up with its task of destroying toxic substances. The kidneys cannot excrete all the leftover chemicals that accumulate in the blood. Slowly we begin to accumulate toxic substances in our body which, in turn, produce further disease. This is a vicious cycle. Fortunately, this aging process can be slowed down by proper nutrition.

Cardiovascular disease speeds up normal body aging. A 50 year old person with advanced atherosclerosis and arteriosclerosis

Cardiovascular Disease

(hardening and obstruction of the arteries) may have the body and mind of an 80 year old person with clean and soft arteries. In other words, disease can add 30 years to your body and mental abilities. Clogging your arteries clogs your mind and slowly kills your brain cells, significantly reducing your mental abilities.

Warning signs of heart disease or stroke

Although a heart attack may occur suddenly, without any apparent warning, it is usually preceded by one or more of the following signs:

- **Shortness of breath**. You get tired more quickly than you used to. You seem to need more air.
- **Dizziness and fainting**. Many cells are not getting enough oxygen because your heart cannot pump enough blood to your body. You feel weak, and sometimes cannot think well.
- **Sweating, nausea or a feeling of fullness in the center of the chest**. You feel as if you have eaten too much.
- **Chest pain**. You have pain around your heart that extends to the shoulders, arms and neck.
- **Temporary muscle weakness and numbness which often affects only one side of the body (either the left or the right)**. This is due to insufficient flow of blood to a part of the brain which effects the control of muscles.
- **Confusion, disorientation and loss of intellectual functions**. This is due to a more drastic reduction in brain blood.

Most of these symptoms may last for only a few minutes and then disappear. You may have these symptoms for brief periods without necessarily having heart disease. They are particularly significant when they get worse during exercise or in cold weather, suggesting that your heart cannot keep up with the demands of your body, and that your blood circulation is impaired.

We need to be slim when our heart or kidneys are ill

The heart is a pump that moves blood in the body. The kidneys act like filters to clean the blood. When they are ill or damaged, they do not work as well as they should. The heart pumps less blood. The kidneys clean less efficiently.

Cardiovascular Disease

Without sufficient pressure, there is not enough oxygenated blood to feed the body and slowly the organs (brain, kidney, liver, even the heart) die. Thus, when the heart is not working well, it causes slow death of other parts of the body. After a heart attack the heart has fewer working parts (because parts of it are dead) and cannot feed itself and the rest of the body. Unless a person loses a lot of weight, another heart attack will usually occur. Soon the person dies.

It is impossible to grow another heart or cure the parts of the heart or kidney that are dead. The only thing to do to help our body is to reduce body size to match the ability of the heart to pump blood, or change diet to reduce atherosclerosis. With kidney disease, we need to reduce body size to reduce the amount of chemicals that must be cleaned from the blood.

There are many drugs that make your heart and kidney work harder. These drugs are effective in increasing the ability of your kidney and heart to meet the demands of your body. However, the increased effort by your kidney and heart often translates into decreased life span: Your organs have to work harder, and they die sooner. You are trading a shorter life span for a better life while you are living. However, there is another choice: You can improve your nutrition so that your organs work better without being exploited to the point of causing premature death. This is the option described in the following chapters.

References and Notes

[1] The heart is an unusual organ. While most organs get blood continuously, the vessels of the heart itself get most of their blood in between pumps of the heart. When the heart pumps, it makes so much pressure that it practically closes many of its own arteries. When it relaxes, the arteries receive the blood. When there is a partial obstruction to the arteries, there is not enough time in between "pumps" for the heart to receive enough blood. When the heart starts pumping harder and faster because of increased demands on your body, such as when you run, exercise, get upset, etc., then there is even less time between pumps for the heart arteries to receive enough blood. This increases the chance that some parts of the heart will die.

[2] This coagulability refers to the ability of the body to form clots or aggregate platelets.

[3] This applies only to hypertension caused by hardening and obstruction of the arteries due to atherosclerosis and arteriosclerosis. This is usually known as "intrinsic" hypertension or hypertension of unknown origin. A small number of people have hypertension caused by hormone imbalance or disease such as a tumor. This analysis is not applicable to those situations.

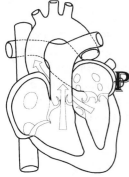

III.2

PEOPLE WITH CORONARY ARTERY DISEASE

"You can prevent heart disease: Take control of your life."

Topics: Case histories. People who are at risk for heart disease. Doctors also have heart disease. Old and sick people can get better.

Summary

Heart disease affects everyone, young and old, rich and poor, people without a high school education and those with PhDs and MDs. Many of us feel immortal and believe that disease will bypass us. Many health professionals behave as if prevention and treatment were necessary only for patients, and that doctors never get ill. But everyone is at risk for heart disease.

Case histories

The reluctance of traditional medicine to consider the role of diet in general, and of vegetable and fish oils in particular, in the prevention and treatment of cardiovascular disease became apparent to me in medical school. I often recommended selected vegetable oils and fish to my patients, to medical students and to other physicians, and stressed the importance of EFAs for health. The reaction generated by my interest was anything but enthusiastic. Professors thought I was nuts for sponsoring theories that were considered "non scientific", for which I had no data to support, and that disagreed with the medical wisdom of that time. Fortunately, my recommendations, though considered useless, were also considered harmless and I was often allowed to prescribe dietary modifications for my patients.

A man with heart disease

An immortal man. My first major break came one day when I met
Mr. G. He was a Latin American worker in his early forties. He had
had two heart attacks, suffered from diabetes and hypertension, was
overweight and smoked. Mr. G had all the factors that indicate a high
risk for heart disease ("**risk factors**"). He was also extremely
uncooperative. He refused to do anything to treat his diabetes, to give
up smoking or to lose weight. His diet was as bad as could be imagined
for his condition: he loved beef & pork(fried), alcohol, pizza, cheese,
sweets and other unhealthy foods which make up the bulk of the
standard American diet. He thought he was strong and would never
die --- an immortal man.

A lost cause. When he was discharged from the Intensive Care Unit
after his second heart attack, the doctors decided that he was a lost
cause: He refused to follow medical advice, and even if he did, given his
medical condition, there was little hope that he would live much longer.
He would soon have either a stroke or another heart attack which
would kill him. Given the weakened condition of his heart and his
oversized body, it was very likely that his heart would soon fail because
of the strain put on it.

Traditional care had failed. I was assigned to treat him because I
spoke Spanish, and because Mr. G was such a lost cause that no other
physician wanted to take care of him. Perhaps my superiors wanted me
to try out my "unusual" ideas about nutrition, cholesterol and how to
treat heart disease on a hopeless case. And when he died, would it not
confirm established wisdom and leave me to face the consequences?

To kill yourself. I went to visit Mr. G in his room, and found there a
classic example of what a person suffering from heart disease should
NOT do. He was sitting up in bed eating a *hearty* breakfast of
sausages, eggs, pancakes and butter. His scheduled lunch included
meat, a fatty dessert, and coffee. The coffee was ordered **with** sugar
and artificial creamer; after all, you can't expect a grown man to drink
bitter coffee! The one concession to dietary sanity was an instruction
that everything be low in salt; however this seemed like a bad joke
considering the rest of the menu. Mr. G was also smoking, even though
patients are usually not allowed to smoke in their rooms.

The dream. I sat down and spoke to Mr. G. He told me that he
wanted to get better and go back to work. BUT he was not willing to

People with heart disease

modify his life style. Not only were his tastes in food hard to change, but his food consumption was a matter of status for him. It had taken him many years to reach a level of prosperity where he could afford meat, cigarettes, and other luxury items. He would not allow me to take them away from him and place him on a poor man's diet. As a token gesture he was willing, occasionally, to eat more vegetables. He also consented to try (but not too hard) to lose some weight.

Factors that increase and decrease the risk of cardiovascular disease.

What is especially interesting is Mr. G's assessment of his health and habits. It is worth examining in detail because his misconceptions are widely held by many victims and potential victims of cardiovascular disease.

- **He claimed to eat very little.** Most overweight people are convinced that they eat very little and that their food intake cannot possibly be responsible for their being too fat. Many patients claim that they are fat because of the drugs they take or because of their "metabolism". But of course he, like most people, was overweight because he ate too much.

- **He maintained that he was already on a restricted diet since he was restricting his salt intake.** Most patients believe that being on a low salt diet is the solution to all their cardiovascular problems and high blood pressure. It is not. It merely tries to prevent the problems from getting worse.

- **He smoked only a few cigarettes per day.** After all, one cigarette was not going to kill him. While one cigarette is almost never fatal, countless repetitions of "just one cigarette" certainly may be.

- **He thought he was THIN.** Most overweight people think they are of average weight or even thin. Mr. G was actually only slightly above average by the charts, but his body was far too big for his damaged heart. Thus, he was very overweight.

- **He was already complying with his treatment.** He was taking "pills" for his high blood pressure and avoiding salt. Like many people who suffer from a serious disease, Mr. G thought that by taking a drug he was curing the illness and therefore removing the risks of heart disease. In fact, drugs often relieve

People with heart disease

symptoms of a disease while leaving the disease untouched. The disease may even progress under medication. Lowering hypertension with drugs may prevent some complications of hypertension, such as the risk that a brain vessel will rupture due to the high pressure of the blood inside the brain arteries, but it does not cure the cause of hypertension.

- **He took care of his diabetes, although he did not like to take insulin shots and was a little careless with sugar.** Patients often do not realize how dangerous it can be to deviate from a prescribed regimen, especially with diabetes and cardiovascular disease. Following the therapy on and off is like breathing every other day: After one day without oxygen many of your brain cells may not live to breathe the next day.

- **He felt he got enough exercise.** He was a truck driver. He walked around a lot on his job and at home, and often had to move things around. It is common for people to overestimate how much exercise they get, because they have no idea what kinds of exercise are necessary for, and beneficial to, cardiovascular functioning. For those suffering from cardiovascular disease, performing normal activities can be so fatiguing that sufferers feel as if they have exercised. Active exercise means running for over one hour per day or its equivalent. Compare yourself to a primitive human chasing after food or being chased by "food". That was exercise! Unless you are an athlete, you probably lead a comparatively sedentary life.

- **Mr. G considered his poor dietary habits as an essential part of the quality of life.** He stated that he preferred to live a few good years, enjoying rich foods, smoking, and ignoring the warnings of his body rather than to extend his life a few years and live without any satisfaction. It is difficult to realize that life can be satisfying without overeating and abusing the body in other ways. Patients often forget what life was like when they were healthy. They may also not realize that their unhealthy regimen may have assumed such importance in their lives because it has gradually removed the possibility of their participating in many rewarding activities. In other words, they do not realize how truly restricting are their habits of overindulgence and eating an unbalanced diet. They can't see the behavior modifications recommended by their physician in their true light, as a way to liberate themselves from their disabilities.

People with heart disease

The real choices are between many alert and healthy years versus a premature death often preceded by many years with partial disability and severe activity restriction.

- **Mr G. said he ate plenty of vegetables.** Because he ate a salad with dinner he felt he was eating his necessary "quota" of vegetables. But in fact fresh, uncooked, green vegetables were an *almost negligible proportion of his total caloric intake* (total food consumed in a day). In his condition, the small amount of vegetables he ate was almost irrelevant.

Drastic action. It was time for drastic action in Mr. G's case. His two heart attacks had left his heart severely damaged, unable to meet the needs of his body. In addition to eliminating cigarettes, he had to reduce the size of his body to match the diminished capacity of his heart. He had to go on a very strict diet. Active exercise was not indicated in his condition as a means of losing weight, because of the weakness of his heart. Thus, reducing food intake was the only answer.

The real choice. Mr. G's assessment of his choices was also mistaken. The choice was not between an average, pleasure-filled life with no food restrictions and a slightly longer, but dull life on a strict diet. The real choice before him was between almost no life at all (early death) and a chance at rebuilding his health and leading a long and full life.

There is hope. I explained to him that the other doctors in the hospital felt that he had no chance of recovering and therefore had little interest in treating him. I expressed my opinion that there was some hope, if he were willing to change his life drastically. Drastic measures were needed, because in his condition, a small change would not be very significant.

> ## *Eat to live well; do not live to eat*

Refusal, negotiation, agreement. Mr. G's first reaction to my suggestions was typical. He refused. Then he began negotiating for concessions. After all, one extra cigarette could not make that much of a difference. A teaspoon of sugar? Have you heard of anyone dying after taking a teaspoon of sugar? A little piece of bacon? What harm can it do? And so on. I realized it was time to be blunt. I told him I felt he would die soon if he didn't follow my advice. I enlisted his wife as an ally in my efforts to convince him to take responsibility for his health.

People with heart disease

We discussed all the wonderful things he could do in life if he were well. I explained how important it was to eat to live and not to live to eat. His initial refusal eventually gave way to a willingness to try to follow my advice. What exactly caused this change in attitude I do not know. Perhaps he sensed that I really cared about him. Perhaps my bluntness forced him to face the inevitability of his own death if he continued to eat as before.

Once he agreed to cooperate, I took the necessary steps to implement the dietary program I had proposed. I arranged a meeting with the dietitian. Mr. G's regular physicians did not interfere; after all, he was going to die soon, so anything I did was all right. Besides, maybe this was what was necessary to show me how unimportant nutrition really was. Acting on my instructions the dietitian arranged for a drastic change in Mr. G's diet. And how radical a change it was for him! He was allowed only vegetables, for a total of 600 to 1000 calories per day. He was of course forbidden to smoke. I also wanted his diet to be supplemented with soybean oil. Unfortunately, nobody had heard about *omega-3* and *omega-6* fatty acids and there was no soybean oil to be found in the hospital kitchen. But there was corn oil and I prescribed a supplement of 1 to 2 tablespoons of raw, unheated, corn oil every day as a source of polyunsaturated fatty acids (PUFAs), in an almost fat-free but otherwise balanced diet.

The miracle. Then a miracle occurred: He stuck to his diet. That was the miracle; getting better was not a miracle, it was just a consequence of the diet. Slowly he began to improve. About a month later, after I had rotated to another section of the hospital, I heard that Mr. G had come to the hospital asking to see me. He had improved, had been discharged and had gone back to his old job. He was able to walk and work for far longer periods of time than before he followed my treatment. He felt more energetic and had no chest pain. There were other cases like Mr. G's and they improved my standing in medical school and helped me to graduate: Perhaps I had an unusual approach to treatment [1], but at least I had given my professors and classmates something to think about.

Doctors who used essential fats to treat heart disease and high cholesterol

I came to Boston for my medical residency to learn more about nutrition, biochemistry, metabolism, and blood tests, and to do research

---
People with heart disease

on fats. One day I was speaking to a chemist in the hospital laboratory and mentioned to him my interest in fats and the use of fats in cardiovascular research. It was a fortunate coincidence. He had worked for many years with Dr. C, an old cardiologist who had recently died. This cardiologist had been feeding his patients oil extracts. I obtained copies of the available records he had left when he died, records that were going to be thrown away. I found that for more than 10 years he had been treating patients with a mixture of essential fats that he had prepared with the help of a chemist. His patients, very severely ill patients with highly elevated cholesterol, were doing extremely well, so well that from time to time I heard that his patients were complaining to the physicians who had replaced Dr. C because the drugs that the physicians were now using were not as effective as the oils. Another famous British researcher, Dr. Sinclair, had written extensively about the benefits of EFAs before his death.

A medical student

The following case is a particularly sad one for me. One of my friends, a world-renowned scientist whom I met in medical school. We spent many hours together learning to survive and cope with the medical system while he recalled his adventures in Africa or lunch with the Queen of England. He told me that he had an apparently slight problem: He was in his late thirties and had what is called "very mild" hypertension. I took the liberty of raising my concern about his condition. He didn't see any cause for concern. After all, he played tennis regularly, had a strong complexion, and appeared to be in good health.

I was less confident, however. I had seen many men like him with a strong complexion and apparently in good health. In fact, my first cadaver in anatomy was a man whose condition was reminiscent of my colleague's: He was very strong, healthy-looking, and muscular, but his arteries were almost closed due to atherosclerosis. Thus, in spite of appearances he had really been quite sick. I believed that my friend should drastically change his diet, lose weight and, of course, eat more EFAs. He thought this was ridiculous. He had been seen by the most famous physicians at the hospital, world known specialists in hypertension and heart disease. According to their evaluations, his blood pressure values were within the "normal range", and he was therefore a normal, healthy man with nothing to worry about. I disagreed. I felt he should not have any hypertension at all. Being

People with heart disease

normal was not satisfactory if by normal we mean "average". He should try to be better than average in order to beat the odds and live longer than the average man. My advice went unheeded. Several years went by and I heard that he died of an apparent heart attack while playing tennis. He was in his early 40's.

Sudden death is often predictable and preventable

Hundreds of thousands of people die every year from a sudden heart attack or a stroke. Sudden death attacks a wide range of people, even those with huge financial resources or great looking bodies. Rich and famous people, professional athletes and people in presumably "excellent" physical shape who exercise every day suddenly die of a heart attack or a stroke. Why? What do they have in common? Could anyone have predicted their deaths? Could they have been prevented? The sad answer is that their deaths were mostly predictable and preventable. What these individuals frequently have in common is a circulatory system that is partially obstructed and cannot keep up with the demands for nutrients by the body. Their blood is often more dense, or more sluggish in its movement, and less "fluid". The platelets, those little cells that form clots, are more likely to form clots inside the blood vessels. The vessels themselves are harder. The heart already suffers because its own blood vessels cannot supply it with enough oxygen and nutrients, and thus it is slowly dying. The brain has a similar problem.

Even when I was in medical school, I developed a dependable ability to predict death. My first patient, as a medical student, had deteriorating kidney function. In my ignorance, I plotted the test results and predicted that he would die within one week. My classmates, interns and professors scoffed at my crude charts and told me that test results often varied and could not be used to make predictions about death. They were generally right, but in my ignorance I continued. Given my background, I could not help it. Before going to medical school I was trained as a physicist-mathematician, and my expertise was in developing predictive models. With some ups and downs, the trend in this patient's tests was downwards. Eventually I told my "medical team" that it was time for drastic treatment measures because I predicted death within 2 days. The team had a good laugh and ordered gastrointestinal X-rays to identify the cause of abdominal pain, further renal tests and various other diagnostic procedures scheduled over a

People with heart disease

period of 4 days. (At that time, patients went to the hospital and spent their days waiting for diagnostic tests to be done.) The patient died before all diagnostic tests were completed. The team criticized me for making predictions.

During the course of my student days I continued to make my "unofficial predictions". Despite my success, my methods were largely ignored due to a combination of factors. My team members constantly changed and every new senior physician thought my scientific methods were not accurate. My approach, to evaluate the nutritional and biochemical status of the patient, was considered practically irrelevant because it was the consensus that nutritional abnormalities were irrelevant to most diseases except for a few cases of iron, B_{12} or folate deficiency anemia. My proposal that the balance of fatty acids was one of the most significant determinants of health and disease was a constant source for laughter.

Three major events caused people to think that perhaps I was right. I was even invited to give several talks on my ideas about nutrition and preventive medicine. As a third year medical student, I suggested to my team that I could improve the treatment of insulin dependent diabetic patients. At that time, elderly diabetic women and men were being subjected to multiple blood drawings to evaluate their glucose and their insulin, and their food intake was constantly adjusted up and down. The patients' arms were always purple from the bruises caused by repeated blood drawings. The team accepted my challenge and gave me several of the most difficult-to-treat cases. In less than one week I had them under control and had eliminated most of the blood drawing. The patients pleaded to have me continue with them when my rotation ended. My "secret" was simple. I did not aim for perfect glucose control, something practically impossible in many diabetics. I also considered it more dangerous to be hypoglycemic (low glucose) than hyperglycemic (high glucose). Being hypoglycemic can kill cells; being slightly hyperglycemic merely makes you urinate more often. I analyzed the glucose in the urine rather than the blood to have broad targets. I imposed strict controls on food intake to match the pattern of blood insulin predicted from the injections, which is perhaps the most significant issue in the control of insulin-dependent diabetics.

The second event involved a patient with inflammatory bowel disease. He was earning about $1,000,000 per year. When I saw him he was lying flat on a bed and told me that he could not get up because of

---

People with heart disease

muscular weakness and other problems. I evaluated his test results, requested several additional ones, and diagnosed him as suffering from severe "selected" nutritional deficiencies caused by huge imbalances in the absorption of nutrients. In simpler words, he had too much of some nutrients, and not enough of others. He was deficient in potassium, other minerals and several vitamins, and deficient in EFAs. I recommended that he eat daily a specially formulated diet that provided the needed supplements. I presented my case in front of my team and a famous "guest" speaker who discussed his approach and my approach. Being already well known and quite talented himself, he was not afraid to recognize the value of my suggestions, which ended up being implemented. The patient got much better, told me how he would now be able to earn even more than he was earning before, said thank you, and left.

The third event began one day during morning rounds, when the team evaluated a 40+ overweight woman with adult onset diabetes. The team found her diabetes under control and recommended that she be discharged that morning. I told the team that I believed that she was going to die soon, probably that same day and she should not be discharged. The students, interns, residents and professor took me aside in the hall and gave me a "lecture" for about 15 minutes. I was told that I should stop making unsound predictions, that I should study more, and learn more before I made outrageous predictions. I was told to practice medicine depending more on X-rays, EKGs and conventional tests rather than blood or nutritional tests. Just at the time when the team leader was preparing to propose his "punishment" for my silly sayings, the patient went into cardiac arrest. The team attempted to resuscitate her but failed The patient was declared dead about 30 minutes later.

While the team stood in the hall, telling me "don't you dare say anything," one classmate who had seen me make accurate predictions before asked me how I did it. Was it pure luck? I told the team that I had examined the patient early that morning, as was my duty before rounds. I had seen that the patient had several risk factors for hardening of the arteries and increased risk of clot formation. The patient was overweight and had a dietary history of very low intake of EFAs. Each morning diabetic patients have blood drawn for analysis. At the site of blood drawing, the tiny wound had not healed well. When I touched it, it started to bleed again. In a healthy person, the small hole from the needle used for blood drawing closes up very quickly and

People with heart disease

does not bleed again. When patients have a disorder of blood clotting called "disseminated intravascular coagulation", the blood forms clots inside most of the vessels and exhausts the supply of platelets. As a result, some parts of the body cannot form clots and bleed. This is a life-threatening condition which can be treated if properly diagnosed. A common sign is bleeding at the site where blood was recently drawn.

The autopsy revealed multiple clots in the body. The team could not dispute the facts, but attributed them to my luck. Just in case, the team never disputed anything I said. From then on they ordered tests or treatment I suggested, and gave me a passing grade. I did not receive any more lectures about my unsuitable prediction models. Instead, I continued to develop methods to identify the causes of cardiovascular disease and how to prevent and treat them. Throughout the years I was guided by colleagues who believed in my approach and helped me to learn about nutritional biochemistry and preventive medicine.

Heart disease is a silent killer

Heart disease, elevated cholesterol and elevated blood pressure are sometimes called the "silent killers" because they have no obvious symptoms. A person may feel quite well, and die suddenly of a heart attack. That is the reason why blood tests, careful medical examination, and good habits are so important. Prevention is easy; treatment is very difficult, since many heart attacks and strokes lead irreversibly to death. The proper medical evaluation will reveal factors that indicate a person is at risk for heart disease. Waiting until one feels chest pain may be waiting too long.

Choose a physician who follows his/her own advice: does not smoke, follows a healthy diet, is thin, has normal blood pressure and cholesterol

Physicians and dentists have heart disease and high cholesterol

Doctors with medical knowledge and with access to the finest medical attention available have the same problems as people without any medical degrees. One of my dentists resembled my former friend. A

People with heart disease

strong man, in apparently good health, he played tennis and felt nothing was wrong with him. I told him I thought he was overweight and that he should drastically change his diet and get proper medical advice. But he too was being seen by famous physicians whose conventional wisdom assured him that he had nothing to worry about. Luckily, he developed warning symptoms: chest pain and some other indications of cardiovascular disease that scared him and his physicians and he was put on a better diet. He lost quite a bit of weight and is much better now.

Several health professionals I know have similar physical appearances. Some are 10% to 20% overweight. I usually suggest that they lose weight, drastically change their lifestyle and improve their balance of EFAs. But these professionals have no symptoms of cardiovascular disease, and, therefore, feel invulnerable. Some of them try to lose weight, but a few "good meals", holidays and parties undo any progress made in losing weight.

Intelligent men and women often feel invulnerable. It is unfortunate that so many intelligent men and women chose to ignore common sense and not take good care of their bodies. My colleagues agree with me, but they cannot take the steps required to change their lifestyle.

Heart disease affects health professionals as well as other people. Physicians and dentists also have a hard time trying to control their lifestyles. Parties, "good" food, sedentary jobs, smoking: they know all too well that those factors lead to heart disease. Yet, somehow, they think that heart disease will overlook them because they know about it.

> *Knowledge does not prevent disease unless one uses that knowledge correctly.*

You are never too old or too sick to improve your health

Aged and sick people can improve their health

Even if you are elderly or sick, you can and should still work to prevent cardiovascular disease. My parents were over 60 when they started a program to prevent heart disease and drastically lowered their cholesterol levels and their need for blood pressure control medication.

People with heart disease

A man with prostate cancer and heart disease.

Mr. H was battling against prostate cancer, and for many years had been suffering from elevated cholesterol and hypertension. He told me he could do nothing about his heart as long as he worried about his prostate cancer. I disagreed. I have written that the best diet for cancer is usually the best one to prevent cardiovascular disease. For his hypertension, Mr. H received a variety of medications that created other problems. He initially refused a prostatectomy and had massive radiation treatment. Working with many physicians and reviewing thousands of scientific articles published across the world, I helped to implement an experimental therapy, which worked quite well and eventually cured his cancer. That treatment is now used with most prostate cancer patients. Treating his cancer was difficult and he would often say to me: "Why bother about my heart if I am going to die of cancer anyway?" I explained to him that his cancer, now under control, might or might not kill him, but even if it did it could be in 10 or perhaps 20 years. Heart disease could kill him tomorrow. I convinced Mr. H to change his diet drastically. He lost over 20 lbs. and began to eat an almost exclusively vegetarian diet, with special vitamin and mineral supplements, egg whites, tofu and fish, and supplementation with vegetable and fish oil. His blood pressure declined from the 140-180 range with medication, to 110 with very little medication. His cholesterol went below 200. In five years he went from being barely able to walk one block, to climbing stairs, and riding my bicycle. Most medications were no longer needed. It is also possible that the new diet helped to cure his cancer.

A woman with Paget's disease and hypertension

Ms. M was 65 years old and had Paget's disease, a disorder that destroys the bones. She also had a heart attack, cardiovascular disease, hypertension and elevated cholesterol. She was more difficult to treat. Mr. H, when he had chest or leg pain, became frightened and was willing to change. In contrast, Ms. M does not have any symptoms, and is therefore less willing to lose weight, but she is trying. I convinced her to change to a low fat high EFA diet. She lost over 20 lbs. Her cholesterol has been dropping steadily even since she began eating more essential fats.

People with heart disease

A diabetic patient with high cholesterol

Mrs. S had diabetes mellitus since she was five. She received insulin every day. She had severe heart problems, major heart surgery, elevated cholesterol, and poorly functioning kidneys; she was also going blind (a typical complication of diabetes). For at least 10 years she had severe limitations of movement. She could not walk up or down stairs. She had difficulties traveling by public transportation because she could not get on a vehicle or even remain standing if the conveyance was crowded, and it was sometimes difficult for her even to get dressed or eat by herself. I placed her on a diet which she reluctantly tried to follow, since she hates fish and does not like vegetables. Using soybean oil we were able, for the first time, to drastically reduce her cholesterol to below 200 in less than two years (a 25% decline). A therapy of vegetables, fish and oils also helped her drastically lower her cholesterol and triglyceride counts, and stopped the deterioration of her eyes and heart. Unfortunately she received little support from her regular physicians who regarded my therapies as unorthodox, or from her family members and friends who invited her to parties and told her that one more sandwich or hot dog was not going to kill her. After some improvement, she returned to her old ways and refused to commit herself to a severely restricted diet. *Her diet had to be extremely low in calories; because she moved so little, she had to eat very little in order to lose weight.* Unfortunately now it is too late; she died of heart disease complications. I find that many patients refuse to follow strict diets to improve their health until it is too late. Lifestyle needs to change at the first symptom of disease. Even better, prevention should begin at an early age.

Scientific Findings

There are a huge number of research articles linking various factors to cardiovascular disease. I will cite only a few. Cigarette smoking greatly increases the risk of coronary heart disease among women as well as men.[2] In men, the following factors increase the risk of a stroke: increased blood pressure (which, if too high, can break vessels and leak blood into the brain), abdominal obesity, increased plasma fibrinogen (a chemical that affects coagulation and is in turn modulated by the levels of EFAs), and a maternal history of stroke.[3]

People with heart disease

There is an increased risk of death from heart attack in the morning, and it is related to the fact that platelets tend to aggregate more easily in the morning.[4] If your tests show that your platelets have a tendency to aggregate and you are concerned about dying from a clot sometime in the morning, increasing the balance of ω3 vs. ω6 fatty acids will decrease the ability of platelets to form clots. Obviously, this is not a do-it-yourself job but requires careful blood testing for EFAs and supervision in the dietary changes you make.

Many people ask me whether it is better to lose weight by increasing exercise or eating less. A study by Wood and coworkers found that "fat loss through dieting or exercising produces comparable and favorable changes in plasma lipoprotein concentrations."[5] In other words, burning calories or eating less calories reduce your risk of heart disease. Exercising more allows you to eat more nutrients. Eating more allows your body to get more nutrients and essential fats. However, keep in mind that you must exercise a lot to burn 200 calories. You can easily eat in one sitting all the calories you burn in one week of exercise, because the body is a very efficient machine. If you eat fewer calories, your diet must be more carefully balanced to assure enough EFAs, vitamins and minerals.

References and Notes

[1] Many physicians considered that nutrition had a very limited role in the treatment of cardiovascular disease. Siguel EN. Triglycerides and HDL cholesterol. Corresp. *N. Engl. J. Med.* 304(7):424, 1981. Siguel EN. Controversial aspects of nutrition (let.). *J.Parent.Ent. Nutr.* 5:169-70, 1981.

[2] Willett WC, Green A, Stampfer MJ et al. Relative and absolute excess risks of coronary heart disease among women who smoke cigarettes. *New Eng. J. Med* 1987; 317:1303-9.

[3] Welin L, Svardsudd K, Wilhelmsen L et al. Analysis of risk factors for stroke in a cohort of men born in 1913. *New Eng. J. Med* 1987; 317:521-6.

[4] Tofler GH, Brezinski MBD, Schafer AI, Czeisler CA, Rutherford JD, Willich MBS, Gleason RE, Williams GH, Muller JE. Concurrent morning increase in platelet aggregability and the risk of myocardial infarction and sudden cardiac death.

[5] Wodd PD, Stefanick ML, Dreon DM et al. Changes in plasma lipids and lipoproteins in overweight men during weight loss through dieting as compared with exercise. *New Eng. J. Med.* 1988; 319:1173-9.

People with heart disease

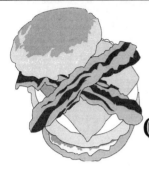

III.3

RISK FACTORS FOR CORONARY ARTERY DISEASE

"Know the factors that increase your risk for heart disease"

Topics: *Risk factors for a heart attack: Smoking, Hypertension, Diabetes, High Cholesterol, Overweight, Stress, Family History. What you can do.*

Summary

Risk factors are the characteristics that make a person more likely to have a heart attack. Research has shown that individuals who have one or more of these "factors" or characteristics have a greater chance of developing heart disease and dying of a heart attack. The risk factors are: smoking; high blood pressure, high total cholesterol and not enough cholesterol in HDL particles; diabetes, high blood glucose (sugar); overweight, lifestyle, a blood-related family member with heart disease at a young age (under 60), and abnormal blood levels of essential fats.

Risk Factors

Risk factors are the characteristics that make a person more likely to have a heart attack. Many years of research have identified habits, physical characteristics and test results that indicate who is more likely to have a heart attack. The most important factors are described below.

Smoking

People who smoke are more likely than those who don't to suffer from cardiovascular disease and cancer, particular lung cancer. They are also likely to have a variety of breathing problems such as emphysema. Smoking interferes with the blood;s ability to carry oxygen and slowly kills the organs of the body. Smoking may act as a heavy oxidant, which, roughly stated, "burns up" nutrients and ultimately body parts.

High blood pressure (Hypertension)

High blood pressure (**hypertension**) is a risk factor because the high pressure inside the arteries may burst a blood vessel and produce internal bleeding. Chronic hypertension forces the vessels to become stronger and thicker to resist the high pressure, which in turns causes the heart to pump harder, causing even higher pressure.

Elevated cholesterol/ HDL cholesterol

The cholesterol in the blood is a major factor in the development of heart disease. The ratio of total cholesterol over the cholesterol in the HDL particles is referred to by clinicians as the total cholesterol/HDL cholesterol ratio. Triglycerides are another type of fat found in the blood. Elevated levels of both total cholesterol/HDL cholesterol and triglycerides lead to fat and cholesterol being deposited in the arteries, which eventually harden and become obstructed. Some of the excessive cholesterol forms crystals, which are chunks of rock-hard cholesterol inside your arteries. Think of a highway scattered with chunks of rock, some as large as a 10 story building, spread all over the road, and then think of trying to drive a car through this obstacle course. This is what blood cells and platelets encounter when moving through a blood vessel with fat and cholesterol obstructions. No wonder the platelets hit them and form clots (clumped platelets), which further obstruct the arteries. The resulting reduced blood flow and poor circulation is insufficient to feed all the cells. Some cells die for lack of oxygen or nutrients.

Research studies have provided guidelines about desirable ratios of cholesterol levels and the amount of risk associated with abnormal cholesterol values. You can compare your own values with those in the chart here and those of several typical groups: Vegetarians = 1.7; Boston Marathon runners 2.0; Males without evidence of Coronary Heart Disease = 3.3; Males with evidence of Coronary Heart Disease = 3.8. Vegetarians have cholesterol levels around 130. In my clinical

Risk Factors for CAD

Risk for heart disease according to Cholesterol ratios[1]

Risk	LDL/HDL	Total Chol /HDL	Total Chol
Low	below 2.0	below 2.5	below 160
Some	2 - 3	2.5-3.5	160 - 200
Significant	3 - 5	3.5-5.0	200 - 240
High	above 5	above 5.0	above 240

experience, very healthy men and women have cholesterol levels between 100 and 130 mg/dl and cholesterol/HDL cholesterol below 2.5.

If you are in good health, a low level of cholesterol does not appear to cause any danger. Many healthy people have cholesterol below 100, particularly in other countries. Cholesterol below 100 is very rare in the USA. Sometimes, however, a very low cholesterol suggests that you may have some disease that you do not know about, or that you are undernourished. If you do not eat for several days, your cholesterol will decline. When I was evaluating the cholesterol of all the patients at the Intensive Care Unit of a large Medical Center in Boston, I found that many patients had very low cholesterol a few days after they were admitted for severe heart disease. The reasons was that these patients had not eaten for several days while in the hospital.

High glucose levels and Diabetes

Individuals with high levels of **glucose** in their blood and diabetes are likely to have a heart attack. The elevated glucose is probably caused by inefficient transport and use. This excess glucose in the blood may lead to the accumulation of saturated fat in the cells and interferes with the ability of the body to use the essential fats.

Overweight

Some parts of the body, like the skin, expand or contract to adapt to the size of the body. Unfortunately, the ability of the heart to adapt to the

Risk Factors for CAD

size of the body is limited. Moreover, small parts of the heart are dying all the time due to the "aging". As a consequence, as we get older we have a smaller working heart (our heart may be larger, but it contains a lot of dead tissue). The only way to compensate is by having a smaller body. Overweight stresses the heart beyond its abilities and causes more cells to die, leading to premature heart disease.

Stress

Stress increases the requirements of the heart. We get more wear and tear of the heart which is equivalent to faster aging. However, stress is not as big a killer as many people think. Some stress is healthy because it increases your metabolism and is equivalent to getting more exercise. Highly motivated and accomplished people are "stressed" but perform well and live very long. Some easy going people are "stressed" because they are not motivated and feel that their lives are meaningless. If your body is healthy and you eat well, stress is unlikely to kill you (except for some diseases specifically affected by stress).

Alcohol

There is great controversy surrounding this topic and huge financial interests behind it. Obviously, people who sell or like to drink alcohol would like it to be "healthy", while those opposed to drinking prefer to find it dangerous to one's health. We will never find one answer because whether or not alcohol is dangerous depends on the balance of many other factors. There is scientific evidence that the equivalent of 4-8 ounces of **red wine** per day may inhibit the formation of clots and thereby act like aspirin, preventing the sudden heart attack or stroke caused by a clot's sudden obstruction of an artery. However, if you are already taking aspirin, or if your blood does not clot easily, one may expect that red wine could be hazardous to your health. The active ingredient in red wine appears to be a chemical found in the skin of the grapes rather than alcohol itself. And you may need to take it almost every day; otherwise its effects may wear off rapidly. However, daily drinking of alcohol also will slowly damage your liver.[2]

There is little doubt that frequent consumption of alcohol causes damage to the liver and possibly other organs. Moderate alcohol consumption also increases the risk of breast cancer.[3] "Moderate" in this study referred to about 5 to 14 grams of pure alcohol per week (less than one tablespoon or about the amount in three to nine drinks). The

Risk Factors for CAD

increase in risk was about 2.5. However, because the overall risk of breast cancer is quite small compared with other causes of death, elderly people who do not have cancer are unlikely to develop cancer from an occasional drink. Incidentally, because prostate and breast cancer are related (both are hormone-related cancers affecting similar types of organs but in different sexes), we can expect that moderate alcohol drinking also increases the chances of prostate cancer.

After considering the pros and cons of alcohol, one could conclude that small amounts of red wine are OK, but that we should stay away from significant drinking of other types of alcohol. However, if you drink less than 4 ounces of wine/day, the protective effects against heart disease are small and apply only to those at high risk of forming clots. If you drink more, you increase your risk of alcohol-related diseases.

Alcohol provides empty calories, that is, calories without nutritional value other than the calories themselves. The calories from alcohol add to the total of calories consumed from other sources. All calories which are not used by the body are converted and stored as SFAs. To avoid becoming obese, people who drink alcohol do not eat foods rich in other nutrients. Others gain weight from the alcohol, which is stored as SFAs and causes hardening of the arteries. Furthermore, alcohol seems to interfere with the optimal use of EFAs by the body. This is so because the liver is involved in the delivery of EFAs to other parts of the body. Alcohol harms the liver and the enzymes of the liver that prepare the EFAs for delivery to the rest of the body.

I do not believe that drinking wine is the solution to heart disease or that it plays a major role in preventing disease. There are numerous reasons that confuse the research findings. For example, if most people were to drink highly polluted water and die of cancer before 60, the death rate of heart disease will plummet (only the most sturdy would survive to die of heart disease). Then researchers would find that polluted water decreases the risk of heart disease. Researchers try to adjust mortality rates to compensate for different "survival", but the adjustment is imprecise and we can only adjust for factors we know. While wine may provide some benefits and in small amounts provides pleasure with minimal risks, I suggest drinking less than one small glass of wine per day, the less the better (particularly if you are young).

Genetics (family factors)

There are great differences from one person to another. We are the result of the factors expressed in our genes. Each person has different physical characteristics: body shape, hair color, facial expressions, etc. Many differences among people cannot be seen by the naked eye. These are differences in the way the physiology or machinery of the body works. Some people have genes that allow them to get rid of toxic chemicals better than others. Others have genes that provide better hearing or vision. And some people have genes that protect against heart disease. Similarly, we have different genes that regulate our needs for vitamins, minerals and essential fats. Some people have genes that allow them to make more efficient use of the essential fats and therefore need less of them. Others probably need more to survive. I suspect that the needs for essential fats of people with dark-skin are quite different from those of light-colored skin.[4]

Scientists are beginning to identify what genes are associated with heart disease. We do not know how they work. For now, the best way to know whether you have good genes is to study the health history of your blood relatives. If most of the people in your family have died after the age of 80, then you have good genes. If any of your family members died before the age of 50 due to heart disease, you may have some bad genes. Your physician can help you to evaluate the cause of death of your family members and the type of genes you may have. Everybody benefits from following a good diet. People with bad genes need to be more careful with their diets if they want to live a long life.

References and Notes

[1.] The numbers presented here are rough approximations. There are many similar tables published in scientific papers. The exact numbers are not important; what is important are the rough categories. In fact, exact numbers do not exist: Each person is different and therefore studies with different groups give different results, but they all agree on the same broad categories. These results are summaries of data published in many scientific journals.

[2] It would be interesting to know if eating red grapes has similar effects to drinking red wine.

[3] Willett WC, Stampfer MJ, Colditz GA et al. Moderate alcohol consumption and the risk of breast cancer. *New Engl. J. of Medicine* 1987; 316:1174-80.

[4] Animals and plants from warm tropical areas have different needs for and metabolism of essential fats than those from cold areas. I believe that individuals who genetically originated in warm parts of the world have different requirements for essential fats than individuals who originated in cold parts of the world. Notice that a dark-skin person born in Alaska has more genes in common with a dark-skin person born in Haiti than with a light-skin person born in Alaska. Genes reflect our body composition which has evolved for hundreds of thousands of years, not just a few generations.

Risk Factors for CAD

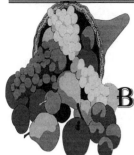

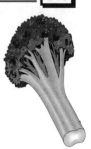

III.4

BASIC PREVENTION
PROGRAM

"Take control of your life"

Topics: *Prevention Program: things to do. Eat a balance of omega-3 and omega-6 fats. Correct for years on a diet high in saturated fats. Exercise. Slowly improve overall health.*

Summary

Most people are likely to have three problems in varying degrees: heart disease, hypertension, and a high risk of getting a stroke or a heart attack. The first step is to prevent the most severe complications, namely the risk of obstructing an artery with a clot. Then, slowly, reduce high blood pressure and soften artery walls. People on my program report improved memory, softer, younger looking skin and other health benefits. The key to preventing cardiovascular disease and lowering hypertension is a diet rich in green vegetables, grains and seeds, containing little animal fat except that in cold water fish. You should eat to maintain your ideal weight. Essential to a health-building diet in an adult is supplementation with oils to ensure a proper balance of ω3 and ω6 fats. This corrects for years on a diet high in calories and low in EFAs. Not all foods are equally valuable in the prevention and treatment of cardiovascular disease and hypertension; the person seeking to improve his or her health must learn to select intelligently among the items that are available. Exercise helps to attain and maintain a healthy body, and allows us to eat more food, and thereby get adequate nutrients. But exercise is rarely enough to lose weight.

You can easily change a few things in your life and greatly improve your chances of living many more healthy years. Health or disease is not a lottery: It is determined by what you do. To improve your health you should be slim, eat a balanced diet, exercise and refrain from smoking. It is important to treat any medical problems as soon as possible, before they become untreatable. And finally, improve your health by improving your diet: Specifically, reduce your intake of calories, saturated fat, and processed foods, and replace them with appropriate amounts of essential fats and natural foods.

How you can improve your health

Prevention of cardiovascular disease means slowing down the process of aging and the deterioration of the cardiovascular system. We will all die, but some of us take longer to do it; others drop dead in middle age, just when they have learned and saved enough to enjoy life. Living longer requires breaking out of a vicious cycle of disease causing more disease, and making your body a partner in your health and your life. You can control your life and preserve your youth. While it is true that from the day we are born our arteries begin to age, we can influence and mitigate the effects of the passing year's on our blood vessels. People who are careful about their bodies and who eat in such a way as to strengthen their cardiovascular systems can greatly slow down the process of aging. Those whose diets place burdens on the arteries age prematurely and increase the danger of an early death.

Everyone has seen people who at age 50 seem to be 35 years old while others at 40 seem to be 55. You could look 10, even 20 years younger than you are, with a proper diet. Of course, some people have "good genes", and this is not a negligible factor. But even good genes will not protect you if you are not careful. People with good genes are quite fortunate. For reasons we do not know, their bodies can take more abuse than the bodies of those with bad genes. However, people with good genes can also become sick through improper diet, and people with bad genes can prevent disease by eating carefully. It just requires more effort and control. Even the best car in the world will wear down quickly if you are careless in the way you care for it.

Treatment is quite simple

What we need to do is simple to state but requires determination to implement. We must reverse the factors that have increased our risk for cardiovascular disease. We must decrease the fat in our blood and also change it so that it contains more essential fats and less saturated fat. We must control diabetes and hypertension. We must soften our arteries. And we must keep our health problems from getting worse. Practically all the excess calories that you eat are stored by the body as saturated and monounsaturated fat. We need to replace a great chunk of that fat with essential fats and the mixture of ω3 and ω6 unique for each one of us.

Do not smoke. Be thin. Eat a balanced diet. Eat less calories and eat more essential fats found in vegetables and oils. Manage stress. Exercise. Eat more natural foods

A basic prevention program

The basic elements of a prevention program are listed below in the order of relative importance:

- 1. **Do not smoke**.
- 2. **Attain and maintain ideal weight**. In case of doubt about what your ideal weight is, err on the slender side; it is better to be thinner than heavier. If necessary, reduce your caloric intake.
- 3. **Eat a diet containing 10-20 different natural foods every week**. This is essential for good health.
  - a) Decrease the amount of foods containing animal fat in the diet and increase the percentage of calories derived from vegetables. This approach also allows you to eat more food and more nutrients.
  - b) Eat as many natural foods in season as possible. Do not overcook vegetables, and, if possible, eat vegetables raw. Emphasize green vegetables.
- 4. **Eat a mixture of ω3 and ω6 fats** (essential = polyunsaturated fat) found in some vegetable oils and seeds.
- 5. **Avoid animal fat and partially hydrogenated fat**, often included in processed foods.
- 6. **Exercise** at least 30 minutes per day, every day.
- 7. Learn to **relax** and **reduce stress**.

Basic Prevention Program

- 8. **Eat less than 300 mg per day of cholesterol**. This is easily accomplished by minimizing your consumption of foods containing animal fat.
- 9. **Do not add sodium to your meals**; instead use other condiments.
- 10. **Control your diabetes and high blood pressure** (which will occur if you follow the above guidelines).

The emphasis of this book is on fats. However, my experience with hundreds of patients has given me many insights about aspects of the prevention program that I will share with you.

> *Health or disease is not a lottery: it is determined by what you do.*

Do not smoke

This is a piece of advice that barely requires any clarification at all. Do not smoke cigarettes and do not inhale the smoke of other people's cigarettes. It seems so simple . . . if you do not smoke you are more likely to live a longer and happier life and save quite a bit of money. It is the most important thing you can do to prevent aging.

Achieve ideal (not normal) weight

If you are like the vast majority of Americans, you are overweight. It is crucial to evaluate your weight accurately in order to be able to plan a diet for yourself. From experience I have found that people tend to have an optimistic picture of themselves. Most people who think they are of average weight are about 5% to 10% overweight. If they tell me they are "plump", it means 10% to 20% overweight. If they think they are overweight, then they really are!

It is safer and healthier to be thinner than fatter. You look better, your clothes fit you better, you are less tired, you put less stress on your body and you are more resistant to disease. We store fat in order to have food during periods when food is not available. In pre-technological societies, when refrigerators and supermarkets were scarce, our ancestors had to hunt for food. In the winter, weeks could go by before food was found. To be fat was not only healthy but essential to

Basic Prevention Program

survival. Today, overweight people stand a better chance of survival if their plane crashes in snow-covered mountains: Fat protects from the cold and provides them with extra energy to survive.

If you are planning to be lost in the Sahara dessert or climb Mount Everest, please EAT. You may be without food for many months and need to store plenty of fat for the occasion. However if you live close to a supermarket, you are unlikely to starve. Even if you live in an area where supermarkets are not open 24 hours per day, and your refrigerator breaks down, you are very *very* unlikely to starve from Sunday until Monday. Therefore you do not need to store extra food in your body: store it in your refrigerator or kitchen cabinets instead.

A big body burdens your heart

Why is overweight such an important contributing factor in cardiovascular disease? A big body imposes extraordinary demands on the cardiovascular system. The heart has to pump more blood. The arteries are longer and the heart has to push harder to get the blood everywhere. All the organs have to work extra to keep up with the needs of your body. Your legs have to carry and move the extra weight: they need to work harder. This increases wear and tear on your joints.

As we get older, our circulatory system becomes less efficient. Therefore we should have a smaller (thinner) bodies. Unfortunately, most people get heavier as they get older. Not only they have a less efficient system, but they make it work even harder. No wonder that their heart collapses prematurely! Most people are overweight when they have their first heart attack or bypass operation.

Activity	Calories
Sleeping	30
Softball	120
Watching TV	30
Calisthenics	140
Office work	80
Golf	130
Slow walking	100
Bicycling	190
Housework	110
Aerobic dance	200
Walking up	200
Tennis singles	210
Walking fast	200
Swimming	220
Jogging	300

Exercise maintains

Basic Prevention Program

your muscle tone and weight

Exercise improves your muscles and increases the efficiency of your circulation. The amount of exercise depends, of course, on your physical condition. While exercise can prevent heart disease, if your heart is too weak, it can also kill you. Spending about 200-300 calories per day on moderate exercise such as rapid walking or a similar activity helps you burn fat and keep your body in good shape. However, exercise does not protect against eating a diet low in EFAs and high in calories and SFAs, as shown in places like eastern Finland where people are very physically active yet have a high rate of coronary artery disease.[1] We must remember that people who rarely exercise and suddenly embark on a strenuous exercise program may drastically increase their chances of a heart attack. If you are not in good shape and do not exercise daily, you should not spend an hour shoveling snow during your first cold and snowy day. Instead, do it slowly, with plenty of breaks. Better yet, be prepared by exercising actively for at least 15 minutes every day.

Some people think that exercise is a good way to lose weight. The truth is that exercise is helpful but is rarely sufficient. The human body is a very efficient machine. The table attached shows the calories spent in various physical activities for about 30 minutes by an average adult.[2] If you are slim, you burn fewer calories. If you are overweight, you burn more calories. If you are very muscular you burn more calories because muscle cells use more energy than fat cells. You can see that even if you spend a whole hour running you will have used only a small amount of calories. Thus, exercise alone will not help you to lose or maintain weight: You must still control your food intake. However, exercise, properly done, will help you in at least two ways:

- It will improve your overall body function and tone, including the blood circulation.
- You will be able to eat more food and therefore obtain all the nutrients you need without gaining weight. In particular, you can store more essential fats and burn more saturated fat.

Reduce stress

Easier said than done! But you should try. Sometimes we worry about unimportant things. Sometimes we fight for things we do not really need. Most Americans have comfortable lives: There is no need to make our lives miserable by driving aggressively on the streets, or pushing people around. Relax, and enjoy what you have rather than worry about what you could have.

Many health organizations and libraries have brochures to help you deal with stress. The key issue is to be in control: Think positively and find solutions to your problems. Think less of the problem and more of what you can do to prevent, avoid or resolve it. Many problems are really not that important. Look at it this way: How will a particular problem affect your life 20 years from now? If it will not, then there is little to worry about it. Slowly change your lifestyle to reduce those situations that are stressful to you.

Treat your medical problems early, before they become a disaster

Treat medical problems

Medical problems that have developed over the years cannot be ignored while you are changing your lifestyle. A better diet will slowly decrease high blood pressure and improve diabetes, making the body better able to handle blood sugar (**improved glucose regulation**). In the meantime you should follow your physician's advice on what drugs to take, if any, to control your disease.

Eat a balanced diet

The next chapters include our Modern Prevention and Treatment Diet, and the newly revised diets by the Federal Government and Public Health Organizations. Regardless of what diet you follow, I suggest that you substitute vegetables, tofu, and egg whites for most animal foods. If you like dairy products, eat those with very low fat and keep their proportion of your total intake of calories low.

Eat natural (uncooked) foods grown in season

Eat natural foods with less added salt

It is important to eat most of your vegetables and fruits in their natural form, that is raw. Nutritional deficiencies are in part caused by an over consumption of processed foods. Cooking alters the chemical

Basic Prevention Program

composition of the food and may destroy some of the vitamins and essential fats. Processed foods are usually low in essential fats. Many processed foods contain partially hydrogenated oil, which contains very few ω3 fatty acids and many *trans* fatty acids (**TFAs**) and other types of unusual fatty acids called "*isomers*" (which technically means a variation of the usual type of chemical molecule). Hydrogenated vegetable oil is a prime example of an originally healthful food that, through processing, has become unhealthy. Hydrogenated oil can even lead to dietary deficiencies. For these reasons, we need to eat oils to compensate for the essential fats that either have been removed or have been chemically changed due to food processing.

Work with nature, not against it in your fight against disease

Eat foods in season grown locally

You should also try to eat food in season, grown in an area with a temperature similar to your area, that is food that grows without artificial conditions in your region. This means eating fewer tropical fruits during the winter --- if you live a in a cold area. We make this recommendation because it has been found that the ambient temperature influences the chemical structure of foods. Foods from cold areas contain essential fats that help people who live in cold areas. Other protective ingredients in foods grown under the same environmental conditions as the people who eat them may include an optimal mixture of vitamins and minerals, optimized for a particular season of the year. Our body needs vary according to the season and ideally we should eat accordingly by eating foods in season. However, in practice this is rarely possible. Still, one should eat more essential fats in the winter than in the summer.

Change your fat:

- Eat less animal fat, less hydrogenated oil, and less tropical oil.

- Eat more vegetables, particularly leafy vegetables. Leaves contain membranes high in essential fats.

- Eat some vegetable oils with a balanced mixture of ω3 and ω6 fatty acids.

Basic Prevention Program

- Eat some oil extracts from fish (ω3) and plants (ω6s) if you have one of the conditions described in later chapters which require that you take EFA derivatives.

- Eat fish oils (high in ω3s) if you need to make your blood more fluid and less likely to form clots, and eat more linolenic acid (ω3), for better long term regulation of blood coagulation.

- Moderately increase your intake of antioxidants (such as vitamins E and C and selenium) if you eat more essential fats.

These issues are discussed in more detail in the following chapters. You should know the mixture of different types of fatty acids in your blood and have them measured periodically to monitor the effects of changes in their diet. Notice that most fruits contain practically no fat and no protein; they are almost pure carbohydrates. Fruits do contain minerals, vitamins, fiber and many other nutrients. However, from the perspective of EFAs, eating more fruit is like eating more SFAs (all excessive calories from fruit are converted by the body to saturated fat). If you are slim, you can eat many fruits as part of a balanced diet. If you need to lose weight, you should reduce your intake of calories from carbohydrates, including fruits.

> ***Eat more natural carbohydrates rather than simple or complex carbohydrates***

Simple vs. Complex Carbohydrates

Practically every nutrition book and article on diets tells you to eat more complex carbohydrates and fewer simple carbohydrates. These authors advocate eating more breads, pasta and cereals and eating less sugar. This is also part of the recent "pyramid" of food choices recommended by the US Department of Agriculture (**USDA**). I believe that these recommendations are misleading and incorrectly represent the research findings. What research has found is that eating natural foods which contain complex carbohydrates together with vitamins, minerals, fiber and essential fats is better than eating processed simple carbohydrates like sugar. However, research has not shown that it is healthy to eat processed complex carbohydrates such as those found in flour (even whole wheat organic flour), breads, pasta and most supermarkets cereals. Quite the contrary, I believe that complex

Basic Prevention Program

Ten ways to improve your chances of dying sooner

- **1. Smoke**. The more the better.

- **2. Gain weight**. The more the better.

- **3.** Eat an **unbalanced diet**.

- **4. Avoid natural foods** and vegetables, eat mostly processed artificial foods.

- **5. Eat/ take excessive extracts from unusual sources**. Take large doses of supplements without knowing whether you have a deficiency or an excess of a specific nutrient or consulting with a specialist. Eat huge amounts of vitamins and minerals and force your body to deal with these abnormal quantities.

- **6. Take unnecessary risks with your life**. Consider yourself immortal and unlikely to get ill. **Do not exercise. Drink and be merry.**

- **7. Eat mostly saturated fatty acids, and lots of calories**.

- **8. Eat little EFAs.**

- **9.** Eat **unbalanced mixtures of EFAs: ω3 and ω6.**

- **10. Guess your abnormalities and try to correct them blindly**. Correct your biochemical abnormalities by guessing what they are rather than by doing the proper tests, because you know your body best, and know how to improve human design, and your mind is the most powerful computer ever invented. You know what your body needs because you have a built in gauge to test for specific deficiencies and you know better than nature how to improve what nature designed for humans.

processed carbohydrates are quite similar to simple sugars because the body digests them very quickly. In fact, I expect that over the next few years diabetes organizations, which have promoted for many years the distinction between simple and complex carbohydrates, will reverse themselves and state that eating sugar is not much worse than eating bread or pasta without fat (fat slows the digestion of carbohydrate).

Basic Prevention Program

Healthy foods are natural foods in their natural state. Complex processed carbohydrates with depleted minerals, vitamins, fiber and essential fat are probably not that much better than sugar. If you like them, eat them but with restraint. Whenever possible, substitute them for natural foods as found in their natural state (rather than as extracts from natural foods).

Other behaviors to consider

What do doctors consider as important **health hints**? In a survey of more than 1,000 physicians [3] they indicated several behaviors (in addition to those listed above) as a way to promote good health:

Wear protective clothing when exposed to harmful substances; use seat belts; limit consumption of caffeine; get enough sleep; know the medicines you take; avoid unnecessary X-rays; and drink alcohol only in moderation, if at all.

> ### Eat less animal fat and fewer calories

References and notes

[1] Keys AB. Seven countries: a multivariate analysis of death and coronary heart disease. Cambridge, Mass: Harvard Univ. Press, 1980.

[2] Remember that these are very rough estimates. The more active you, are the more calories you use. If you barely move, you barely burn calories.

[3.] Reported in the December 1985 issue of the *American Journal of Public Health*.

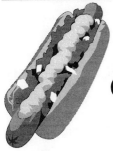
III.5

CURRENT AMERICAN DIET

"To eat or not to eat is not the question. The question is what to eat"

Topics: *Typical American Diet. What is wrong with it. Where do you stand. How to improve your meals. Eat more natural foods, omega-3 and omega-6 essential fats, complex carbohydrates and fiber.*

Summary

The typical American diet is very high in saturated fat and processed carbohydrates and low in ω3 and ω6 EFAs, complex natural carbohydrates and fiber. Americans obtain most of their calories from processed and cooked foods instead of natural unprocessed food, and eat large quantities of sugar and related syrups (used to sweeten processed foods). You find saturated fat derived from lard and partially hydrogenated fats in pastries, cookies, pizza, bread and many other processed foods. These fats contain many *trans* fatty acids which interfere with the EFAs. Keep a daily record of all the food you eat. You will use this record to identify foods that should be replaced.

Typical American Diet

The average American eats a diet rich in calories, saturated fat and simple carbohydrates.[1] The amount of individual nutrients as a percent of total calories is: protein (13%-15%), carbohydrate (40%-50%), fat (35%-45%), cholesterol (450-600 mg/day). More than half of all carbohydrates comes from sugar and simple starches. Less than 5% of total fat is polyunsaturated fat from EFAs. Most Americans eat very little ω6 and almost no ω3 fats. Moreover, many individuals drink large quantities of alcohol and eat far too many calories, leading to overweight. See tables in the appendix for further description.

What is wrong with our usual diet

Nutritionists agree that Americans eat too much fat and too many calories. The people of many European and Oriental countries have a significantly smaller incidence of heart disease and overall mortality. This is most likely due to meals which have:

- Less food, thus a smaller total caloric intake.
- Far less saturated fat and cholesterol.
- More vegetables and complex natural carbohydrates. [1]
- A much higher proportion of essential fats in their diet.

Too much saturated fat and processed foods.

Most Americans eat animal products and processed foods high in fat. Processed foods contain large amounts of saturated or hydrogenated fat. These fats replace the EFAs naturally present in the original substance with "artificial" (mostly human-made) fats which may lead to heart disease and cancer.

Fried foods contain fats called isomers and *trans* which have been altered by the intense heat and may lead to heart disease or cancer. Many companies advertise the use of vegetable shortening and low cholesterol in their products. Some people are misled into thinking that because shortening is a vegetable, it is healthy. Unfortunately, most vegetable shortening is high in saturated fat and other chemical derivatives of natural oils which research has shown to be harmful. Chemically produced shortening may be more harmful than natural butter.

> **The American Diet: Too many calories, too much fat. Not enough vegetables and EFAs.**

Other "hidden" sources of saturated fat are dairy products and cheese. Many patients proudly tell me that they rarely eat red meat but eat cheese and high fat dairy products. Even if dairy foods are low in cholesterol, they are high in saturated fat. And remember: The major "culprit" in heart disease is excessive fat and calories, not cholesterol. Actually, the major culprit is excessive calories, but most people who

Current American Diet

eat too many calories do so by eating too many fats. However, quite a few people manage to eat huge amounts of calories from low fat foods such as breads and pasta.

Furthermore, a diet high in processed foods supplies calories derived from nutritionally imbalanced ingredients, that is to say, from ingredients that do not furnish us with a balanced mixture of vitamins and minerals.

Where do you stand

Most qualified nutritionists can analyze the foods you eat and tell you how to improve your meals. You can keep a diary and find out what you really eat each week. Be honest and be ready for a big surprise. You can analyze the food yourself by recording how much you eat and the amount of protein, carbohydrate, fat and calories usually indicated in the labels or found in many books.

How to make it better

Nutrition authors agree that people should eat less processed food, including simple carbohydrates, and eat more vegetables, grains and fruits. In the last decade many Americans have been eating less saturated fat and more EFAs from vegetable oils. The results have been a decline in cardiovascular deaths and lower cholesterol. The decline in cholesterol has been greater in whites than in blacks, and it is usually highest among the better educated.[2]

Change towards a vegetarian diet

Eating more of your calories from natural vegetables and fewer from processed foods and animal fat will help you in several ways. This dietary program will naturally reduce your caloric intake (and help you to lose weight), increase your intake of key nutrients including vitamins, minerals, and EFAs. You can continue to eat animal meat or fish, but you should reduce the size of your servings and the amount of fat in them. In particular, beware of animal products like cream and cheese that are very high in animal fat.[3]

Natural complex carbohydrates contain EFAs

Vegetables and some seeds are excellent sources of EFAs, a fact often overlooked. The membranes of cells, found in vegetables, are rich in

Current American Diet

Complete Vegetarian vs. Typical American Diet

Characteristic	Vegetarian	American
Type of food	Mostly natural	Mostly processed
Chewing	Slowly	Fast
Eating Time	Long	Short
Concentrated Calories	No	Yes
Total Calories	Few	Many
Carbohydrates	Complex	Simple
Sweets	Rare	Common
Protein	Adequate	High
EFAs	Adequate	Deficient
Saturated Fat	Rare	Common
Hydrogenated Fat	Rare	Common
Vitamins + Minerals	Many	Few
Other nutrients	Plenty	Often deleted

lecithin and other phospholipids high in EFAs. Seeds, such as pumpkin, flax, safflower and various nuts are high in EFAs. Therefore, eating more natural carbohydrates increases the amount of essential fats in the diet. Of course, most processed carbohydrates, like many refined products, contain no EFAs. The original EFAs are either removed by processing, or are hydrogenated.

What you can do: hints to eat better

Thousands of Americans are already changing their diets. These hints may help you:

- **Prepare your own meals**: Processed meals are more expensive and less healthy. Simple meals are easy to prepare and do not take more time than prepared meals such as frozen foods. You can start by taking your own lunch to work or school.

Current American Diet

- **Use a timer to eat slowly**: Eat for a few minutes; rest; eat again, rest, and so on.

- **Chew more times**: Chewing helps your digestion and decreases your appetite. Do not put more food in your mouth until you have finished swallowing.

- **Eat with silverware**: Using a fork, knife or spoon stops you from eating unhealthy snacks with your fingers.

- **Make eating a formal time**: Eating at a table will reduce eating between meals, while watching TV, etc.

- **Do not eat all the available food**: Get up and leave when you are no longer hungry. In fact, being a bit hungry is just right. Store leftover food.

- **Pay yourself for eating well**: Give yourself money each time you eat well and remain hungry, and take it away when you "cheat". Once a month buy a gift (not junk food) to reward your good behavior.

Easy rules

The following **five tongue-in-cheek rules** help people to focus on better foods and eating habits.

- 1. **If it is not green, yellow or red, it is probably not good for you** (emphasize green vegetables).

- 2. **If you are not hungry, you are eating too much.** After a meal it takes time for the body to feel satiated or full; if you do not feel hungry is because you ate too much.

- 3. **If you are very hungry, wait; exercise instead.** Eating while very hungry leads to eating bad foods.

- 4. **Fat and calories leads to fat.** If you eat a lot of fat and calories, you'll get a lot of fat, where you do not want it.

- 5. **Eat not for pleasure but for need.** If you make a habit of eating just because it tastes and feels good, or you are depressed, you transform food into a habit rather than a need.

Current American Diet

Easily lose 25 pounds and 50 units of cholesterol

You can easily lose two pounds per week and make your cholesterol decline more than 20% in six months. Follow our proposed diets with only modest deviations. Strict following could help you lose over 25 lbs. in two months, reduce your cholesterol by over 50 points and drastically lower your chances of a heart attack, particularly if you correct your imbalance of EFAs.

References and notes

1 Schaefer EJ, Rees DG, Siguel, EN. Nutrition, Lipoproteins, and Atherosclerosis. *Clinical Nutrition*, Vol. 5, No 3, pages 99-111, May/June 1986. Siguel EN, Schaefer EJ. Aging and Nutritional Requirements of Essential Fatty Acids. In: Beare J, ed. Dietary Fats, Champaign, Il. American Oil Chemists Society, Chapter 13. (1989).

2 Trends in Serum Cholesterol Levels among US Adults aged 20 to 74 years. National Center for Health Statistics, *J American Medical Assoc.*, Vol. 257, pages 937-942, Feb. 20, 1987.

3 Not all vegetarians eat a healthy diet. Some vegetarians eat too many high fat dairy products, some with *trans* fatty acids. Some eat too many processed carbohydrates and not enough vegetables in their natural state.

Table

Mean Daily Intake[a] of Food Energy, Nutrients, and Food Components for Men, Women, and Young Children from the Continuing Survey of Food Intakes by Individuals (CSFII), 1985[b]*

	Men	Women	Children
Total Food Energy (% REI)[c]	(94)	(82)	(100)
Fat [% total energy]			
Total fat	[36]	[37]	[34]
Saturated fatty acids	[13]	[13]	[14]
Monounsaturated fatty acids	[14]	[14]	[12]
Polyunsaturated fatty acids	[7]	[7]	[6]
Cholesterol mg	435	304	254
Protein			
[% total energy]	[16]	[16]	[16]
(% RDA)[d]	(175)	(144)	(222)
Carbohydrates [% total energy]	[45]	[46]	[52]
Dietary Fiber g	18	12	10
Vitamins (% RDA)			
Vitamin A	(122)	(127)	(215)
Vitamin E	(98)	(97)	(108)
Vitamin C	(182)	(133)	(186)
Thiamin	(124)	(110)	(153)
Riboflavin	(129)	(115)	(197)
Niacin	(146)	(130)	(151)
Vitamin B_6	(85)	(61)	(127)
Vitamin B_{12}	(245)	(156)	(192)
Folacin	(76)[f]	(51)[f]	(157)[f]
Minerals (% RDA)			
Calcium	(115)	(78)	(105)
Phosphorus	(192)	(126)	(132)
Iron	(159)	(61)[f]	(88)[f]
Zinc	(94)[f]	(60)	(84)
Magnesium	(94)	(72)	(121)
Minerals (ESADDI)[e]			
Sodium	(exceeds)	(within)	(exceeds)
Potassium	(within)	(within)	(1-3 years exceeds) (4-5 years within)
Copper	(below)	(below)	(below)

* The Surgeon General's Report on Nutrition and Health. U.S. Department of Health and Human Services. Public Health Service USDHHS (PHS)Publication No. 88-50210, 1988.[410]

[a] Estimated mean daily intake is expressed in several ways: amount of intake, percent of total energy intake, percent of 1980 Recommended Dietary Allowance, or comparison with Estimated Safe and Adequate Daily Dietary Intake.

[b] Data based on 1-day dietary recalls obtained by personal interview for 658 men 19 to 50 years of age, for 1,459 women 19 to 50 years of age, and for 489 of their children 1 to 5 years of age in 1985 (unweighted numbers). Nutrient intakes do not include vitamin and mineral supplements or sodium from salt added at the table.

[c] Recommended Energy Intake;[411] Source of percentages: NFCS, CSFII Report Nos. 85-1 and 85-3.[14,15]

[d] Recommended Dietary Allowance;[411] Source of percentages: NFCS, CSFII Report Nos. 85-1 and 85-3.[14,15]

[e] Estimated Safe and Adequate Daily Dietary Intake.[411]

[f] Figures given are based upon 1980 RDA's; the 1989 RDA's for these nutrients are substantially lower.

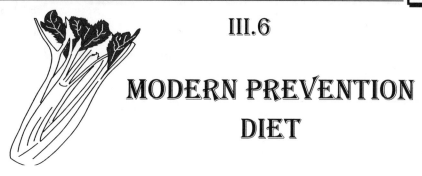

III.6

MODERN PREVENTION DIET

"Hard fat is out; vegetables and essential fats are in"

Topics: *The basic food groups.* **Plants**: *Vegetables, Grains, Fruits, Seeds.* **Animals**: *Fish, Cattle, Poultry, Pork, Dairy. Vegetarian diets. Nutritional supplements. Achieve ideal weight and remain slender. Eat less cholesterol and saturated fat. Eat more Essential Fats.*

Summary

To prevent disease you must eat a diet with a good balance of ω3 and ω6 fats (and, of course, minerals, vitamins and fiber). Strive to achieve ideal weight and remain slender. A *balanced* vegetable diet will provide all the proper nutrients. If your diet is deficient, you need to compensate for missing vitamins and minerals by taking supplements. Although most people are aware of the need for vitamins, very few people know that they may be deficient in essential fats. After all, with most of the US population overweight, who can conceive of deliberately consuming more fat? Yet, many victims and potential victims of cardiovascular disease have deficiencies or imbalances of ω3 and ω6 fatty acids. Ironically, we consume diets so high in saturated fat as to produce disease yet we have deficiencies of the nutritionally essential fats.

The basic meal

To prevent cardiovascular disease you must follow a diet high in vegetables (particularly green vegetables), grains and seeds and low in all animal fat (i.e., dairy, red meat, and poultry). The exception is cold water fish which contains ω3 derivatives. If you are an adult, your meals may need to be supplemented with one or more tablespoons per day of a mixture of uncooked oils, until you correct your deficiency. The oils compensate for years of eating foods high in saturated fats and calories, and also will compensate for occasional meals high in saturated fat (cookies, pizza, beer, etc.).

To treat cardiovascular disease: Follow the same diet but supplement it with fish oils and more vegetable oils. This diet is addressed specifically in later chapters.

Guidelines to plan your meals:

- **1. Eat to achieve ideal weight.** If you are gaining weight, you are eating too much (unless you want to gain weight). Eat more food or less food to achieve and maintain your ideal weight. Counting calories can help, but scales and waist measurement are simpler and better indicators of your status. You can cheat with calories but you cannot cheat the scale.

- **2. Eat proportionately less fat.** Among equal weights of fat, carbohydrate and protein, fat has approximately twice as many calories as protein or carbohydrates. Thus, you can eat twice as much low fat food as high fat food. To gain weight eat more fat; to lose weight eat less fat. Beware of fat hidden inside foods.

- **3. Eat two to four ounces of protein per day.** It helps to vary the amount of protein you eat each day.[1] Limiting animal food to less than three ounces per day (average) automatically reduces protein intake.

- **4. Eat a variety of different foods.** Eat at least twenty different foods each week, and more than 10 on a given day. Eat foods of different colors from all healthy categories. Do not worry about keeping track of vitamins and minerals.[2] If you eat many different types of natural foods, your body keeps what you need and discards the excess. This does not apply to fats: The body does not discard excessive fats, it stores them.[3]

- **5. Eat more essential fats and less saturated fat.** Eat more vegetables and fewer animal foods.

- **6. Eat uncooked food in season.** Cook food as little as possible, and choose foods grown in season according to your local area. In this manner your body gets the nutrients that

Modern Prevention Diet

are needed in your particularly area. Depending on temperature and humidity, we may need more of some nutrients and less of others. However, note that some foods are dangerous when eaten raw because they may contain bacteria. Meat cut into small pieces is most vulnerable to bacteria. Thus, you must cook some foods, especially animal foods, to kill infectious organisms.

- **7. Exercise to lose or maintain weight.** Exercise allows you to eat more food and get more nutrients without gaining weight and burns the hard, saturated fat in your body.

Comparison of recommendations

Most health organizations agree on the following recommendations:

- Less than 30% of all calories should come from fat.

- People should eat 10% of total calories (or 1/3 of calories from fat) as SFA, 10% as MUFA and 10% as PUFA. In other words, most health organizations recommend that you eat approximately equal proportions of each type of fat, with the calories from fat not to exceed 1/3 of your total calories. For example, if you eat 2,000 calories per day, you should eat less than 600 calories as fat, with 200 as SFA, 200 as MUFA and 200 as PUFA. If you can, eating even less SFA per day is recommended.

- Total daily cholesterol should be below 300 mg.

- People should eat about 25 to 30 grams of fiber daily.

- Every day people should eat foods rich in carotene, vitamins and minerals, such as cruciferous vegetables and fruits.[4]

Many public health groups now recommend that people eat more calories from MUFA and eat more carbohydrates instead of fat. In the way that most public health recommendations are written, people are allowed to replace their calories from fat with calories from carbohydrates. Because the emphasis is on avoiding SFA rather than eating fewer calories, many people replace their fat with carbohydrates, but eat so many carbohydrates than their total caloric intake increases. Because excess calories are converted to SFAs, their bodies still make too many SFAs.

My recommendations are different. I agree that people should eat more natural foods, and avoid processed foods rich in fat. I also agree that people should eat less food high in animal fat. However, *my research indicates that the two most important factors in a healthy diet are total calories and calories from essential fats*. As long as a person is slim and eats a balanced diet which consists of many different natural foods, he/she does not need to be too concerned about keeping track of total fat or saturated fat or cholesterol. Most natural foods do not contain too much cholesterol. The key is to maintain ideal weight. If a person gains weight, he/she is eating too much. It does not matter where the calories come from. Saturated fat, monounsaturated fat, carbohydrates, and protein contribute calories which, in excess, will be converted to the same thing in the body: saturated fat. It is easier to maintain ideal weight if one avoids foods high in fat and eats more natural foods high in carbohydrates and fiber.

In addition, a person should eat a minimum amount of essential fats every day. This minimum amount depends on the size of the body, that is, how many cells the body has. This minimum amount increases when one has to compensate for many years of bad eating (especially eating foods low in essential fats), or one has a disease that requires supplements of essential fats.

> **If you are slim and otherwise eating a healthy diet, a pizza is often as healthy as bread or pasta. It depends on the amounts of EFAs and TFAs rather than SFAs in the food, which vary from one brand to another.**

The basic food groups

The table in this chapter presents the foods that help you to prevent and treat cardiovascular disease. We have included some excellent foods in the category of "neutral" foods. These foods have relatively little effect on heart disease, but are needed for a balanced diet. The sections which describe the specific foods for which intake should increase, or decrease, are the critical ones. These are the areas of a person's diet that require immediate modification.

Vegetables, Grains, Fruits, Seeds, nuts

Eat mostly green vegetables and raw vegetables. It is possible to eat only uncooked foods, but it takes considerable effort.[5] Most seeds and sprouts are also an excellent source of nutrients and essential fats.[6]

Modern Prevention Diet

Fish, Poultry, Pork, Cattle, Dairy

Cold water fish is the preferred animal food. Unfortunately, many fish are full of pesticides and other pollutants. Moreover, soon we will kill most of the fish in the oceans because of overfishing.[7] You can eat uncontaminated cold water fish almost every day (if you can find it). On the other hand, poultry, pork and beef should be eaten in small portions for a total of less than one pound per week. Your total intake of animal meat should be under 3 ounces per day. Dairy products, particularly those from skimmed milk, are permissible every day, as long as the total fat content is under 2 grams/day. Of course, these are average values; you can eat a little bit more or less each day.

What can you do

The best diet --- for most healthy people --- consists of balanced vegetarian meals with *occasional small amounts of meat and fish*. When you eat animal products, select them in this order: *fish preferred to poultry preferred to pork preferred to beef*.[8] Select low fat animal products over those which are high in fat. These recommendations regarding meat are subject to change because the meat industry is changing the way it raises animals. Future beef may be higher in polyunsaturated fat because of dietary changes. Also some chickens are now fed ω3 fatty acids. Soon we may have chicken that smell like fish and has fat similar to fish fat. This, of course, follows the trend of tomatoes that look or taste like potatoes, and so on. The difference is that this is not change due to genetic engineering but to diet. When this happens, beware that animals fed EFA rich foods, particularly ω3 foods (like flax seeds) have fat that deteriorates quickly, and consequently needs better refrigeration and cooking at lower temperatures. And do not forget to have your hammer ready to kill the bacteria left alive by low temperature cooking! As you can see, tampering with nature provides no simple solutions.

Plan your meals using foods, not nutrients

Many educated people attempt to plan their diet to ensure that they get enough of each type of nutrient: protein, carbohydrate, fat, vitamins, minerals and fiber. This is the idea reinforced by consumer groups and the Food and Drug Administration that requires food labeling. Apparently, these organizations believe that humans carry portable computers with them to keep track of food composition, and then

Modern Prevention Diet

Examples of Nutrients vs. Foods

Nutrients	Foods
Fat (ω3)	Salmon
Fat (ω6)	Corn oil
Fat (Saturated)	Butter
Protein	Tofu, egg white
Carbohydrate	Potato, oats
Vitamins (i.e., C)	Orange
Minerals (Copper, Zinc, etc.)	Molasses
Fiber	Green beans
Water	Water

update their data every time they eat anything.[9] To me this approach is a huge waste of government and corporate money.

Keeping track every day of every food you eat is far too complicated. Even with the aid of a computer and extensive tables, food analysis by nutrient is not exact and is only useful in research or as a very rough guide to identify nutritional deficiencies. Furthermore, every year we discover new substances in natural foods that are found to be useful to maintain good health. There are thousands of such chemicals in natural foods and they could never be listed on food labels. It is for this reason that I do not believe food labels are very useful. They will never be able to describe all chemical constituents of every food. The most useful information, the amount of calories from different types of essential fats vs. total calories, or TFAs, or the amount of toxic contaminants like pesticides, is not listed. Food labels should indicate only the natural foods used and any additives incorporated, including the amount of toxic pesticides.

A better way to plan meals is by type of food. Even though you need nutrients, you buy foods. Hence it is easier to plan your meals around foods rather than nutrients. Because we know relatively little about the biochemical structure of foods, and the optimal combination of foods is not known, I believe that it is best to eat a variety of foods. Eating well naturally provides the proper mixture of vitamins and minerals.

Excess calories are converted to saturated fat

All the excess protein and carbohydrate you eat eventually becomes saturated fat. *Fat is the most efficient way to store energy in the body.*

Modern Prevention Diet

One gram of fat stores more than twice as many calories as one gram of protein or carbohydrate. *Saturated fat is the most efficient way to store fat in the body.* Saturated fatty acids (**SFAs**) are straight molecules that form very tight, packed, substances. Monounsaturated (MUFAs) and polyunsaturated (PUFAs) fatty acids are twisted and take more space to store. Thus, the body can pack more energy per unit of volume using SFAs than MUFAs or PUFAs. Because animal bodies are efficiently designed, they use the least amount of space to store the extra fat. Whenever it is necessary, the body converts SFAs to MUFAs. Now, remember that we are talking here about storage of extra fat in adipose tissue. We are not talking about the fat that is in other organ systems like the brain or breast.

Complex natural carbohydrates are a good replacement for saturated fat because you can eat more food quantity while actually eating fewer calories. Moreover, foods high in complex carbohydrates contain more fiber (no calories), water, vitamins, minerals and essential fats. But replacement of saturated fat with simple carbohydrates like sugar, refined flour, grains and syrup does not improve your nutritional status. Eating large quantities of carbohydrates is as bad as eating saturated fat.[10] Unfortunately, this conversion of calories to fat and their storage as saturated fat is a well known biochemical fact often overlooked by nutritionists.

If you were to replace all the foods you eat that contain fat, such as beef or pizza, with processed carbohydrate foods (and assuming that you neither lose nor gain weight), you would not be better off. The reason for this is that beef and many pizzas contain some essential fats, while pure carbohydrates do not contain any. Thus, many foods containing processed oats or cereals, and hydrogenated, coconut, or palm oil plus sweeteners are probably more dangerous than beef or pizza.

Technical explanation for the role of MUFAs

The body is very efficient. The amount of monounsaturated fatty acids (**MUFAs**) that the body makes is primarily dependent on the amount of PUFAs in the body. Maintenance of the "fluidity" of cell membranes is very important to the body. My research has shown that humans closely regulate the production of MUFAs to maintain plasma levels inversely proportional to polyunsaturated fatty acid levels. In other words, when PUFA levels go down, MUFA levels go up. MUFAs are made by the body from SFAs. The opposite is not true: the body cannot make PUFA from MUFA or SFA; you must eat them. This mechanism likely evolved as a way to maintain membrane fluidity.[11] My research indicates that the body can make as much MUFA as it needs. Eating more MUFAs will not prevent heart disease but could cause it!.

Remember that a MUFA has one kink while a SFA has none. Thus, a MUFA can make cell membranes softer (more fluid) than a SFA. A MUFA is closer to a PUFA than a SFA in terms of how soft or fluid it makes the membranes of a cell. Because humans cannot make PUFA, when faced with too much saturated fat and the possibility that the cell membranes will become hard, the body makes more MUFAs and more cholesterol. Cholesterol is inserted between molecules of SFAs in cell membranes; moving SFAs further apart makes cell membranes more fluid. This is one reason why excess saturated fat in the body turns on the mechanisms for making cholesterol.

Many researchers have studied Mediterranean countries where people have a lower incidence of heart disease. It appears that they eat more MUFAs. For that reason, some researchers think that MUFAs protect against heart disease. I believe that such research is misleading because it relies on dietary intake data, which is highly inaccurate. Most researchers have failed to study the fatty acid composition of the blood and adipose tissue in the manner I have reported in my published research. When this is done, I predict that we will find that individuals who have less incidence of heart disease eat more essential fats.

Eat less cholesterol and fewer calories

Cholesterol is a special type of fat found primarily in animal foods. It is important because it helps to form membranes and hormones that the body needs. However, humans do not need to eat cholesterol. Our body can fabricate it from other foods we eat. Vegetables have very little cholesterol. Like most scientists, I recommend that you eat less than 300 mg per day of cholesterol, if any. This is done easily by reducing your intake of animal fat. Animal fat is high in SFAs and cholesterol, both of which lead to increased body cholesterol. To reduce dietary intake of cholesterol below 300 mg, you must consume less animal fat: less meat, fewer dairy products, fewer egg yolks.

Eating less cholesterol is NOT the only modification of your fat intake that is necessary in order to reduce the risk of cardiovascular disease. In fact, eating less cholesterol is not critical if you eat plenty of polyunsaturated fat. The answer is not to eat NO fat; it is to eat the right kinds of fat.

Modern Prevention Diet

Beware of many commercial products which use modified vegetable fat and then advertise themselves as low in cholesterol. Often, they use a type of processed vegetable fat called hydrogenated oil, which is high in saturated fats and low in essential fats, and quite often high in the undesirable *trans* fatty acids. Thus, the food itself may be low in cholesterol, but it still has the opposite impact in your body, namely it increases your blood cholesterol.

> *Eat less animal fat except for cold water fish. Eat more vegetables especially green vegetables.*

High fat dairy products are another source of saturated fat. Skim milk (lower in fat than low fat milk) and cheese made with skim milk are good substitutes for those who like dairy products. Other alternatives are soy products, which contain EFAs.

Eat more Essential Fats

You remember that there are three main types of fat: saturated, monounsaturated and polyunsaturated fat. We refer to the polyunsaturated fatty acids (**PUFA**) as the **essential fats** because humans need them to survive. The essential fats consist of the essential fatty acids (**EFAs**) and fatty acids derived from them, either made by the body or found in nature. PUFA is a term which includes two different types of fat: ω3 and ω6 fats, both of which are essential to the body. As a general rule, humans only need to eat the EFAs. From the EFAs, human bodies can make the EFA derivatives. However, it is healthy to eat some EFA derivatives such as those found in fish.

The rule of thumb for a healthy heart states that eating saturated fat or too many calories leads to hardening of the arteries while polyunsaturated, essential, fat softens the arteries and reduces high blood pressure. To plan an adequate diet you must mix foods that contain both ω3s and ω6s. For instance, animal fat is rich in derivatives of linoleic acid or ω6 fats while fish is rich in derivatives of linolenic acid or ω3 fats. Vegetables and vegetable oils contain both linoleic and linolenic acid (the EFAs), but not their derivatives. Safflower, sunflower and corn oil contain linoleic but have little linolenic acid. Soybean and walnut oils are rich in linoleic (ω6) <u>and</u> linolenic (ω3) acids.

Modern Prevention Diet

In general, people who have been eating healthy meals most of their lives should continue to eat natural foods. However, those who have been eating too much saturated fat and not enough essential fats will most likely need to eat oil supplements to compensate for years of neglect. The essential fats can be obtained from several sources: vegetables, nuts, seeds and some and animal products. Fruits contain practically zero fat.

Recommended Daily Allowances are not established for EFAs.

For many years, nutrition and medical textbooks have stated that humans need about 1-2% of their calories as $\omega6$ (linoleic) essential fatty acids. No requirement for $\omega3$ has been established. Most researchers have proposed that 2% of calories be linoleic and 0.5%-1% be linolenic acid. However, my data on healthy humans suggest that at least 5%-10% of calories should be PUFA, with $\omega6/\omega3$ ratios between 10:1 to 2:1 (see below). Public health groups recommend that no more than 30% of calories per day be fat, with approximately equal proportions of saturated (**SFA**), monounsaturated (**MUFA**), and polyunsaturated (**PUFA**) fat. That is, 10% of calories should be SFA, 10% MUFA and 10% PUFA. These numbers are based on a 2,000 calories/day diet. However, these recommendations are misleading. As interpreted by most people, the same percentages would apply to diets with any number of calories. This is incorrect. The amount of essential fats (PUFA) that a person needs depends on the number of cells in the body, disease status and metabolism, but is only marginally related to the amount of calories that a person eats. Thus, the percent of calories as PUFAs is not the same for diets with different calories. For example, a woman who eats 1,500 calories per day requires the same amount (in grams or ounces) of PUFA as an "identical" woman who exercises more and eats 2,500 calories per day.

To avoid this confusion, which has resulted in advocacy of EFA deficient diets, I recommend that dietary requirements for PUFA be specified in absolute terms: as grams of PUFA per kilogram of body weight per day.

Requirements for essential fats

Due to frequent eating of processed foods low in EFAs (such as cereals, breads, pasta, TFAs and animal fat, most individuals have a dietary

Precursor (parent) or EFAs

Fat	Foods	Examples
ω3 Linolenic	Vegetables	Green beans, sprouts; Soybeans
	Oils	Soybean, Walnut, Flax
	Seeds & nuts	Flax seeds, walnuts
ω6 Linoleic	Vegetables	Leafy greens, corn
	Oils	Corn, Soybean, Olive; Safflower, Sunflower
	Seeds & nuts	Safflower, sesame, pumpkin seeds. Walnuts.

history of reduced intake of ω6 and ω3. Because excess calories are stored by the body as SFA or MUFA, *the factors most relevant for preventive medicine are total EFAs and total calories.*

My research, based on the body composition of people, indicates that people eating 2000 calories per day should eat 6% to 8% of their calories as ω6 and 2% to 4% as ω3 fatty acids. Total PUFA (essential fats) should be around 200 calories or 10% of calories for a 2,000 calorie diet. The 200 calories amount to about 22 grams of PUFA per day. For an average 150 pound man it means 20 to 25 grams/day.

The above recommendations are consistent with the recommendations of most public health organizations, that is, on a 2000 calorie/day diet,

Derivatives (daughter) of EFAs

Fat	Foods	Examples
ω3 EPA, DHA	Oils	Fish oil, cod liver
	Fish	Cold water fish
	Extracts	Fish oil extracts sold in capsules.
ω6 DGLA	Animal fat	Chicken, liver (high in arachidonic)
	Oils	Primrose, borage oil. sold in capsules

Modern Prevention Diet

the average 150 pound person should eat 10% of calories from PUFA. However, these similarities are something of an artifact; I have significant differences with the way these recommendations are implemented by other health organizations. *My research has shown that people need to eat a minimum amount of essential fat every day.* Because essential fats are needed to maintain and repair body cells, the amount of EFA needed by an individual depends on how many cells that individual has. Thus, minimum daily requirements are related to body size. In addition, some medical conditions increase the need for more essential fats. Such conditions include pregnancy (where you are feeding two bodies), burns (where many cells need to be formed), gastrointestinal disease (where the intestine needs to be repaired and food is poorly absorbed), and several related conditions.

> *We recommend a minimum daily EFA requirement of 1/3 gram per Kg of body weight (about 1/6 gram per pound) for an adult, with an ω6:ω3 ratio between 10:1 and 4:1.*[12]

EFA requirements are expressed as minimum daily requirements of 1/3 gram/Kg body weight for adults (approximately). This is equivalent to 1/6 gram per pound of body weight. For a healthy 70 Kg (154 pounds) man this represents about 22 grams of PUFA per day, or slightly more than 2 tablespoons of soybean oil per day. For a healthy 110 lb. woman, this represents about 18 grams of PUFA per day. Menstruating women may need more EFAs. People eating more than 2000 calories per day should eat the same amount of essential fats (in grams), which is a *smaller percent of total calories.*

The amount of EFAs that a person needs depends primarily on the number of cell membranes in the body that need to be repaired or replaced. This depends on body weight and state of health rather than percent of calories from fats. Larger bodies have more cells, so require more EFAs. Growing bodies (i.e., children and pregnant women) need more EFAs, as do people recovering from surgery or burns. Eating a low fat diet does not by itself make your body smaller, and therefore your EFA needs do not change. On a low fat diet you ought to eat, proportionately, more EFAs. On a high fat diet, the proportion of EFAs out of the total fat should be smaller than on a low fat diet, if you exercise to burn the extra calories.

Modern Prevention Diet

Individual genetic and sex differences are also significant to EFA metabolism. Future research is likely to find a wide range of variability in the enzymes that form EFA derivatives, and those that incorporate EFAs into cells. In simple terms, some people may use EFAs more efficiently than others and therefore require a smaller amount of them. The fatty acid profile **EFA-SR** measures not only individual fatty acids, but markers of the ability of the body to use EFAs. If the test shows that your body is "stressed" and has biochemical signs of EFA deficiency, you probably need more EFAs.

Warning: Intake of PUFA above 15% of calories may be toxic for a person eating a high calorie diet (more than 2,500 calories per day), particularly without adequate amounts of antioxidants. Intake below 5% may contribute to hyperlipidemia, cardiovascular disease and other disorders. Again, in both situations, it would be useful to establish daily requirements for PUFAs according to body weight rather than percentage of calories.

How foods are rated

Traditionally, nutritionists have described the EFA content of foods using the PUFA/SFA (**P/S ratio**) without distinguishing EFA from EFA derivatives, or ω3 from ω6. According to this "wisdom," an ideal P/S ratio for a food is high, that is, its content of polyunsaturated fat is high in relation to its content of saturated fat. However, the P/S ratio is a confusing and misleading term. A high P/S ratio can be achieved by a food low in both PUFA and saturated fat, but high in monounsaturates, carbohydrate and/or protein. Even though such a food has a desirably high P/S ratio according to conventional wisdom, it is deficient in EFAs. Moreover, in the body, its effect will be similar to a food with a larger amount of saturated fat. Thus, *forget about "P/S" ratios of food*. Just look at the actual amounts of each essential fat.

How essential fats have evolved

Essential fats were discovered during the 30s in experiments performed on animals and infants. However, because most adult people are overweight (i.e., have too much fat), scientists felt that nobody lacked essential fat. Over 20 years ago, a few scientists suggested that cardiovascular disease and related diseases (diabetes, hypertension, stroke) were a consequence of eating too much saturated fat and not enough essential fats (see the Introduction). However, scientists were only able to document a deficiency of essential fat in less than 1/100,000

Modern Prevention Diet

persons, making this deficiency a very rare condition in the western population. Therefore, the link between essential fats and cardiovascular disease was placed in doubt and theories about the need for essential fats were forgotten or ignored. In 1994 my research showed that patients with heart disease have biochemical evidence of EFA insufficiency (**EFAI**) caused by insufficient levels of EFAs.

During the 80's, research confirmed that eating vegetable and fish oils (rich in essential fats) decreases cholesterol and high blood pressure. Furthermore, it was also found that lowering cholesterol and high blood pressure reduced the risk of cardiovascular disease. As a result, most nutritionists recommended that people eat fish oils. Recently, my research found that many Americans have a deficiency of essential fats because they eat relatively too much saturated fat compared to the amounts of EFAs. I named this disorder **Relative *Essential Fatty Acid Insufficiency*** (**EFAI**).[13] In relative EFA insufficiency (**REFAI**) (described in chapter I.3), people have plenty of EFAs in adipose tissue (body fat) but not enough in their blood and organs. The reason for this is that excessive saturated fat makes it difficult for EFAs to reach the cells that need them. As in a traffic jam, the police or ambulances have a difficult time going where they have to go.

Replacing saturated fat in the body with essential fats prevents and treats cardiovascular disease. Unfortunately, old ideas take a long time to die, even when they are ideas held in the face of massive scientific evidence to the contrary. Even now many respected physicians believe that nutrition has little to do with cholesterol or heart disease.[14] Whether a theory is fashionable or not also plays a role in determining how much attention it will get from researchers. For many years nutrition in general, and essential fats in particular, have not been considered important factors in heart disease. This way of thinking makes it difficult to obtain research funds. Research results, no matter how accurate and instructive, are difficult to publish. Emphasis has been placed on high technology medicine and on drugs. This remains the case. People are looking and waiting for miraculous drugs and genetic engineering to save them from their bad eating habits. People want to eat their cake, and then have it removed from their arteries by a magic pill so that they can eat more cake (and doughnuts, beer, pasta, . . . the list is endless). They hear about new drugs for strange diseases and hope that the same drugs will help them too. People hope to avoid responsibility for their physical health by blaming their genes for their body's composition, or the environment for their bad eating habits.

Modern Prevention Diet

Fortunately, or unfortunately, we still have quite a bit of control over how much we eat. We cannot blame the government or our ancestors for eating too much.

The lack of familiarity of many physicians with the role of essential fats in health and disease goes back to deficiencies in medical education. Essential fats are barely covered in the traditional curriculum that medical students follow. Most textbooks devote at most a few pages to a description of essential fatty acids. Medical education and medicine are primarily concerned with drugs and procedures. As a medical student, I took many courses and spent thousands of hours learning about drugs (most of which no longer exist), X-rays, EKGs, and other complex procedures. My medical education devoted less than 10 minutes to essential fats.

The publicity that accompanied the research in ω3 fats in the 1980s encouraged companies to sell fish oil extracts and tout the benefits of ω3 fatty acids. However, when miraculous cures did not occur immediately, people forgot about them. When current research on the benefits of ω6 fats becomes more widespread, we can expect a large number of companies to sell ω6 fatty acids. However, remember that it is the proper balance of ω3 and ω6 that matters.

Vegetarian diets

A balanced vegetarian meal requires careful planning. Some vitamins and minerals are not plentiful in non-animal products (such as Calcium and Iron or B_{12}). These vitamins or minerals may need to be supplemented. For new vegetarians, planning meals to obtain an adequate protein balance can be difficult. However, once a few simple combinations are understood, planning becomes easy. In general, a combination of a grain and a legume will result in an adequate protein balance (i.e., sufficient amounts of each needed amino acid). If a variety of whole grains, vegetables, legumes, and nuts are consumed during the day, it is not at all difficult to have appropriate protein intake. For people who are looking for a simple way to manage protein intake, I have prepared a list of easy sources to supplement your meals. You may prefer mostly a vegetarian diet with occasional animal food supplements. Most people obtain some protein from vegetables and a small protein supplement of 2 egg whites per day is sufficient, together with a multivitamin with minerals two to four times per week.

Egg Whites or Tofu. Egg white, Tofu, or soybean protein replaces animal protein. About 6 large size egg whites per day or the equivalent amount in Tofu (depending on the type, 1 ½ ounce Tofu = 1 large size egg white) provide most of your required daily protein.

Fish. Alternatively, use fish according to this formula: One large size egg white = ½ ounce of fish.

Vitamin and Mineral supplements

People who eat well rarely need supplements.[15] Unfortunately, very few people eat well and therefore most of us need supplements to correct likely deficiencies. I suggest you avoid fortified foods unless they merely replace vitamins and minerals removed during processing. Fortification may enhance nutritional imbalances because if you eat 100% of your daily needs in one food, you are likely to exceed your daily requirements with the other foods you eat. Balance is the key, and eating too much of something the body needs hurts rather than helps (for example, water is essential to human health, but drowning in water is not going to make you healthier).

The labels of vitamin and mineral supplements indicate their content. Use the **RDA** (Recommended Daily Allowance) as your guide. Choose a product which is closest to the RDA for most vitamins and minerals. Take one tablet 2 to 4 times per week; more could be toxic because you already eat vitamins and minerals with your foods. An adequate product contains 100% of the RDA for most of these vitamins and minerals:

- **Vitamins water soluble**: C, B_1 (thiamin), B_2 (riboflavin), B_6 (pyridoxine), B_{12} (cobalamin), Niacinamide (Niacin), Folate (folic acid, folacin), biotin, pantothenic acid.
- **Vitamins fat soluble**: A, D, E.
- Minerals: Iron, Zinc, Copper, Magnesium, Manganese, Selenium, Chromium, Molybdenum, Sodium, Phosphorus.

Not usually required in a multivitamin supplement: Vitamin K, Biotin (made by intestinal bacteria), Iodine (included with most salts), Calcium (requires separate capsules because you need far greater quantities), Phosphorus. Most other ingredients in multivitamins are not needed or are present in such small quantities as to be useless. Very few people need Sodium or Iodine, which are incorporated in table

Modern Prevention Diet

salt and many foods. Multivitamin tablets that list Calcium, Potassium, and Phosphorus rarely contain useful amounts.

- **Potassium, magnesium, manganese, calcium, iron**

Almost everyone gets adequate potassium unless they have a disease or take drugs that make them lose potassium. Some people may not be eating enough magnesium or manganese. Magnesium supplements help if you are often constipated, because magnesium is a primary ingredient in products that soften your bowels (like Milk of Magnesia). However, taking these products every day could make your problem worse because the body loses its ability to regulate itself. Manganese is more difficult to find, but it is now available at most health food stores. Most animal products contain plenty of magnesium, manganese, potassium and iron. Manganese is found in tea, nuts, unrefined grains and some fruits and cereals.[16]

People who eat only a few green leafy vegetables and dairy products may require calcium supplements. A single tablet with 500 mg of Calcium per day is sufficient as a supplement. Iron is particularly important for menstruating women who eat little red meat. Contrary to popular belief, the content of a typical vitamin supplement, 18 mg of Iron, is enough for several days. Therefore, one capsule two to four times per week is sufficient.

Vitamin B$_{12}$, A, C, D, E

Vitamin B$_{12}$ supplements are often required by individuals who eat very little animal meat. People who eat plenty of vegetables and fruits, as we recommend, get all the vitamin A and C they need. I believe that very few people need to take more than 200 mg/day of vitamin C. Vitamin D is found in fortified products like milk, or is made by the body after exposure to the sun. Sun requirements, of course, depend on the intensity of the sun and your skin exposure, but a few hours per day is usually sufficient (too much sun may lead to skin cancer).

Vitamin E Supplements. If you drink oil supplements you should take approximately 100 IU of vitamin E per day for every tablespoon of oil. We suggest a maximum of two tablespoons of oil per day and no more than 200 IU of vitamin E per day.[17]

Prevention vs. Treatment

To prevent disease we must eat a diet that *maintains* our good health. If we start early enough in life eating healthy diets, our bodies eliminate excesses and retain key nutrients in the appropriate balance. If we start as adults, we must treat existing disease. Even if we do not feel it, most of us have hardening and narrowing of the arteries. For some, the problem is minor; for others it is life-threatening. A 40 year old man cannot afford to wait 30 years until a preventive, healthy diet corrects for 40 years of bad eating. Most people have not eaten enough EFAs during their lifetimes, and have accumulated too much saturated fat in their bodies. The only way to know how many EFAs we need, and the proper balance of ω3 and ω6s, is to have our blood analyzed.

To treat existing disease and prevent problems from getting worse, we must usually lose weight and eat large amounts of oils, probably 1 to 3 tablespoons per day (130 to 400 calories per day). Eating such large amounts of oil requires that we eliminate other foods, or exercise quite a bit more. One reason many diets do not lower cholesterol or high blood pressure is that the amount of EFAs that people eat are not enough to change the body's EFA composition.

There is a fundamental difference between prevention and treatment. In prevention you do not know what disease you are going to get in the future. Therefore, the diet must be balanced to prevent the most likely diseases. It is impossible to prevent every disease and sometimes the diets and behaviors to prevent one disease may be different than those to prevent another. Thus, it seems wise to change your behavior to prevent the diseases most likely to affect you. If you smoke a pack a day, and roller skate without a helmet at 30 miles per hour on the wrong side of the road, and get drunk every week, you might as well eat anything. Long before you die of heart disease, you will be killed by a car, die of lung cancer, or from the complications of alcoholism.

In treatment, you know what problems you have. Therefore, your diet must be optimized to treat what you have rather than what you could get in the future. If you already have heart disease, the chances of dying of heart disease are far greater than the chances of getting cancer and dying from it. You should treat the heart disease even though the treatment may increase your chances of getting cancer. If you have an infection, your chances of dying from it are far greater than the chances of dying from the side effects of the antibiotic you take to treat the infection. "Balance" in general is no longer very important; instead, you

Modern Prevention Diet

want to treat the existing disease. You need to balance the risk of *existing* disease vs. the potential risk of a ***possible*** disease in the future. You may have to eat a diet that emphasizes supplements plus foods containing oils in order to treat an existing disease. This is needed even though that diet would not be a "balanced" diet. This diet would be different from the diet you would follow if you were trying to prevent other diseases.

References and notes

1 Varying the amount of daily protein may protect your kidneys. Eating small amounts of daily protein prevents excessive protein waste and overwork of kidneys. Occasionally eating large amounts of protein helps to maintain the function of the whole kidney by having it work harder, like periodic exercise maintains the tone and function of your heart and muscles. It is possible that primitive humans used to eat large protein meals from time to time. When they caught an animal, they ate a large meal; other days they ate less meat, if any at all. This approach may be healthiest for us. If we always eat about the same amount of protein, parts of the kidney that are not used slowly atrophy (die).

2 When you eat a wide range of natural foods, the body automatically accumulates the vitamins and minerals you need and excretes those you do not need. I find food labels practically useless (except when they list ingredients that I want to avoid). Trying to keep track of how many vitamins and minerals I eat every single day is practically impossible. I know that if I eat a wide variety of foods, my body will do a better job than the job I could do. Besides, even if I kept track of vitamins and minerals, I do not know what my body needs. Natural balancing works best when the foods are not fortified.

The situation is quite different with carbohydrates and saturated fats. The body cannot eliminate excessive calories and instead accumulates them as saturated fat. Therefore, you must be careful not to eat too many calories.

3 The reason to store excessive fat is that our ancestors found it difficult to find food. Sometimes the food run too fast; sometimes it ran after our ancestors!. Thus, storing surplus food as fat helped our ancestors survive during difficult winter times.

4 Shapiro DV, Kumar NB. Disease Prevention. A link missing. *Arch. Internal Med.*, 1989; 149: 1253-54. Reviews common nutritional recommendations.

5 Section V presents a vegetarian plan consisting primarily of raw foods. Although quite different from traditional American meals, you may want to use these guidelines for preparation of raw foods.

6 Eat most of your fruits in the summer, consistent with the recommendation of eating foods in season according to the temperature of the area where you live. This means that if you live in Boston, during the winter you should avoid winter foods from California: The California winter is different from the Boston winter.

7 You should write to your government to insist that it prohibit fishing in the oceans and dumping of garbage in the ocean. Instead we should establish large fish farms. In this manner we could eat safer fish while protecting the environment.

8 The Food and Nutrition News, March/April, 1987, indicates that the polyunsaturated content of muscular lipids (fats) of various animals follows this

order (approximate percent of total fat as ω6 polyunsaturated in parentheses; there are practically no ω3 fatty acids):

Turkey (29%) > Chicken (23%) > Pork (12%) > Veal/Lamb (8%) > Beef (4%).

This is the basis for our recommendations of the order of preference of animal foods. There is one important exception. Some animals are now fed foods high in ω3, particularly chicken. We may soon have chicken high in ω3 fatty acids. If not fresh, it may taste a bit like outdated fish.

9   I suppose the government assumes that you carry your portable computer with a phone and fax machine to the supermarket. In that way you can keep up with frequent press releases and news concerning labels, recalls, etc.

10   Research has shown that many people, particularly diabetics and hypertensives, should not eat too many calories as carbohydrates (Science, Vol. 235. page 164, January 9, 1987). Dr. Siguel's research suggests that the key factor in good health is the amount of essential fatty acids in the diet; calories from carbohydrates are converted to saturated fat and decrease the body ratio of PUFA / (SFA + MUFA).

11   Siguel, EN, Lerman, RH.   Fatty Acid Patterns In Patients With Angiographically Documented Coronary Artery Disease. *Metabolism*, 9/1994.

12   These numbers are rough guidelines until further research is completed. Some authors suggest ω6/ω3 = 2:1 The ratios vary according to age (children probably need more ω3s for the brain), disease and sex.

13   Using sophisticated instrumentation, Dr. Siguel developed a sensitive technique to measure essential fats and deficiencies of essential fats and found that many people with cardiovascular disease have deficiencies of the essential fats

14   For several years I assisted in the preparation of exhibits on cholesterol and heart disease at the annual meetings of the Massachusetts Medical Society. During those meetings physicians came to talk to me and told me that they did not believe that diet played a significant role in the etiology (cause) of heart disease.

15   This is only an outline of the major issues because we are primarily concerned with fat. If this matter interests you I suggest you consult with your nutritionist or read another book.

16   Vitamins and minerals are not discussed in this book. Furthermore, it is impractical for people to eat foods just because they are high in a particular vitamin or mineral. People who have a disease with a documented nutritional abnormality will most likely need supplements; healthy people should eat a variety of foods. Otherwise they may correct one deficiency and cause another.

17   But follow your doctor's advice.

Modern Prevention Diet

PRUDENT DIET

To prevent or treat cardiovascular disease

These foods are primarily for the treatment of cardiovascular disease

Decreased Intake Recommended

Animal foods products such as beef, meat, cheese, milk, butter, cream.
Foods containing partially hydrogenated oils and processed fat (i.e.,
most pastry, non dairy creamers). Fried foods. Nuts and seeds high in
saturated fat. Fruits high in saturated fat, such as avocados, coconut.
These foods provide nutrients and dense calories. They are high in
saturated fat and even small servings would make you gain weight. If
you are slim, they are OK.

Neutral Foods

These are foods that have important nutrients. They have a relatively
neutral effect on cardiovascular disease from the perspective of fat.
Olive oil (has some ω6 fatty acids) (use only for flavor). Peanut oil (use
only for flavor). Low fat products (skim milk, skim cheese. Fruits.
Carbohydrates and grains. Alcohol (less than one ounce per day or one
small glass of wine). Most condiments. Protein sources such as egg
whites, fish. These foods provide nutrients and calories, but practically
zero EFAs.

Increased intake recommenced

Uncooked oils such as sunflower, safflower, soybean, walnut, cod liver,
corn, sesame seed, flax. Fresh nuts. Most vegetable products,
particularly green leafy vegetables. Cold water fish (i.e., mackerel,
salmon). These are foods high in EFAs. Vegetables have very low
caloric intake and high bulk.

Foods whose benefits and risks are debated

Avoid them as much as possible. Margarine. sugar. Cocoa, coffee, tea,
food additives, such as colorants.

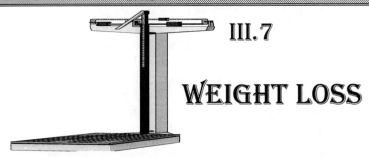

III.7

WEIGHT LOSS

"If you are never hungry you are probably eating too much"

Topics: *The key to weight loss is a diet of foods low in calories and high in volume. Exercise. Eat low calorie snacks several times per day. Start your meals with a big salad. Low fat diets and EFAs. Recent research. Boston Egg white diet.*

Summary

The key to weight loss is foods low in calories and high in volume. Eating a substantial amount of the right foods makes you less hungry and less likely to eat "bad" foods. Preface your meals with exercise. Eat low calorie snacks (i.e. vegetables) several times per day. Start your meals with a big salad. During phase I of our weight reduction program you follow a rigid diet for two to three weeks to prepare your body. During this first phase your appetite will be reduced and you can lose more than 10 pounds. During phase II you are allowed a wide variety of foods and will continue to lose 1 to 3 pounds per week. During phase III you are allowed most foods and will either continue to lose weight or maintain your weight. It is not difficult to lose weight while eating tempting, healthful meals. The secret is the right diet, combined with perseverance. The Boston Egg white diet: optimal diet to lose weight.

Introduction

Being mildly overweight is not necessarily a dangerous problem. There are many reasons why one might need to lose weight. You may want to consider weight loss if you are concerned about your self-image. If you have a muscle-skeletal problem such as arthritis, you may need to weigh less because your joints cannot support you at an overly heavy weight. You should also lose weight if you have abnormal cholesterol levels, high blood pressure, diabetes, or any other reason to suspect cardiovascular disease, such as fatigue from mild exercise. If you choose not to lose weight you can drastically reduce your risk of heart disease by improving the balance of essential fatty acids (**EFAs**) in your body. My research has shown that most overweight people have insufficient amounts of EFAs and what they do have is not balanced; that is, the amounts of ω3 vs. ω6 **are not in the right proportion**.

There exists a multitude of weight reduction diets and nearly every month brings forth a new rash of magazine articles about weight loss erupts. What I discuss here are the basic components of a medically safe diet. This dietary program is effective in reducing the fat in your body, without damaging your organs like so many crash diets do. After you reach your ideal weight, change to a Prevention or Treatment program as described in Parts III and IV, respectively. You can find further discussion of weight reduction in the excellent publications reviewed in Part V or in the appendix that lists selected references.

What is overweight?

There is not a fixed definition of overweight. We do know, from animal experiments, that lean animals, those who are allowed to eat only the smallest amount of calories needed to live, live the longest. Several hundred thousand years ago, when supermarkets were closed on weekends, humans needed to store food as fat in reserve for long periods of starvation. Today, when many supermarkets are open every day, we can store food in the refrigerator or shelves rather than in adipose tissue, and we can replenish it when needed. When I tell patients what I consider to be the "ideal weight", they tell me it is impossible for them to be so thin. They claim that they need to be as they are or else they do not have "energy," "creativity," "aura," etc. Many tell me they will die because their body cannot possibly become that thin. Obviously, I cannot argue against such subjective feelings. However, most patients can be far slimmer than they are. At times I suspect that the way patients speak to me about "genetics" and "individual metabolic needs", implies that these scientific labels have become excuses for not facing the challenge of losing excess weight.

The sad truth is that, unless you have conclusive evidence that you were born on another planet, or are the direct descendant of a genetically obese alien invader, you will not die if you lose weight.

Weight Loss

Quite the contrary. Excessive body weight causes fat to accumulate, eventually clogging arteries and the brain. Excessive body weight is one of the most significant factors in cardiovascular disease, early loss of brain cells and early death.

Your "ideal weight" is the weight that allows your arteries and heart to supply enough food and oxygen to the brain, kidneys and other parts of the body. Many of the tables of "ideal body weight" have been prepared using averages of people of different height and age. Because most people are overweight in the USA, it is not surprising that the average table contains inflated numbers for ideal weight. Practically all studies linking weight to health and disease have found that slimmer people have less cardiovascular disease and live longer. The exception to this rule is the person who is slim *because* of illness.

How to make a diet work

People often lose weight on a crash diet and gain it back because they have not changed their dietary habits. What you need is not just a new diet, but a program for weight control. "Most people who lose weight successfully do so on their own initiative without the aid of commercial products or medical intervention."[1] Therefore, I suggest you make a list of the foods you can eat, design your own meals using these foods, and begin your own personalized weight loss program.

Steps to follow

1.   *Prepare your own meals*
By making your own meals you expend more energy (i.e., burn calories), and you eat healthier and better tasting foods. You also save money because commercially prepared meals cost more than those you make.

2.   *Make a plan and keep records*
Plan your activities and meals, and record what you eat. Keep a record of exercise. Use your records to monitor your progress, and note when you deviate from your plan. Records will help you to find out what you are doing right and wrong, allowing you to eliminate negative behavior.

3.   *Analyze what you are doing*
Analyze when and where you indulge in fattening foods or eat unnecessarily. These are the extra calories that turn into unwanted

Instead of	Do this
Eating junk food snacks	Replace with healthy snacks
High calorie food	Low calorie food
Take the elevator	Walk up a few flights
Park close by	Park far and walk
Watch TV	Walk to the library; play a game
Talk on the phone	Meet a friend for a walk
Have paper delivered	Purchase paper at a store; walk
Have a sedentary life	Exercise as much as you can
Walk	Run
Buy prepared foods	Design and cook your own meals
Continue with routines	Experiment and make changes

pounds. For instance, do you eat while watching TV? Then substitute a different activity, one incompatible with eating, such as writing a letter or working on a crafts project. Or read something that requires your full attention. Select activities that engage your hands and attention fully. TV viewing is a passive activity that encourages you to eat even without thinking about what you are eating. Do not watch TV commercials about food. And if you must eat, eat a healthy snack.

4. Avoid "social eating": Eat only if hungry

Be on guard against eating as a social activity. Learn to say no to offers of fattening foods at parties. Avoid hunger at social situations where you know you are going to be tempted with high-calorie treats by eating your snacks before the event.

5. Change your habits

You may also want to try some basic behavior modification. Many of our bad habits make us overweight but with conscious efforts, habits can be modified. Bad habits can be replaced by good ones. Quite often a few simple steps pay big dividends in improving your lifestyle. Find ways to increase the amount you exercise in anything you do. A few minutes of exercise added here and there can mean 25 pounds lost in one year!. The following table shows some behaviors you can change.

Other hints to change your eating habits

- As you chew slowly, count how many times you chew and try to chew a little bit longer.

- Sit when you eat and eat slowly. Take a rest after eating for a few minutes to let the food reach your brain.

- Put food in your mouth, and leave the fork or spoon on the table while you are chewing the food.

- Limit your food to food that you need to eat with a fork, knife or spoon. In this way you will eat fewer finger foods like candy snacks and potato chips.

- Every time you limit the amount of food you eat and avoid temptation, put some money in a piggy-bank. Then use it to buy something you like (besides foods!).

6. *Do not go hungry and be tempted*

You can also plan your intake of food so that your eating schedule contributes to weight loss and weight maintenance. Rather than eating three big meals, spread your consumption of food out into several small meals a day. This will remove some of the temptation for snacks consisting of sweets and other high calorie foods. Eat slowly, so you will feel satisfied.

Ideal weight

A concern for one's "ideal weight" is common among people who are too heavy. They set for themselves the goal of reaching this magical number, and consult many different tables of ideal weight in order to refine their goal as much as possible. However, the concept of "ideal weight" is not necessarily a constructive one for the dieter. More practical is the goal of changing your habits of food intake. For optimal results, develop a plan to change your behavior patterns and follow it.

If in doubt, be thin

There are many tables of "ideal weight", most of them derived from insurance data which is not applicable to you. The weight ranges given in these tables are quite broad. They classify people as having a small, medium or large frame. As a result, most people like to think of themselves as having a medium or large frame; that way their weight is "normal". My impression is that most of the tables mislead people into

Weight Loss

thinking that they have the proper weight. To use these tables properly people should select the lower figure of each range, not the higher one, as the ideal weight they are aiming for. Also read the footnotes on ideal weight charts carefully to determine whether you should subtract 1" or 2" for your shoes. And be honest. Practically everybody I meet thinks he/she is taller than he/she really is.

Suggested ideal weight tables

As one gets older, it is better to become slimmer rather than heavier. The heart and kidney and other organs shrink due to aging, and they are unable to feed a body as large as they could feed when one was 20 years old. Because you cannot make your heart or kidneys younger, you must reduce your body size. This suggestion contradicts guidelines that allow people to gain weight as they get older.

Get slimmer as you get older

In 1994 I received an advertisement from Consumer Reports On Health that listed three separate tables for recommended weights (by height, sex and age). One set of weights was recommended by Metropolitan Life, another set from an obesity panel from the National Institutes of Health (defined obesity), and another was an age-adjusted recommendation from the Gerontology Research Center. The last one showed that recommended weight increases with age.

Most of those recommendations are misleading. The general rule is that the organs and the body do not get better with age. As we get older, our heart, lungs and kidneys become less efficient and they can no longer manage a large body. To compensate for loss of organ efficiency, we must maintain or decrease our weight. The combination of increased weight and decreased organ efficiency is deadly.

Furthermore, most studies have shown that longevity is not associated with increased weight. Overweight and fat are only useful to protect us during long periods of starvation and cold. [1] In modern times, the chance that we will not be able to find food for several weeks is very small. Thus, my position is that people should be as slim as possible given their height and frame. An exception to this recommendation is during pregnancy, when women must eat more, because they have to feed two bodies. In a recent study published in *JAMA*, the authors found significant methodological errors in many of the studies relating body weight to longevity, and concluded by stating that "available

---

Weight Loss

evidence suggests that minimum mortality occurs at relative weights at least 10% below the US average".[2]

Approximate Men's formula (adults)[3]
Ideal Weight (in pounds) = 110 + 5 x Height (in inches after 5')

Approximate Women's formula (adults)
Ideal Weight (in pounds) = 95 + 5 x Height (in inches after 5')

How thin is thin?

Most scientific studies have shown that thin animals live longer than overweight animals. In the USA very few people die of starvation. Even malnourished people do not die of starvation, they suffer from *malnutrition* rather than insufficient calories. Most people eat too much rather than too little. Unless you plan to get lost in the Himalayans or at the North Pole, you do not need to store in your body enough food for 60 days. Food for two days should be plenty.

Reconsider your image: try to be as thin as possible as long as you are comfortable with yourself. The thinner you are, the less work your heart and other organs must perform, and the less likely it is for fat to clog your arteries and brain.

Wait for body fat to redistribute

If you suddenly lose weight it will take a while for the body fat and muscle to redistribute. For a while your face and some parts of your body may look too thin. DO NOT EAT to correct your facial appearance. PLEASE WAIT: That look will go away soon.

Science vs. Psychology

Most scientists agree on how to lose weight. There are basically very few significant discoveries regarding weight loss. Some scientists speak about fat cells and state that some people accumulate fat more easily than others. Some people have a faster metabolism which burns fat. But none of this is very significant. There is really one fundamental truth that underlies almost all weight problems: Anyone who is overweight is overweight because he or she eats too much.

Of course, it is true that if two people eat two pounds of food per day, one may gain one pound of weight every week and the other may lose

Weight Loss

one pound. That is due to differences in body composition, metabolism, exercise, genetics, etc. But the truth is that the one who gains weight needs to eat less, and the one who loses weight needs to eat more. Thus, how much food one needs to eat depends on the amount of exercise he or she does, and on the speed of one's metabolism. The most difficult aspects of losing weight are not scientific but psychological. Almost all proper diets have a similar scientific basis but approach the subject with a different psychological tactic.

Estimated minimum calories needed every day

Men = 1.0 Calories x ideal weight (pounds)/2.2 x 24.

Women = 0.95 Calories x ideal weight (pounds)/2.2 x 24.

Substract **0.1 Calories x ideal weight (pounds)/2.2 x # hours sleep.**

To this you must add additional calories for exercise.

The secret to weight loss: scientific basis

This book is not about psychological tactics to lose weight. We assume that you are well motivated and that you want to be thin and live longer. Therefore we present the scientific basis for losing weight. However, we will mention one psychological factor that is essential to the success of your diet: **Family support.**

Your family and friends must cooperate

Everybody in your household should follow a similar diet, or respect and support your efforts. Family members should avoid organizing social gatherings at which fattening foods will be served that will weaken your resolve. Parties and outside meals with people who like to eat should be avoided: The temptation may become too great to resist.

Lose fat, not water or protein

The diets presented here are both short and long-term diets. It is easy to design a diet that will appear to make you lose a lot of weight by burning muscle or losing water. But the secret is to lose fat, not water or protein. Losing fat is not difficult if you eat well. Water lost is eventually recovered. If it were not, you would remain dehydrated and that eventually could be fatal. Protein lost is lost from muscle and cell tissue. It is almost like cutting off a limb in order to see a lower number of pounds register on the scale. The dieter weighs less, but his/her body has been damaged. Losing weight means keeping your muscle and cells, but eliminating unnecessary fat.

Goals

A reasonable goal is to lose one to two pounds per week of fat, not water. In fact, it is practically impossible to lose one pound of fat per day and you should be happy if you lose two pounds every week.

You must continue on the weight reduction program until you reach your ideal weight. Under strict medical supervision it is possible to engage in a more restrictive program (very low calories) that will help you lose more pounds each week, but only severely obese people should attempt such a program. Beware of fads that make you lose several pounds each day: it is likely to be water, eventually to be recovered when you drink water. Playing tennis for 6 hours on a hot and sunny day could make you lose 6 pounds, of which 5 or more are water.

Losing weight means eating better foods

Losing weight means eating healthful foods with few calories. It is that simple. The average adult man requires about 1500 to 2500 calories per day. The average adult woman requires 1200 to 2000 calories per day. Those who exercise vigorously (see below) require more calories. Elderly people often require less than 1500 calories, depending on their activity. Of course, if your lifestyle requires a great deal of physical effort, you need more calories. A high-powered job in an air-conditioned office may be stressful, but it is not physically demanding.

One pound of fat = 3500 calories

There is a simple rule of thumb that can guide you in planning a program of weight loss for yourself. For every 3500 calories of food that you DO NOT EAT (or burn as exercise), you lose approximately one pound of fat. Therefore, if you cut your daily intake by 500 calories, you can lose one pound per week. If you exercise the equivalent of another 500 calories per day (over one hour per day of exercise) you will lose another pound per week.

Role of exercise

More exercise means using more calories, and thus losing weight. But for most people exercise is not an effective way to lose weight. The body is very efficient and you usually need to exercise one hour to expend over 300 calories. It is very easy to recover all the calories lost in one hour of exercise with one soft drink or half a sandwich. And some people are so hungry after exercising that they eat more calories in junk food than they just lost while exercising! So while exercise is very important, it is not as effective as proper eating to lose a lot of weight.

Typical plan (weight loss)

Total caloric intake: 800 to 1200 calories per day

Weight loss: 1 to 3 pounds/week; "save" 3500 to 7000 calories/ week. With active exercise you can safely lose more than 6 pounds per week.

Balanced diet

Protein: 40 to 60 grams per day. About 0.8 grams/kg of ideal body weight, higher for a tall man, lower one for a short woman.[4]

Carbohydrate: 100 grams per day (about 3-4 ounces).

Fat: as little as possible, outside the necessary amount of essential fats. Beware of hidden fat in bread, processed foods, dairy supplements, etc. Eat 1 teaspoon to 1 tablespoon of oil (such as soybean oil) per day as indicated in other chapters.

Minerals and Vitamins: one multivitamin with minerals 3-5 times per week. This is one of the few times when a multivitamin with minerals is appropriate. Choose the one that has the recommended daily allowance (RDA) for the vitamins A, C, D, E and many of the B's (see vitamin chapter), and iron. Calcium supplements come in a different tablet. Take about 1000 mg/day of calcium, about 100 I.U of Vitamin E. per day or about 600-800 per week. You do not need to take the supplements every day.

Fiber and vegetables. Eat as much fiber-rich foods (leafy vegetables) as you can tolerate; this will fill you up and it is generally healthful.

Water: Drink plenty of water, about 1 to 2 quarts per day. Drink less if you eat watery foods.[5]

Foods to avoid: high calorie, low volume

Many foods pack a large number of calories into a small volume. Many dry cereals do not fill you up because they have a small volume. You

Weight Loss

may end up eating a lot of them and they are almost pure calories. Most vegetables and many fruits contain lots of water and fiber which have no calories. In contrast, fruit juices have little fiber but many calories. **Hint**: Eat dry cereals, like oats, with plenty of water. Other ideas about foods to avoid:

- Foods of animal origin such as meats, milk, cheese, dairy, which are high in saturated fat.
- Pastries, cookies, ice cream, breads, pizza, processed foods.
- Hard fat, hydrogenated oils, fried foods.
- Sugars, sweets, syrups, alcohol, fruit juices, beverages.
- Dried foods, dried fruits, dry cereals/grains, high salt (sodium) foods or smoked foods.

Foods to eat: low calorie, high volume, high fiber

For weight reduction you should eat foods that are high in fiber but low in calories, thus eating a lot of food with little weight gain. Ex: Apple with skin. Other ideas about foods to eat:

- Water or very low calorie drinks.
- Foods with a large bulk and ratio of weight to calories, such as those high in fiber like whole grains, legumes, and vegetables.
- Whole fruits, not just the juice.
- Cereals prepared with plenty of water (such as oatmeal).
- Skim milk (1% fat), low calorie yogurt, low fat foods.
- Foods cooked by broiling, baking or microwaving; not by frying.
- Foods "fried" without fat or oil using non-stick pans.
- Spices such as herbs, lemon juice, and garlic, but NOT salt.

The Boston Egg White Diet: A diet for weight loss

Several years ago I designed a diet using natural foods that contained the necessary nutrients and had the smallest number of calories. The result is the **Boston Egg White Diet**. It is practically impossible to

Weight Loss

design a better diet using regular inexpensive foods. I tried this diet myself, with family members and friends. The results were terrific: Everybody lost fat and remained thin. And everyone liked the food.

Phase I. First two to three weeks

Objectives: (a) *Prompt weight loss; (b) Shift to get your body accustomed to little food*

Nutrients:

Protein: 6 large size egg whites per day (about 36 grams per day). You may substitute fish for up to 2 egg whites, approximately one ounce of fish for every large size egg white. You may also substitute Tofu for 2 Egg whites; read the food label for the Tofu you use to get about 12 grams of protein from Tofu. You can prepare the egg whites, Tofu or fish anyway you want, as long as no additional fat is used with it. The reason we use 1 ½ times more fish than egg white is that the protein in egg white is more efficient at meeting body needs than the protein in fish. Egg whites are preferred because they are pure protein while fish contains fat and thus it has more calories. Although fish helps to prevent cardiovascular disease, the first step is to be thin, and egg whites will help you to get thin quickly. You may also use skim milk for some of the protein and carbohydrate; just read the label to decide how much protein and carbohydrate you are getting.

You may cook and eat the eggs anyway you want, and at any time. I suggest that you hard boil them and eat them over the day. Egg whites are especially valuable as snacks when you are feeling hungry because of their ability to reduce appetite.

Carbohydrate: the equivalent of 100 grams (3 ounces) of dry carbohydrate (excluding water) on a daily basis. For example, 3 ounces of dry rice per day. Cook the rice with plenty of water and seasoning. Eat wild or whole grain rice. **But** beware: some people get constipated by eating rice. Should this happen to you, replace the rice with other cereal, or eat more fiber.

Another good source of carbohydrates is the potato. Potatoes have approximately 80% water. Therefore, a 10 ounce potato is approximately 2 ounces of carbohydrate. Fruits also provide carbohydrates. You should consume at most one fruit per day as part of your carbohydrate count. Fruits also contain quite a bit of water. One pound of apples has about 60 grams of carbohydrate; one pound of

Weight Loss

oranges has about 40 grams of carbohydrate, less than apples because the skin is not edible.

Vegetables play a crucial role in a weight-loss program. Vegetables are the ideal snack food for the hungry dieter. Low in calories, high in fiber and volume, they require much chewing and you CAN eat a great deal. The best vegetables to use as snacks are those with green leaves, such as lettuce, spinach, green beans, celery, or broccoli.

Supplements: one teaspoon of soybean oil, one multivitamin with minerals, and plenty of spices and herbs to make the food more palatable.[6]

Snacks: Good snacks to take to work: celery, whole apple, one raw carrot. They are very sturdy, require no refrigeration, and are easy to carry. Just chewing them keeps you away from tempting foods.

Avoid all other foods, including sweets, juices, etc. Although you should learn to drink water instead of soft drinks, if you must have soda use very low calorie soft drinks. Ahh, one small secret: you can eat one egg yolk or two per week. Egg yolks have EFAs even though they also have cholesterol. I find that they give flavor to the egg whites.

Scientific basis

In order for a diet to be successful in producing weight loss and building health rather than harming the body, it has to have a scientific basis. What this means is that the weight-loss program must be designed to provide *balanced nutrition* with a minimum amount of calories. The diet we are proposing here was planned in just this way. Let's look at the different essential nutrients and how they are provided in my weight reduction program. Then you can judge its scientific basis.

- **Protein.** Egg whites are one of the most balanced proteins. You obtain the protein you need from six large size eggs whites per day. Because egg whites are almost pure protein, they contain no unnecessary calories. It is practically impossible to find a natural food that contains more protein and provides fewer calories.

- **Carbohydrate.** Approximately 3 ounces (80 to 100 grams) of carbohydrate are required each day to properly metabolize (burn and use) your fat. The carbohydrate is obtained from vegetables which also provide fiber. Vegetables contain very little fat, mostly EFAs. Hence you get few unnecessary

calories. Eating dry cereals or sugar also provides
carbohydrates but with less bulk or fiber; therefore you are
more hungry.

- **Fat**. The essential fatty acids come from one teaspoon of oil
per day. Additional fats come from your own body fat which is
released by this diet. Soybean or walnut oil gives you a
balanced mixture of ω3 and ω6. It is best to have a blood test
for fatty acids before you start losing weight because you may
need one tablespoon or more per day.

- **Vitamins and minerals**. Because it is very difficult to eat
foods containing adequate amounts of vitamins and minerals,
while on this very low calorie diet we recommend that you
take a multivitamin with minerals 3 to 6 times per week. You
do not need it every day because vegetables provide some of
the required vitamins and minerals.

Procedure: Suggestions for implementing this diet

1.   Start the diet slowly.

Take several days to one week to shift to this diet. Otherwise you may
have too much variation in food intake, and this might create
constipation. If constipated, take any of the fiber supplements
available in the drugstore. Alternatively, take ½ teaspoon of
Magnesium sulfate in 50% solution, 1 to 4 times per day. Your
pharmacist can prepare this inexpensive solution for you. This gives
you more magnesium and helps your bowels move.

2.   Eat only when you are very hungry.

When hungry try to do something active (i.e., not watching TV); write a
letter to a friend; talk to someone; or go for a walk. When you do eat,
always eat a salad first, preferably with plenty of green vegetables. Eat
several healthy snacks during the day.

3.   Exercise for 15 minutes before you eat, to reduce your appetite.

A little exercise before each meal shifts your blood towards your
muscles and away from your stomach.

Weight Loss

Example of a typical day

Breakfast: 10-15 min. exercise (before the meal). A bowl of very soft mushy oatmeal. Apple with skin or peeled orange (if bearable, wait until phase II for the fruit). Caffeine-free tea/coffee.

Snack: 5 min. exercise; ½ carrot; one or two sticks of celery; Broccoli. Water.

Lunch: 10-15 min. exercise. Big green leaf salad with lettuce, spinach, etc. 2 Egg whites (hard boiled whites are easy to separate and carry with your lunch). Many spices (garlic, pepper, oregano, etc.). Rice (about one ounce dry) or 1/2 potato. Low calorie soft drink.

Snack: 5 min. exercise; ½ carrot; one or two sticks of celery; broccoli. Low calorie soft drink. 1 Egg white.

Dinner: 10-15 min. exercise. Salad: Use oil + vinegar + lemon for dressing (in any combination). 2 Egg whites. Perhaps an "omelet" with egg whites and a little yolk or vegetables fried without oil. Rice or baked/boiled potato or 1/2 tomato. Main vegetable dish (lots of leafy green vegetables). Water, low calorie soft drink or caffeine-free tea/coffee.

Bedtime snack: Exercise 10 minutes. Celery, 1 egg white. This high protein food helps you sleep.

Appetite loss

You will find that after about two weeks on this diet you will not be as hungry as you used to be. The first two weeks are the worst. Remember: Eat celery and egg whites to curb your appetite. If you are not hungry, reserve the egg whites for hungrier times, but always eat about 6 per day or equivalent protein from other comprehensive sources such as milk, Tofu, fish, very low fat beef, or pork.

Phase II. Week 3-5 and subsequent weeks until you reach your ideal weight

By now you know how much weight you have been losing. If you have lost more than 2 pounds per week, add more food to maintain your loss at 2 pounds per week. If you have lost less than 2 pounds per week, you need to eat less food, "cheat" less or exercise more.

Weight Loss

Modifications

The ultimate objective of any diet is to achieve a balanced nutritional status and to improve health. While this is the end, the means can vary. Being thin in itself may not be healthy. In fact, some very thin people have very poor nutritional status and are not healthy. Thus, you can try other books and other diets as long as you eat enough EFAs and other nutrients.

You can add more green vegetables and vegetables of other colors. For variety add a little bit of fish. Most cereals sold in boxes are "dry" cereals. A wet cereal is oatmeal made with plenty of water. Other cereals and grains can be prepared in this way. Preferably use water instead of milk with your cereals, but you can use a bit of skim milk if you desire.

Phase III.   Graduation

During the first three weeks you should have lost more than 6 pounds. You may continue at that rate or reduce it to one pound per week. It is easy to remain on this diet for long periods of time. Slowly add more foods, including once a week servings of very lean meat, poultry or fish. On this program you will not be hungry, you can eat as much as you like of low calorie foods and have occasional "treats" of meat, poultry, cakes, pastries, and even pizza and beer.

Medical supervision

Have a complete exam before you start this diet to make sure you don't have a medical problem that can be compounded by the diet. This recommendation applies to any significant weight loss program. Some people become hypotensive (their blood pressure declines substantially) during this diet. You can tell if this has happened to you if you feel dizzy upon getting up suddenly, particularly when you get out of bed in the morning. This is not very serious; it is often caused by sodium deficiency. Increase your fluid intake; some physicians suggest that you eat a dill pickle spear or some bouillon soup to correct this deficiency. In fact, lowering your blood pressure could be beneficial, but you should check with your doctor for possible side effects of rapid weight loss. Sudden weight loss is often accompanied by mineral abnormalities that can be dangerous.

If you are doing quite well with Phase I of the diet, you should continue, but you may need medical supervision if you continue for more than

Weight Loss

four weeks. If you need to follow a more stringent diet or exercise much more, you definitely need medical supervision to evaluate your condition and prevent complications.

Are low fat diets dangerous for you?

Everybody seems to recommend low fat diets. Companies are changing most of their foods to "low fat" or "zero fat". Through the miracles of modern technology, it is now possible to produce foods with almost no fat. Companies are making them and we eat them. But, are they good or bad for you?

The answer depends on three main issues: (1) the amount of EFAs in your body, (2) whether you are eating foods without EFAs; (3) and whether you are eating low fat foods for a short period of time.

Do you have enough EFAs in your body?

If you are overweight and have adequate stores of EFAs in your body fat, losing weight will mobilize those EFAs and bring them to your organs. A low fat diet will burn the excess of saturated, useless fat in your body and bring you more into balance. If you do not have adequate stores of EFAs, you need to eat more of them in your diet. A low fat diet will not provide you with enough EFAs. Foods such as processed grains and cereals, breads, pasta and fruits have practically no EFAs. Foods without fat have no EFAs, because EFAs are fat!

Without an appropriate test it is impossible for you to know whether or not you have enough EFAs in your body. If a fatty acid profile shows that your have enough EFAs, then you can eat low fat foods. If you do not have enough, you must supplement your diet with EFAs if you plan to diet for more than four weeks. My research has shown that many overweight people have enough ω6 but not enough ω3 fatty acids. If necessary, you can meet your need for EFAs with vegetable oils such as soybean or walnut oil (ω3+ω6), or flax (ω3) seeds.

Ideally you want to eat natural foods high in EFAs, such as leafy vegetables. Leafy vegetables are high in EFAs and fiber and low in calories. Natural foods are cheaper and healthier, and provide you with an optimal balance of vitamins and minerals.

Weight Loss

Are you eating foods without EFAs?

People who routinely follow a low calorie, low fat diet rarely get enough EFAs from their usual diet. Under these circumstances you need to eat supplements rich in EFAs, such as vegetable oils. This is particularly important if most of your calories come from pasta, breads and cereals that have practically zero EFAs. If virtually all your calories come from vegetables and you eat mostly leafy vegetables (i.e. several pounds daily), you would be getting many EFAs because leafy vegetables have cell membranes with EFAs.

Are you dieting for only a few weeks?

If you are dieting for only a few weeks and plan to return to a diet high in EFAs, you may not need EFA supplements. However, very few people can maintain their ideal weight on 3,000 calories per day (the calories that humans were designed to eat). Moreover, very few of us get most of our calories from natural foods. Instead, we eat mostly processed foods that have been deprived of their EFAs. Therefore, practically all adults need some oil supplement for their entire lives. For most people this means eating both ω3 and ω6, but usually more ω3s than ω6s because it is more common to have insufficient levels of ω3 than ω6 fatty acids.

The future of overweight and obesity

My father told me: "You will get rich only when you discover a pill that I can take and eat whatever I want". Is there hope for such a pill? Will science be able to develop it?

For years there has been discussion about the roles of genetics vs. behavior in overweight and obesity.[7] The answer depends on the form of the question, a trick often used by pollsters to get the answer they want. If you ask the question: Do genetics play a role in overweight?, the answer is yes. If you ask the question: Do environment or behavior play a role in overweight?, the answer is also yes. The reason for this apparent contradiction is the form of the question. Practically everything in life is interrelated, but not everything is equally important. One may ask: what are the relative roles of genetics vs. behavior in overweight? Unfortunately, the answer to this question is also misleading, because it groups different types of people. There are many people, perhaps as many as 5%, who have significant genetic

Weight Loss

differences that cause very abnormal cholesterol, or heart disease, or overweight. There are people living in arctic climates who need extra body fat to protect against the cold.

A better question to ask is: What are the relative roles of genetics vs. behavior in the majority of overweight humans in the USA, except Alaska? In mathematical terms, one asks what variable, genetics vs. behavior, is responsible for the largest amount of variability in weight. My research indicates that behavior is responsible for overweight in most people. Sorry about that, folks. You cannot blame your parents because you eat too much junk food. Genetics determines your body metabolism. However, you can decide whether to eat more or less food.

Recent Research

For many years researchers have been looking for a chemical in the body that makes people stop eating, the "satiety factor". They have also looked for a way to make people burn more fat. There are two basic types of "fat" in adipose tissue: "brown" and "white" fat. **Brown fat** contains a large number of tiny organelles found inside cells called mitochondria; brown cells have far more mitochondria than white cells and therefore have a darker color. Mitochondria have many functions, one of which is to burn fatty acids, the main component of fat. Thus, within brown adipose tissue is the equipment to burn fat. However, humans have very little brown fat. Contrary to some published reports, brown adipose tissue plays a minor role in heat and weight control. Instead, for most people, muscle is the part of the body that uses most energy.[8] Thus, if you want to burn fat, you need to exercise more. Sitting in front of the TV hoping to burn excess weight through your brown fat is wishful thinking.

The body burns fat to maintain body temperature. When the body senses that it is cold, it burns fat to generate heat; when the body senses that it has reached the proper temperature, it stops burning fat. In the 1990s researchers found a protein called "uncoupling protein" (UCP). This protein helps to regulate the burning of fat. Researchers found that mice without brown fat became obese even when they ate the same amount of food as mice that have brown fat. Apparently, animals and perhaps people with an abnormal type of UCP tend to become obese. Since the 1940s, researchers have realized that animals and humans need to maintain body heat (what we call "**temperature**") within a very narrow range or else the body gets sick. The body maintains temperature constantly by changing the amount of fuel (fat)

Weight Loss

burnt, just like the heating system in your home. When the temperature declines, we burn more fat; when the temperature increases, we stop burning fat. Similarly, scientists have hypothesized that we generate heat when we eat. When we have generated enough heat, that turns on a signal to stop eating. The idea was that animals and humans ate enough to generate heat and stopped eating when they had enough food to meet their body needs or get enough heat. Obviously, this was a very simple theory, but scientists were looking for simple explanations.

If we could identify the chemical that sends the signal that we ate enough, we could have people eat more of that "chemical" and they would not be hungry. However, what works perfectly well for an animal may be useless for a person because our genetics and physiology are quite different. While a bear may hibernate, sleep, and live without food for months, such behavior may not be possible for humans (contrary to some sightings of lazy people sleeping on sofas).

Small variations in the efficiency of generation of body heat and metabolism allow one person to eat more than another without gaining weight. However, for most people, the desire to eat is derived from our culture and behavior rather than our genes. For instance, in recent years I have developed a "sweet tooth" for chocolate and candy which I did not have as a child.

Currently researchers are trying to find a drug that decreases appetite or makes the body use more energy. Similar drugs were tested may years ago without much success. The problem is that if one increases body heat too much, or one "uncouples" the process that regulates body heat and allows the body to produce heat even if there is no need for it, the body temperature increases substantially and brain cells die. If we increase body heat, we must find a way to help the body dissipate the heat (for example, by placing people inside refrigerators). Scientists tried placing people in cold water or with ice, but this did not substantially dissipate heat. The human body is very efficient at generating heat. When we burn a lot of fat, we generate a lot of heat. If we generate a lot of heat, we must find a way to quickly cool-off or we fry our brains. Nobody has found the answer to this dilemma. Moreover, even if chemicals were found that make brown fat burn more fat, humans have very few brown fat cells compared with white cells.

Thus, the possibility that we can find a chemical that will burn substantial amounts of fat is small, and if such chemical is found, we

Weight Loss

must find a way to prevent body temperature from increasing and burning the brain. This is a difficult task because body temperature raises very quickly when we burn fat for heat. Finally, if both problems are solved, we must still burn a lot of fat to make a difference, and we must burn more fat than the amount people eat in one day. Humans have such marvelous ability to adapt and eat food that we will find that people who burn more fat simply eat more fat to compensate. More hope can be placed on finding a chemical that will make us stop eating, but probably the body would adapt to it and people would start to eat again. Of course, there are other approaches, such as mouth surgery or hanging people from their toes for a week at a time (despite claims to the contrary, humans do not gain weight from breathing alone). As far as we can tell, you cannot eat a cake and then eat another and another without keeping them in your body. My advice is not to sell your exercise equipment yet.[9]

Is there hope in the new fats and fat substitutes?

Fat replacement products are in the market and soon there will be many more. "Simpless™" is marketed by the same company that makes Nutrasweet™. Scientists discovered that a protein extracted from egg white and milk can be processed so that it resembles and tastes like fat. Clearly, this is a major discovery. Tricking the taste buds into thinking that protein is fat may be useful. From the point of view of calories, because protein has only 4 calories per gram while fat has 9 calories per gram, merely replacing fat with protein would lead to less calories in food. However, the question still remains whether people will eat more calories anyway. My theory is that people look at themselves in the mirror and decide whether or not they look OK. If they look like they could add a few more pounds, they eat more. They stop eating not because they are not hungry, but because they fear being too overweight. Otherwise, we are always hungry for good tasting foods as a way to relieve stress, anxiety, boredom, etc.

Other companies are marketing alternative products that work on different principles. Some produce a fat that is formed with fats rarely found in foods and for which humans have relatively little absorption capacity. People eating those "fats" would feel like they are eating fat, but they would not absorb it. In this manner, you could eat your cake and lose it too.

Unfortunately, there are additional issues. Tricking the mouth is not the same as tricking the stomach or the mind. Fat containing foods

Weight Loss

take more time to be digested and therefore may produce a feeling of fullness for a longer period of time than foods that contain a fat substitute.

There is a danger that people will eat fewer EFAs because they are eating less fat. If you are deficient in EFAs, your body sends a signal that you need to eat more food. Scientists like myself believe that the signal to stop eating food ("**satiety signal**") is a signal that your body does not need more nutrients. If you eat a balanced diet, you are less likely to feel hungry. Because my research has shown that a huge number of people have EFA insufficiency, that is, the body cells do not get enough EFAs, these people receive regular signals from their bodies to eat more EFAs. Because people rarely do, they are always hungry.

According to my research, fat substitutes will fail in making people lose weight. People will remain hungry, or become even hungrier because they do not eat enough EFAs. The only solution to this hunger would be to find what type of EFAs people need and eat EFA supplements. Fortunately, this can easily be done by having a blood test and eating polyunsaturated oils or more natural vegetables and fish.

Excessive intake of protein (from fat substitutes), particularly of protein that overemphasizes certain amino acids, may lead to new diseases caused by the imbalance of amino acids, or may alter the body physiology and make it more vulnerable to cancer and other diseases. Remember that any nutritional imbalance may be hazardous.

Does this means that you must stop eating fat substitutes? Definitely not. Life involves a series of decisions among alternatives with different risks vs. benefits. Statistics suggest that overweight leads to cardiovascular disease, the current major cause of mortality and disability. If fat substitutes are the only way that some people can lose weight, then most likely the benefits of fat substitutes outweigh their disadvantages. Judging by the number of mildly to severely overweight people, it is obvious that millions find it hard to maintain healthy body weight. Fat substitutes provide an approach which could be the needed extra help for such people.

Should we eat more monounsaturated fats?

There are many scientists who believe that monounsaturated fatty acids (**MUFAs**) and even some specific types of saturated fatty acids (**SFAs**) are good for you. I disagree. It is well known that humans can make both SFAs and MUFAs from carbohydrates and protein. My

Weight Loss

research conclusively has shown that the body carefully regulates the amounts of MUFAs. The amount of MUFAs is inversely proportional to the amount of PUFAs. If you do not have enough PUFAs, there are only two choices for the body: to have more SFAs or to have more MUFAs. If you have less PUFA, the body makes more MUFA to compensate, in part, for the deficiency in PUFA. Because MUFAs are more "fluid" (softer) than SFAs, the body finds it better to make structures from MUFAs rather than SFAs.

Eating more or less MUFAs does not make a big difference in their relative amounts in the body. If you eat more MUFAs, your body makes fewer of them. If you eat less MUFAs, the body makes more of them.

There are some uses for high MUFA oils. They are more stable for cooking. However, you might as well use butter, which is even more stable. My research suggests that eating MUFAs has similar effects to eating SFAs.

Medium Chain Triglyceride fats do not decrease weight

Medium Chain Triglycerides, recently promoted as a weight loss supplement and source of "quick energy", actually are almost 100% saturated fat. They burn and metabolize like saturated fat. They are an excellent source of calories, like saturated fat, and are very useful for people who need fat for protection against cold and starvation, such as explorers. All calories from medium chain triglycerides are mixed with all other calories in the body. Calories not used for exercise or heat end up being stored as saturated and monounsaturated fat. The myth that Medium Chain Triglycerides do not increase weight arose because Medium Chain Triglycerides are digested and metabolized much faster by the intestine than the other types of fats we usually eat. These other types are called long chain triglycerides because the molecules are much longer. However, even if the body burns them faster or preferentially to other fat, you are merely substituting one source or calories for another. If your body were actually burning more fat, you would get "warmer", as discussed before. Thus, this is another meaningless extrapolation from an experiment to a completely different situation. Medium chain triglycerides are a source of calories like fat, with no EFAs and no redeeming value. If you need calories, eat pizza which often has some EFAs. Medium chain triglycerides are used in

Weight Loss

very thin patients who have difficulties absorbing regular fat. That condition excludes most of us.

Eating more carbohydrates does not help you burn more fat

The body needs only a small amount of carbohydrates (about 3 ounces per day) to burn fat. Eating more carbohydrates will not help you burn more fat. All calories, whether from carbohydrates or other sources, contribute to your total caloric intake. If you do not use all the calories you eat in one day, you store the excess as fat in your body. This is another example of a misinterpreted scientific principle.

Consumer Reports had an article titled "Losing Weight: what works, what doesn't" in its June, 1993 issue. Although some of the concepts were good ones, I disagree with its fundamental view on what causes overweight and disagree with many of the statements made in the article. In discussing the issue that some people are overweight and others are not, Consumer Reports states: "What makes for the difference? Primarily, it's the genes" (p. 347). I disagree. Primarily, it is human behavior, how we perceive ourselves, how we eat and what we are willing to consider as our "desirable" body weight. Consumer Reports also states (p. 351, bottom) that "the body's ability to store carbohydrates is limited, so when people eat more than their bodies can use, the excess is burned". Calories from carbohydrates, which are not used by the body, are converted to SFAs or MUFAs. You can gain weight from eating a pure carbohydrate diet. Moreover, you can become EFA deficient, thereby increasing your chances of dying of heart disease or stroke.

EFAs do not make you burn more fat but can make you less hungry

My research has now been presented at many scientific meetings and published in many journals. I found that many authors are writing about my ideas, but have misunderstood them. I have proposed that when people have a deficiency of EFAs, they remain hungry for the EFAs. This "hunger" makes people want to eat more food and more fat, and contributes to weight gain. Correction of EFA abnormalities may produce satiety, that is, not being hungry. I say "may", because in

Weight Loss

humans the *need* to eat is in great part determined by psychological rather than physiological reasons.

I have also stated that some people cannot form enough EFA derivatives from the EFA precursors, probably due to some nutritional abnormality, disease, old age or genetic differences. In those individuals, eating EFA derivatives such as GLA (see chapters in EFAs and oils), may increase the amounts of EFA derivatives in the body and turn off hunger.

Authors have confused these statements and have written that eating GLA will burn "brown fat" and make you lose weight. This is not true. Humans have very little brown fat. Most of the studies about "brown fat" were conducted in animals, and thus are not applicable to humans. My research has shown that the fatty acid metabolism of rats and many animals used in research is so different from human metabolism that it is very difficult to interpret animal research in terms of human results.

10 reasons to avoid eating well

Doctors hear the most amazing stories from patients who are overweight. The most common one is the "vegetable man" (or woman). The **vegetable person** can convert air into food, like plants do. The vegetable person is overweight and claims to eat only an apple a day, supplemented, on occasion, with a small carrot and a few other vegetables. He or she rarely eats anything else. He/she does drink lots of water, exercises every day, does not smoke, takes all prescribed medications, and neither smokes nor drinks alcohol. He/she admits that, sometimes, for important events, he may eat a small slice of pizza or taste a little bit of ice cream, but, when asked, the last time was at least one year ago. The vegetable person is a an archeologist's dream. He/she is the missing link in evolution. He/she has the genes leftover from 2 billion years ago when plants dominated and mammals did not exist. He/she can convert air and oxygen into carbohydrate, protein and fat, particularly fat. He/she can gain weight by breathing air. If you know this person you could make as much money as finding the famous "talking frog" (the one you do not want to kiss because princes are a dime a dozen, but talking frogs are priceless.)

In honor of these vegetable men and women, here are 10 of the 99 reasons why some find it difficult to lose weight, and cannot eat a healthy diet:

- 1. It rained and I grew.

Weight Loss

- 2. We had so much sun that I could not stop growing.

- 3. I took a deep breath and I gained 5 pounds. You do not want me to stop breathing, do you Doc?

- 4. I found a bear (thief, alien, space invader, politician, tax collector, _____) in my kitchen and we had to order pizzas.

- 5. I was captured by aliens who force-fed me.

- 6. The supermarket was all out of spinach and vegetables and I could only find beer and pizza.

- 7. There was a tornado warning and we were left with food for 240 days and no electricity, so we had to eat it all in one week.

- 8. My mother forced me to stop eating vegetables.

- 9. The President declared vegetables dangerous to our health.

- 10. The Government found poisonous chemicals in vegetables (this may be true, but most foods are contaminated today).

References and notes

[1] H.S. Solomon, *N Eng J. Medicine*, Letters to the Editor, p.831, 1984.

[2] Manson SE, Stampfer MJ, Hennekens CH, Willett WC. Body weight and longevity. A reassessment. *JAMA* (Journal of the Am. Medical Assoc.), 1987; 257:353-358.

[3] The formulas must be adjusted for people who are muscular. Muscle weighs more than fat.

[4] The amount of protein depends on body size. You may want to eat a minimum of 50 grams of protein per day if you strickly follow this low calorie diet.

[5] A simple trick is to look at the urine: it should be lightly yellow, almost transparent.

[6] Oils are discussed in other chapters.

[7] Remember that obesity refers to greatly increased overweight, more than 20% above the usual recommended weight for height, which is already higher than the numbers I suggest.

[8] Balon TW. Flesh or Bones? *The Journal of NIH Research*, 1994; 6:14 (letter to advice and dissent).

[9] For a recent review see Ezzell C. Getting the Skinny on Obesity. *J. of NIH Research*, April 1994, 4:71-75. Has an excellent diagram on heat generation by uncoupling protein in brown adipose tissue (for medical students).

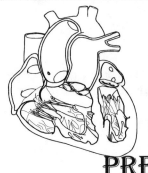

IV.1

FATS THAT LOWER CHOLESTEROL AND PREVENT HEART DISEASE

"Lower your cholesterol, prevent clots and soften your arteries."

Topics: *Basic principles. Key therapeutic factors. Exercise, meals and oil supplements.*

Summary

The objective of nutritional therapy is to improve your health. When your health improves you will feel better. Over time, you will notice that your blood pressure and high cholesterol decrease, indicating that your body is healthier. The key therapeutic factors are: a thin body to match the decreased function of the heart as you get older, and a diet based on natural foods high in essential fats and low in total calories.

Basic Treatment Principles

This chapter provides the principles of nutritional therapy for cardiovascular disease. While the **prevention diet** helps maintain good health, the **treatment diet** corrects for the dietary abuses that led to disease. The treatment must correct for years of abuse to your body, and thus must be tailored to match each person's history. Treatment consists of balanced meals and oil supplements aimed at replacing body fat with essential fats. Occasional animal and fish foods are also indicated. Your age, sex, environment and type of medical problem determines how much you must eat of each type of fat.

Lowering your cholesterol with balanced consumption of essential fats will usually normalize your blood pressure, soften your vessels, and prevent vessel obstruction. Cholesterol generally increases with age. Therefore, many physicians still consider it "normal" for a person to increase his cholesterol as he gets older. We encourage people to remain young; therefore they should seek the body weight and cholesterol levels of a healthy young adult. Additionally, EFA balance could make your skin softer and younger looking.

Treatment Objectives

The objective of therapy is threefold: (1) to modify the fluidity and ability of your body to form clots according to your own risk factors; (2) to make your vessels softer and thereby reduce high blood pressure and total cholesterol; and (3) to decrease the ratio total/ HDL cholesterol. These objectives are consistent with recent updated cholesterol treatment guidelines which emphasize diet and weight loss and lower goals for LDL cholesterol.[1] Older adults (over 60 years old) should realize that their levels of cholesterol are not good indicators or predictors of their risk of death from coronary heart disease.[2] **Adults over 60 years of age cannot rely on cholesterol testing to measure their risk of heart disease**. Unfortunately, these findings are so recent that most people are not informed about them. My research has found that a fatty acid profile such as the test **EFA-SR** is the best blood test both to predict risk of coronary death and to tell you what foods to eat or avoid.

Make your blood less likely to form clots

In treating cardiovascular disease, we often begin with **fish oils**, which have the immediate effect of making your blood less likely to form **clots**. This change prevents a heart attack while you work on improving the quality of your blood vessels. In terms of blood tests, the objective is to increase your **bleeding time** to 6-10 minutes, depending on your medical condition (this test is described in Part II). However, before you start, your doctor may want to determine whether your body can make enough ω3 derivatives (found in fish oils) from the ω3 precursor linolenic acid found in vegetable oils. This information may be found by analysis of blood before and after eating linolenic acid for 10-20 weeks and analyzing your blood to see if you have an increase in the ω3 derivatives.

Results obtained from taking fish oils can be obtained by eating fish itself; however this would require large quantities of fish. Sick people without enough ω3 need to increase their body levels of linolenic (ω3) derivatives quickly without gaining weight; and they can do this by eating fish and vegetable oils rich in ω3s. In contrast, healthy people with adequate amounts of ω3 fats in their body can maintain ω3 balance by eating fish because they only need to maintain or slightly increase their body stores of ω3.

Reducing your blood fat

The next step in treatment of cardiovascular disease is the elimination of unhealthy fats from your blood. In medical terms, you want to reduce your total cholesterol and triglycerides and increase your HDL. For optimal health your cholesterol count should be below 150, considerably lower than the figures usually considered "normal". However, a level below 200 is still a significant step in reducing your risk.

Softening your vessels and normalizing blood pressure

Concurrently, you change your meals to increase the amounts of linoleic acid (ω6) to make your vessels softer, thus reducing their resistance to blood blow and decreasing blood pressure to desirable limits for a healthy person. Generally, a blood pressure lessl than 140/90 is considered "normal". However, I believe that a desirable range is between 110/55 and 120/75. Values are different for men and women and depend on your body type.

Normalizing blood sugar (glucose)

Many people with cardiovascular disease have elevated glucose ("hyperglycemia"), a sign of Diabetes. Eliminating concentrated sweets, losing excess body weight, eating less saturated fats and more essential fat will help normalize your fasting glucose. It will also reduce strong ups and downs in blood sugar that can make you feel tired or dizzy.

Fats that lower cholesterol

Creating healthy blood cells

Another goal of treatment is to improve the health of your blood cells by eating the mixture of EFAs that brings your fatty acid profile within desirable levels. When your body has optimal composition, you should have no anemia and no evidence of premature red cell destruction. Your reticulocyte count (an index of red cell turnover or destruction) should be normal. **Anemia** or inappropriate **reticulocyte count** indicates that your body is not in nutritional balance. You may often hear a doctor tell you that you have "mild chronic anemia" or you have the anemia "normally" found in women. This implies that because many people have this type of mild anemia, it is OK for you to have it too. I disagree. You should not have anemia if you are in good health. Correcting nutritional abnormalities and your EFA balance has virtually no risk and could help improve the health of your blood cells.

Improving organ function

Ultimately, all other blood tests should be normal and the function of your organs should improve. Blood tests of kidney function should show that they are working better to filter and excrete unnecessary chemicals. Also, you will be able to enjoy your body more during physical activity because your heart can keep up with your body's needs.

Symptoms vs. Disease

In treating cardiovascular disease we must emphasize treatment of the disease itself, not just **symptoms**. If your car is making a strange noise, you could buy ear plugs so that you no longer hear the noise (symptom elimination) or you could fix the car (treatment). Our approach is to fix the car. However, remember that many test results identify or monitor a symptom, not the disease. Sometimes you can "fix" the symptom without changing the disease. This can occur when you lower high cholesterol or high blood pressure with medications.

High cholesterol and high blood pressure are symptoms that indicate that the body is not functioning properly. If we treat the disease the symptoms will disappear. It is possible to treat the symptoms: Many drugs do that. Treating the symptoms, such as reducing your high blood pressure with drugs, prevents some of the complications of hypertension but does not cure the basic cause of hypertension. **Our**

Fats that lower cholesterol

objective with nutritional therapy is to cure the
fundamental causes of the disease, not to eliminate the
symptoms.

Drugs vs. Nutrition

Many medical problems can be treated with this approach:

- First let nature cure the problem. Often, natural means,
  including good nutrition, will solve the problem. But
  sometimes nature can use help. Intervention is particularly
  important when the body has suffered trauma (such as a
  broken bone, severe cut or infection), or is in the midst of
  severe breakdown (such as a heart attack).
- If the disease is severe or does not improve by natural means,
  then more drastic approaches such as surgery or drugs may be
  needed. But remember that surgery and drugs have side
  effects; the dangers of the disease and the dangers of the
  surgery or drug must be balanced.[3]

Virtually all cardiovascular disease improves with nutritional therapy.
However, many drugs are sold to treat high blood pressure and elevated
cholesterol. These drugs reduce high blood pressure and elevated
cholesterol. However, such treatment begs the question: Do these
drugs successfully treat underlying cardiovascular disease, or are they
merely treating symptoms? Do they actually improve life expectancy?
No one knows the answer. My research has defined the major
nutritional imbalance present in cardiovascular disease: a deficiency in
essential fats. Because drugs do not change the fat composition of the
body, they cannot successfully treat the disease. They may alter
cholesterol or lower blood pressure, but EFA deficiency remains.

What to expect from treatment

Nutritional treatment is different from what we have come to expect
(but don't always get) from medication. The patient who goes from
doctor to doctor looking for a drug for heart and circulation problems
expects relatively quick results. The patient undertaking nutritional
therapy knows that he or she is responsible for getting well, and that
the consequences of decades of unhealthy eating cannot be undone in a
few weeks. In fact, treatment never stops unless you have reached the

---

Fats that lower cholesterol

goals outlined above. In essence, you will be "in treatment" (i.e., eating healthy foods) for the rest of your life. If you do quite well, and you improve substantially, you can deviate slightly from "treatment" and still remain healthy. If you are quite sick, you need to adhere rigorously to your "treatment". A marvelous side effect of nutritional therapy is that you will find a healthy diet is as satisfying and delicious as an unhealthy one. And what's more, it brings other benefits. Losing weight will give you more energy to do all the things you want to do. You should also notice an increase in your mental alertness. And, most important, you will feel better and be more hopeful about the future.

> ***Eat to live; do not live to eat.***

Dietary treatment

The basic rule in any kind of effective treatment is that each person is different. Even though we provide guidelines in this book, they need to be modified to meet your particular needs. The average American wears a size 8 shoe, but a size 8 shoe may not be the right one for you. Again, common sense and your physician are the best guides.

The more severe the disease, the stricter your diet must be. Sick people have smaller working hearts. Therefore they should have smaller bodies. Moreover, sick people have accumulated, through years of bad eating, much hard fat in their arteries. To clean those arteries and replace the hard fat with soft, polyunsaturated fat requires years of careful work; it is sometimes impossible unless the patient is willing to undertake a radical nutritional treatment, which we will discuss below.

An occasional "feast" is acceptable if you are meeting your health goals

Occasional feasts

If you follow a healthy diet you can occasionally deviate from it and have some of the foods you crave: ice cream, pizza, cake, chocolate, etc. You can use almost any condiment or spice, in moderation. (We say in moderation because some people can eat a whole bottle of condiment at one meal!). Once you reach your desirable health goals, you can deviate once per week and still maintain your good health. Of course, moderation still counts! Eating 6 pizzas once a month is too much.

Fats that lower cholesterol

Participation in an eating contest once per year to prove that you can eat 257 hot dogs in one sitting is not moderation. Eating 2 slices of pizza or 1 hot dog once a week may not be unreasonable if your weight and EFA balance are adequate otherwise.

Basic treatment

Improving your health is not too hard. There is no need to follow exotic diets, or rotate foods in mysterious ways such as eating apples on Tuesdays, grapefruits on Wednesdays, or bananas on Sundays. The treatment for cardiovascular disease is similar to the preventive approach, but requires a more aggressive and restrictive strategy.

More vegetables; less animal fat; some oil supplements

Becoming thin

Attaining the ideal weight for your height is the single most important thing you can do for your heart. Monitor your weight about once per week. Your body must adapt to your weakened heart, becoming smaller so that the remaining healthy portions of your heart are not overworked. The objective is to become as thin as possible without becoming sick or malnourished.

Decrease unneeded clot formation

A nutritional program takes many months before improvements are noticed. In the meantime, to prevent a clot from obstructing an artery, you should eat fish and fish oils which decrease the formation of clots. In the next chapters we explain how the ω3 fats reduce clot formation. But beware: This is not something you should do alone; you must have appropriate blood tests and be under the guidance of a doctor. Because ω3 fats reduce clot formation, you may be more susceptible to bleeding. This must be monitored closely; internal bleeding can have catastrophic results, including stroke.

Eat more essential fats

A diet high in essential fats and low in saturated fat, together with a weight reduction program (i.e., fewer calories) will improve the function of your cells and decrease your Cholesterol/HDL ratio. The objective is to improve the function of your cells; the consequence is a decrease in

Fats that lower cholesterol

your LDL cholesterol and in Cholesterol/HDL ratio. To accomplish
these objectives will probably require supplementation with vegetable
oils. Very healthy people may not need to correct for years of dietary
deficiency, and do not need vegetable oil supplements. But those
wanting to successfully treat cardiovascular disease must correct for
years of poor eating habits.

Case studies: The care of two patients with signs of heart disease[4]

Dr. P, a 43 year old clinical psychologist

Dr. P is on his feet most of the day. He exercises frequently and rides a
bicycle about one hour each day. He says that his diet consists of
mostly vegetables and little red meat. His weight is OK, his total
cholesterol is about 230, and his mild hypertension is controlled with
drugs. His problem is that he cannot bring his cholesterol down. He
does not like the side effects of the drugs prescribed by his physician to
decrease his cholesterol.

Everybody tells him he follows a terrific diet and looks great. But he is
not dumb. He knows something is wrong. His cholesterol is high. He
has hypertension. He is likely to have a heart attack in 10 years. But
he is too young to die. What can he do?

When I saw him I discovered "holes" in his story.

Overweight: Dr. P is 5' 7" without shoes[5] and weighs 172 lbs. He told
me that in his 20's he weighed under 140 lbs. and felt great. Thus, 140
lbs. would be Dr. P's healthy weight; 145 lbs. may be OK, but certainly
not 172 lbs.!

Too much food: Dr. P's exercise program is adequate. Therefore he is
simply eating too much food. Careful questioning reveals that his *low*
fat diet (under 35% of calories as fat, which is low compared with 35%-
40% for most Americans) is actually very high in pure carbohydrates.
In the body, these foods are equivalent to saturated fat when eaten in
excess. Dr. P eats too many sherbets, fruits, and whole grain foods
which he mistakenly thinks are healthy in any amount.

Few essential fats: Dr. P's diet is high in saturated fat and pure
carbohydrates, but very low in essential fats. All the excess

---

Fats that lower cholesterol

carbohydrates he eats get converted by his body into saturated fat. As revealed by the blood test **EFA-SR**, we learn that: (a) he has reduced levels of both ω3 and ω6 in his body, and high levels of SFAs and MUFAs; (b) his ratio of ω3/ω6 is below normal levels (he is more deficient in ω3 than ω6); (c) the ratio of **eicosapentaenoic to arachidonic acid** (**EPA/AA** = 20:5ω3/20:4ω6) is about average; (d) he has plenty of ω3 derivatives given his levels of linolenic acid.[6] We know from the clinical history that he is the type of patient who can form clots that cause heart attacks or strokes.

Recommendations: Lose over 15 lbs., 2 lbs./week by elimination of sweets and limiting to one fruit per day; eat more green vegetables and less processed food; eat one tablespoon of soybean oil/day. This mixture will provide appropriate amounts and ratios of ω3 and ω6. In addition, about 2 fish oil capsules per day to quickly increase the EPA/AA ratio (fish oils are rich in EPA).[7] After several months we will test his blood again and decide whether he needs more soybean oil, more safflower oil (high in ω6), or flax seeds (even higher in ω3 than soybean oil), and whether to increase or decrease the fish oil capsules (depending on achieving a target goal for EPA/AA).

Dr. M, a 58 year old. rehabilitation specialist

Dr. M is 5'10", 160 lbs. He follows mainly a vegetarian's diet and exercises daily. He feels great, with no health problems. His fear? His last cholesterol was 190. He wants it to be below 150 but cannot get it there. He wants to decrease his Total/ HDL cholesterol ratio. What is he doing wrong?

A few questions identified the problem. Dr. M followed a traditional diet high in complex carbohydrates and low in fat as recommended by practically all medical and public health organizations. He had done what he was told to do by his physicians and their advice echoed what he had learned in medical school. Most of his meals consisted of processed breads, cereals, grains, pasta, and fruits.

I explained to Dr. M that his diet was very low in EFAs because most of his calories came from carbohydrates, SFAs and MUFAs. He had been eating virtually no ω3s. His blood test results showed low-normal levels of ω6 and very low levels of ω3 when compared with ideal levels. We developed a plan to his EFA profiles towards his ideal goal. In his case, his ideal goal was not to be average; instead he wanted to have

Fats that lower cholesterol

values similar to those of subjects that appear to be in very good health. He was willing to follow a more extreme diet in order to significantly increase the ratio of PUFA/NoPUFA in his plasma to about 1.2. This ratio is the proportion of total fat which consists of PUFA over the proportion which is not PUFA (SFA + MUFA). The average value is about 1.0, with values below 0.9 as abnormally low. However, I have found that very healthy subjects have values around 1.2.

His treatment required a shift to more foods in their natural state, green vegetables, 1/2 tablespoon of soybean oil/day and 1 tbsp/day flax seed oil until his cholesterol declined to below 130, and perhaps losing 5 lbs. (to be on the thin side). The fat analysis **EFA-SR** was repeated 3 months later. Based on the test results, he reduced the amount of soybean oil to 1/2 tbsp/day. Because he liked fruits, he replaced the calories from oils no longer needed with fruits. One year after this treatment Dr. M's cholesterol was below 150 and he said he felt great.

References and notes

[1] The guidelines are available from NIH. Also see: National Cholesterol Education Program. Detection, evaluation, and treatment of high blood cholesterol in adults (Adult Treatment Panel II). *Circulation* 1994 March; 89:1329-445.

[2] Grover SA et al. Serum lipid screening to identify high-risk individuals for coronary death. *Arch Intern Med* 1994; 154:679-84.

[3] For example, if you have a cold, most antibiotics will not work Antibiotics work against bacteria, not viruses such as the virus that produces the common cold. Using antibiotics may in fact harm the body's defenses and prolong the disease. Many people can't wait and insist on taking antibiotics to fight a viral infection. Because most viral infections go away on their own, they get cured even with antibiotics. On the other hand, a severe bacterial infection could kill you and antibiotics would be a definite help in this case. Cancer is another disease where aggressive therapy is often required. Cancer usually grows unless it is stopped with surgery or drugs.

[4] These stories are composites and do not represent actual people. Any similarity with a person is a coincidence. The advice given here may not apply to you.

[5] Many people are not as tall as they think they are. More than 80% of the people I measure are shorter than they think they are.

[6] The EFA Status Report shows that the ratios of derivatives to precursors, DFA/PFA for both ω6 and ω3 are normal to elevated, and the levels of linoleic (ω6) and linolenic (ω3) are decreased. This indicates that the patient can form derivatives and that the reason he does not have enough is because he does not have enough of the essential fatty acids linoleic and linolenic acid.

[7] The actual number depends on your blood test results and your clinical condition. In this case, 2 were enough. He does not have angina or an imminent risk of a heart attack. The 2 oil capsules will increase his EPA/AA ratio which will continue to increase slowly as a result of eating more linolenic (ω3) acid.

Fats that lower cholesterol

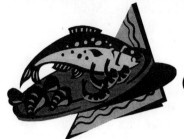

IV.2

OILS AND FATS

"Vegetable oils are liquid fats"

Topics: *Vegetable oils. Sources of the essential fats ω3 and ω6. Uncooked vs. cooked oils. Oil storage.*

Summary

Vegetables oils are the best source of the parent essential fats ω3 and ω6. For many people the proper vegetable oil may provide all their required EFAs. Oils must be used raw (uncooked); cooking changes the chemical structure of the essential fats. Store polyunsaturated oils in the refrigerator.

Essential fat content of common fats and oils

Vegetable oils consist of a mixture of SFAs, MUFAs and EFAs. They rarely contain EFA derivatives. However, healthy humans can manufacture most of the EFA derivatives it needs. Oils from animal sources may contain EFA derivatives (see tables in the appendix).

- **High in ω6:** Safflower, Sunflower, and Corn oils.
- **High in ω3 and ω6:** Soybean and Walnut oils.
- **Very high in ω3:** Linseed (flax) oil (ω3 precursor) and fish oils (ω3 derivatives).
- **Some ω6's:** Almond, Cottonseed, and Peanut oils.
- **High in MUFAs, some ω6:** Olive oil.

- **Mainly SFAs:** Butter, lard, coconut, and palm oils. Most hydrogenated oils.

- **High in *trans* fatty acids:** Hydrogenated oils (such as those found in commercial cookies, doughnuts and cakes), beef fat, many margarines, "dairy" creamers.

- **Mixtures:** Some of the new margarines in the market have practically no *trans* fatty acids and many ω6s, and some ω3s.

Because of the increased awareness about cholesterol and heart disease, companies are introducing new products which are low in cholesterol and SFAs, high in MUFA and TFAs and low in EFAs. When you read food labels, remember:

- **Some cholesterol causes no harm.** Remember most of the cholesterol in your body is manufactured by the body itself in response to high levels of SFAs and low levels of EFAs. It is not required that a product be extremely low in cholesterol, in order to keep the body healthy or return the body to health. Foods with less than 50 mg of cholesterol per serving are low; eating less than 20 mg is like saving pennies to buy a house. It is not necessary to eat zero cholesterol foods.[1]

- **Vegetable foods and oils have practically no cholesterol.** Therefore, their cholesterol content is usually irrelevant. Advertising some oils as low in cholesterol is like telling you that some water is wet.

- **Polyunsaturated fat = Essential fats ω3 + ω6.** Choose products that have a mixture of both fats.

- **Select foods low in total fat and calories, and with a high percentage of polyunsaturated fat.** Beware that some oils are high in monounsaturated fats, and low in saturated fat and polyunsaturated fat. Advertised as low in saturated fat and cholesterol, they are actually less desirable than the oils higher in both EFAs and SFAs.

- **Read labels carefully.** The label on the oil should state its fatty acid composition (unfortunately, not all do). It should also indicate whether it is "partially hydrogenated". Do not buy oils that say "partially hydrogenated". Partial hydrogenation destroys most of the ω3 and some of the ω6 fats

---

that are important to your good health. Also, read the label for the date: Choose the freshest oil.

Oil quality

The quality of the oil depends on the brand. Try several brands until you find one that gives you consistent results. Oils preserve better when they are vacuum packed and stored in dark bottles. Health food stores often have better quality oils but at slightly higher prices.

Fresh oils high in essential fats (polyunsaturated oils) are liquid when stored in the refrigerator. When the chemical characteristics of the important essential fats change, the oil becomes mushy and hardens. Discard oil high in PUFAs when it becomes cloudy, mushy or solid (or use it only for cooking but not for eating). A polyunsaturated oil should remain liquid in the refrigerator.

Some oils become cloudy or partially solid in the refrigerator because they contain low amounts of PUFA. Olive and peanut oils may solidify in the refrigerator. This does not mean that they are rancid; it merely means that they are high in MUFAs which solidify in the refrigerator. Olive oil is not dangerous in small quantities, and has a strong flavor for those who like it. For those fond of this flavor, I recommend mixing it with other oils high in PUFA.

Some cold pressed oils are not refined, look cloudy (but not solid) and have a strong taste. We do not know whether these oils are better than the transparent, almost tasteless refined oils. Because pesticides dissolve quite well in oil, extraction of these pesticides is important. Apparently some companies extract the pesticides from the oil using chemicals. Other companies make oil with organically-grown foods, presumably with few pesticides. But even organically grown foods may be contaminated with pesticides found in water and air. Proper labeling, including pesticide and chemical content in oils, should be mandated by the government.[2]

How to use oils

Eat oils raw. You can pour oil on most foods: salads, breads, pizza, mashed potatoes, pastry, vegetables. If you must fry or bake, choose corn oil, palm oil, or butter. These oils are more stable and less likely to deteriorate or burn at high temperatures. The issue here is a balance of several risks. The best choice is to avoid fried or baked foods containing oil. But if you choose to eat baked foods with oils, those cooked with

Oils and Fat

PUFA oils may have additional chemicals produced by the cooking process which could increase your chances of getting cancer or heart disease. Saturated fat changes little when cooked. The best answer is still not known. Buy a **mayonnaise or dressing** that is made primarily of oil recommended previously. Avoid those made with partially hydrogenated oils.

Fatty acid composition of common foods

High in PUFAs: Almonds, walnuts, filberts, pecans, pumpkin seeds, some mayonnaise and salad dressings, fish, and oils such as corn, soybean, cottonseed, sunflower, and safflower. Seeds from which the above oils are made.

High in MUFAs: Avocados, olives, peanuts, cashews.

High in SFAs: Butter, cheese, meat fat, chocolate (but not cocoa), lard, coconut and palm oils.

Oil Effects: what EFAs do

Many important functions of essential fats are still under investigation. The best known functions are:

1. **ω3 fatty acids** decrease cholesterol and triglycerides, lower high blood pressure, make it more difficult to form clots, modify the immune system, and improve eye function.

2. **ω6 fatty acids** decrease cholesterol and triglycerides, lower high blood pressure, modify the immune system, improve skin function, and soften vessels.

3. **Increased ratio of** ω3/ω6 causes a decrease in platelet aggregation, an increase in bleeding time (a special test to measure platelet aggregation); a very high value of ω3/ω6 can cause an increase in bleeding. A very low value can cause harmful clotting.

Precautions

Oil is a plant extract. Like all extracts, it is concentrated beyond nature's intention; it is possible to eat too much. Because life is a balance of risks and benefits, if you have cardiovascular disease the risk

Oils and Fat

of dying from the disease is much greater than the risk of dying from eating too much oil. Thin, healthy people can eat a little bit of butter and saturated fat without ill effects; sick people would most likely get worse after eating saturated fat. Remember: There is no "free lunch"; a free lunch is usually too salty or too fatty.

Approximate Fatty acid composition of common oils

Oil	18:2ω6	18:3ω6	18:3ω3	SFA	MUFA
Borage	34	44	0	?	?
Black Currant	?	18	9 (ω3)	?	?
Corn	59	0	0	12	24
Canola	24	0	10	6%	60
Flax	18	0	57	9	16
Grapeseed	70	0	0	10	16
Olive	8	0	0	10	82
Peanut	32	0	0	17	46
Primrose	72	9	0	8	11
Pumpkin	57	0	0-15	9	34
Safflower	75	0	0.4	9	12
Sesame	42	0	0.3	14	40
Sunflower	66	0	0	10	20
Soybean	58	0	7	14	23
Walnut	53	0	10	9	23

References and notes

[1] Unless you eat many foods with 50 mg cholesterol per serving or many servings.

[2] In case of doubt the best strategy consists of two parts: First, avoid a doubtful product, and second, write to the government and Congress to insist on proper labeling and the reduction of pesticides and toxic chemicals in food.

Oils and Fat

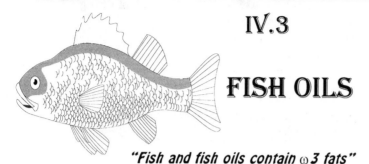

IV.3

FISH OILS

"Fish and fish oils contain ω3 fats"

Topics: *Fish and Fish Oils. Effects. Fish oils instead of fish. Types of fish oils. Buying and storing. Checking quality. How to use.*

Summary

Fish oils are derived from the fat found in cold water fish. Further processing produces an extract that is very high in special types of ω3 fats. Vegetable oils contain the precursor ω3, linolenic acid, which is then used by the body to make other complex ω3 fats. Fish oils already contain these *complex* ω3 fats and therefore produce stronger and quicker effects than vegetable oils.

Many companies manufacture and sell extracts of fish oils. The most traditional and inexpensive one, cod liver oil, is high in ω3 fats but also contains potentially dangerous amounts of vitamins A and D, and other undesirable natural fats and chemicals. It has a very strong flavor, and like other fish oils, becomes rancid very quickly when exposed to heat, light or air. Most commercial companies have found a way to extract fish fat and produce oils with more ω3 fats than cod liver oil, but without the extra vitamin A and D and the other harmful fats. Of course, you pay a much higher price for them. People who do not get enough vitamin A or D in their meals could benefit from their presence in cod liver oil. Most people need less than half a teaspoon of cod liver oil per day; that amount is not likely to produce harmful effects.

Fish oils produce several desirable effects: They lower high cholesterol and triglycerides, reduce hypertension and make the blood less likely to form the clots that obstruct arteries. For the same reasons, they may increase bleeding, produce anemia or make an ulcer worse. Most people may obtain all the ω3 fats they need from the ω3 fatty acid in vegetables and vegetable oils. Therefore, fish oils are to be used under medical supervision and only by those individuals who cannot improve their cardiovascular condition using vegetable oils.

Fish versus Fish Oils

Fish oils quickly reduce the likelihood that a clot will obstruct an artery, giving you time for the rest of your diet to improve your arteries. Fish oils contain the ω3 fats that we call derivatives or daughters of linolenic acid. Derivatives have a more complex chemical structure than their precursor; the derivatives are more polyunsaturated in form.[1] Derivatives also act faster than the precursor linolenic acid found in vegetable oils because the body does not have to spend time producing them.

Research has shown that most people have the enzymes to make the ω3 fats found in fish oils from the ω3 fats found in vegetable oils.[2] However, vegetable oils usually must be taken for several weeks before they begin to have the same effects as fish oils.[3]

Fish fat contains Eicosapentaenoic acid (**EPA** = 20:5ω3) [4] and docosahexaenoic acid (**DHA** = 22:6ω3) [5]. Both of these fatty acids have long carbon chains with multiple double bonds (many kinks). Fish fat also contains a small amount of linolenic acid, 18:3ω3, and various other derivatives of the ω3 family[6]. Research indicates that many of these very long chain fatty acids are essential for proper brain function.

The ratio of eicosapentaenoic/ arachidonic acid (**EPA/AA** = 20:5ω3/20:4ω6) is proportional to the amount of time it takes the platelets to form a clot. As we stated before, **EPA** is derived from linolenic (ω3) and arachidonic acid (**AA)** from linoleic (ω6) acid.

Desirable effects

The ω3 fats are very polyunsaturated. They appear to improve the flexibility and softness of vessels and improve the overall utilization of glucose ("blood sugar") in diabetes. These changes result in a variety of beneficial effects, the most important of which are explained below.

The ω3 fats in fish oils decrease the amount of total fat in the blood. They decrease elevated cholesterol and elevated triglyceride levels.

Fish Oils

They may increase HDL cholesterol, a desirable effect. These effects may be due to the fact that many people have a deficiency of ω3s and the body compensates by releasing more fat and cholesterol into the blood in an attempt to have enough ω3s to feed the hungry cells. When you eat more ω3s, the body is no longer so "hungry," and it stops releasing so much fat into your blood. This is the fat and cholesterol which eventually would have accumulated in your vessels and made them hard.

Fish oils may be more beneficial than vegetable oils for the few individuals who have extremely high cholesterol or triglycerides ("hyperlipidemia", a condition discussed in later chapters).

Eating more ω3 fats makes it more difficult for the blood to form clots; technically, ω3 fats prevent platelet aggregation.[7] The prevention of clot formation is a desirable effect for most people who have a tendency to form clots inside the arteries. About 20% to 50% of the US adult population, particularly men, fall into this category: You can find out by having the proper blood tests done, which include the fatty acid profile **EFA-SR** and a bleeding time test.

The ω3 fats also decrease high blood pressure, prevent or slow some complications of diabetes such as blindness, reduce headaches, and improve kidney function. They may improve the well being of asthmatics and people with allergies, and also facilitate the movement of arthritic joints because they alter the function of the immune system and reduce inflammation. Many diseases caused by *undesirable* alterations of the immune system may be improved by the use of fish oils.

Many of the benefits of ω3 and ω6 oils occur because proper consumption of essential fats improves the functioning of all cells in the body, from the perspective of people who do not have enough to begin with. If you already have adequate essential fats, eating more could make you sick. Because most people lack adequate dietary intake of EFAs, they likely can benefit from supplementation, especially if unwilling to change their diets dramatically.

Side effects

Fish oils must be taken almost every day; if you stop taking them their effects disappear within a few weeks. Fish oils increase bleeding

Fish Oils

because the ω3 fats make it more difficult for the body to form clots. The increased tendency to bleed could make you bruise more easily, or worse, make you more susceptible to a stroke. Even a minor stroke caused by bleeding in the brain could cause considerable damage if your blood does not coagulate promptly. (However, most people are more likely to suffer a stroke caused by a clot obstructing an artery than a stroke caused by a blood vessel breaking and leaking blood). If you have an ulcer, diverticulitis or any other disease that makes you bleed easily, a cut could cause substantial blood loss and consequently, anemia. We do not know whether women who have long menstrual periods become anemic after taking fish oils for many months.

Because more research on side effects of fish oils is necessary to answer these questions thoroughly, **it is essential that fish oils only be eaten under the careful supervision of a doctor**. Many of the worst side effects, including bleeding inside the brain, become more likely over time. Fish oils can be a very useful part of a treatment plan for cardiovascular disease or diabetes, but must be included only with caution and as a temporary measure while waiting for vegetable oil supplementation and dietary change to have their effects. Incidentally, taking *large* amounts of ω3s from ω3 concentrated foods such as flax seeds could have similar effects.[8]

Fish oils alter the production of many important hormones known as eicosanoids.[9] The consequence is that they modify the immune system and most other physiological processes. We do not know what happens when physiological processes are altered by eating large quantities of fish oils, but we suspect that pregnancy and delivery may be substantially affected. Therefore pregnant women should not take fish oils except under close medical supervision. In addition, some fish oils contain natural chemicals and rare and possible toxic fatty acids whose effects are not known. However, most of the encapsulated oils on the market are refined, and the toxic fatty acids removed. There is tremendous variability in chemical composition among the various brands on the market. Moreover, the oils are very unstable and often deteriorate after a few weeks on the shelf. Deterioration is even faster once the protective capsules and seals are broken.[10] Fish oils deteriorate faster than vegetable oils. They have a strong smell and taste. They cost more than vegetable oils.

Fish Oils

Why fish oils instead of fish

If cold water fish has ω3 fats, why eat fish oils when one can eat a small amount of fish? The reason is that you need more ω3s to prevent or treat heart disease, you need to eat much more ω3s that fish can provide. A small amount of fish oil extracts will provide ω3s without a harmful increase in calories. Some fish may be polluted with industrial chemicals, which are often removed when fish oils are extracted. Most oil capsules are healthier than cod liver oil because they do not contain some potentially toxic fatty acids and other chemicals naturally found in cod liver oil. People who must lose weight or who require large quantities of ω3 fats will find it more practical to take a small amount of fish oil rather than eat a large amount of fish. The major drawback is that supplementing the diet with fish oil capsules costs more money than just incorporating fish into one's diet.

As a general rule, fish oil contains 10 to 50 times more ω3 fats than an equal amount of fish. People trying to lose weight may find that egg whites or tofu and fish oil extracts provide protein and ω3 fats with fewer calories than fish. On the other hand, fish alone is a good source of protein and ω3 fats, and may be used as a replacement for other sources of protein in my "EGG WHITE" diet (see weight loss chapter).

Cold water fish

Cold water fish contain more ω3 fats than warm water fish. Studies have shown that fish which migrate from warm to cold waters produce more ω3 fats. One reason is that the ω3 fats protect the fish from the cold. Because these fats are very polyunsaturated, they can stand very low temperatures without freezing or solidifying.

For many people, fish is a pleasant way to get both fish oils and protein. For people who are not at a stage of sickness where fish oils could be useful or even necessary, fish itself is also healthier than fish oil supplements. Again, our bodies have evolved to respond best to natural foods, that is, foods found in nature and eaten without any significant processing. **Warning**: Because of polluted waters, some fish contain toxins and in this case fish oils are definitely better. Until the government mandates that fish state the amount of toxic chemicals, we have not way to know which fish are dangerous to our health.

Fish Oils

The following fish are high in ω3 fats (see tables in Appendix for more information). They are ordered according to the approximate amount of ω3 fats they contain:

- **sardines (Norway), mackerel (Atlantic), tuna (bluefin), herring (Atlantic), salmon, bluefish, whiting, pollock, rainbow trout, king crab, mussels, lobster or shrimp, scallops, cod, flounder.**

Types of fish oils

Oils are made from different fish. Cod liver oil is found in most health food stores. These oils can last two to four weeks in the refrigerator after they are opened. You can find capsules made from different types of fish in many health food and nutrition stores and catalogs. Because fish oils are perceived as a profitable market, many companies are introducing new products or renaming old products. Capsules vary in a number of ways: the amounts of different types of ω3 fatty acids they contain, the source of the oil (salmon, mackerel, etc.), the amount of antioxidants (vitamin E), and the level of refinement.

Purchasing fish oil

It is difficult to tell which brand of fish oil is best. Several companies market enhanced fish oil extracts that contain more ω3 fats and less of the other fats. We do not know whether this is a desirable or undesirable formula. But it appears that individuals with severe abnormalities of fat metabolism (called severe "hyperlipidemia", particularly triglycerides over 300 mg/dl) may benefit from these oils. Most other people can use any brand.

Claims that one product has more ω3 than another may not be justifiable or even relevant. It is not just the amount of ω3 that matters, but the actual chemical composition of the ω3 present. This is impossible to determine without sophisticated equipment, and the manufacturers do not even disclose this information. Moreover, manufacturers may have more than one supplier, each one using a different process and different chemical formula. The origin of the oil, its chemical composition, and the manufacturing process are often considered trade secrets.

Fish Oils

As a general rule, fish oil capsules have the following advantages over bottled fish oil such as cod liver oil: They contain a higher percent of ω3; they contain lesser amounts of some potentially dangerous types of fats , they contain higher amounts of antioxidants and their encapsulation better preserves them. The amount of fish oil to take depends on the particular brand you use. Follow the recommendations given by the brand manufacturer or your physician. Different brands have different amounts of ω3 fats, and even the same ω3 fat may be in a different chemical form from brand to brand. This will have a different effect on different people.

To complicate matters, many companies actually buy from the same manufacturer and change the label! It is impossible for the consumer to know exactly what kind of a product he or she is buying. Unfortunately, the government is more concerned with preventing the sale of these products than in assuring that those sold meet established and uniform quality standards.

In general, your doctor will tell you how many milligrams (mg) of ω3 you need to take per day. You can take many capsules low in ω3, or fewer capsules of the more concentrated oil. You can purchase the least expensive brand (assuming that it satisfies the quality criteria mentioned below). If you are required to eat a large number of capsules, you may prefer the more concentrated type. Otherwise, choose the cheapest. You can have your blood tested to determine how much you have of each type of ω3 fatty acid.

Quality and storage

Store the oils and capsules in the refrigerator or freezer. If they become cloudy or smell very "fishy" it means that they have began to deteriorate. You should smell the bottle the first time you open it: It should have only a mild fish aroma. If the oil comes in capsules, you should chew a few capsules to determine if there is only a mild fish flavor. If the flavor is very strong, it usually means that the oil has gone bad. If the capsule or oil solidifies in the refrigerator, the oil is not good. (It will solidify in the freezer even if it is good oil.)

Most manufacturers claim that they add antioxidants (chemicals such as Vitamin E) to prevent the oil from going bad. The only way to judge the effectiveness of the antioxidant is to buy several brands and determine which one tastes better after you chew the capsules.

Fish Oils

Heat, room temperature, cooking, light, and oxygen, are among the many factors that quickly destroy fish oils. The best way to prevent their quick deterioration is by keeping them in a dark part of the refrigerator (or in a bag), or even better, in the freezer. But before you freeze all the capsules, freeze only a few to test the results: The outer lining of the capsule may break at low temperatures.

How to use fish oils

Using fish oils is tricky. It is not recommended as a do-it-yourself treatment. Although many manufacturers include instructions on the recommended dosage, the amount to be taken is unique for each person. Fish oils are like a very powerful drug. Too little may not be enough; too much may be dangerous. **It is important that you start a program under medical supervision. Blood tests, particularly a fatty acid profile, must be done before you start the program, and repeated periodically from then on.**

Eat the oils and capsules raw (not cooked). If you cannot stand the taste, they can be mixed with almost any food. You need not chew the capsule (which often tastes "fishy", particularly if not very fresh), but can swallow it like a vitamin. Cod liver oil is available with different flavors. Cherry flavor is one of the best because it is very strong. Or you can flavor the oil yourself. I have found that a little bit of cocoa and honey alter the flavor enough to make it edible. The other flavors should be mixed with food unless you can swallow them rapidly. Because of the strong smell you should drink it quickly; otherwise the smell alone makes it difficult to swallow the oil.

A couple of general rules will help you make better use of the fish oils:

- 1.   Oils and water or milk do not mix well.

- 2.   Fish oils have a very strong taste. Mix them with products that have a strong taste and smell. Examples include cocoa, many spices, cherry, port (wine), cola.

- 3.   The capsules are easy to swallow. They have no taste when swallowed whole. You can chew them or mix them with food.

- 4.   If you take cod liver oil, swallow it quickly to avoid the smell and flavor. Drink a glass of water afterwards to remove the aftertaste from your mouth.

Fish Oils

A few more caveats

Some of the results on fish oils come from studies of Eskimos or populations outside the USA. Most of us do not live in the arctic. For the same reason that you need different clothes in the arctic you need different foods in the arctic. The question is whether taking fish oils in non arctic regions is like wearing a ski jacket and two sweaters during the Florida summer. It is possible that a person living in Florida requires different foods from those that are good for a person who lives in Alaska. Because one of the benefits of ω3 fats is protection against the freezing temperatures, people who live in a warm environment could be harmed from eating too many ω3 fats.

References and notes

[1] Technically this means that the ω3 fats in fish and fish oils are more polyunsaturated. The molecules have more "kinks" or "bends" and produce more liquid-like structures.

[2] Section I and the appendix presents the different families of essential fats.

[3] Some studies have shown that eating the ω3 fats in vegetable oils will produce effects similar to those of fish oils when eaten for at least 15-20 weeks. For immediate effects (within a few days), fish oils act far more quickly than vegetable oils because they almost immediately increase EPA (= 20:5ω3, the active fatty acid that prevents blood clots). Eating linolenic acid (ω3) from vegetable oils takes many weeks before it is converted to EPA. However, linolenic acid appears to be a safer way to increase the total ω3 in your body over the long run. You can accumulate linolenic acid in your body while, apparently, you cannot accumulate EPA. However, there are great individual variations and more research is needed to understand the clinical differences between the ω3s in vegetable and fish oils.

[4] This means that it is 20 carbons long, and has 5 double bonds.

[5] This means that it is 22 carbons long, and has 6 double bonds.

[6] Including 18:4ω3, 20:4ω3, 22:5ω3.

[7] Platelets are small cells in blood that form clots and prevent bleeding.

[8] Fish oils often have more ω3s than equal amounts of flax seed oil; however people usually eat more flax or flax seed oil than fish oil.

[9] The eicosanoids are hormones that help regulate the body. They include the prostaglandins, the thromboxanes and the leukotrienes. A balance of each type is very important for the functioning of the immune system, for maintenance of blood coagulation, for normal pregnancy, and for a wide range of other physiological processes.

[10] Chee K.M, Gong J.X., Rees D.M.G., Meydani M., Ausman L, Johnson J, Siguel E.N, Schaefer E.J. Fatty acid content of marine oil capsules. *Lipids*, 1990,25:523-527.

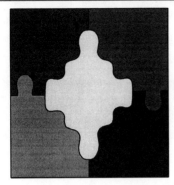

IV.4

PUTTING IT ALL TOGETHER

"Oils supplements soften body fat and correct for past abuses"

Topics: *Fish oils prevent dangerous clotting. Blood tests help you to determine whether you form clots too quickly or too slowly. Supplements of vegetable oils: Mix ω3 and ω6. Omega-3's regulate clotting. Omega-6's soften vessels.*

Summary

Modern nutrition research has produced a significant breakthrough in our understanding of the cause and treatment of cardiovascular disease. Research has shown that the type of fat we eat is a major factor in elevated cholesterol, hardening of the arteries, high blood pressure, heart attacks and stroke. Eating a mixture of ω3 and ω6 fatty acids from vegetables and vegetable oils, and avoiding saturated fats will: 1) lower cholesterol and triglycerides (the elevated fats in blood); 2) soften the arteries; 3) lower high blood pressure; 4) prevent the formation of clots that obstruct arteries and cause heart attacks.

Research has shown that extracts from fish oils have similar effects and act faster than ω3 vegetable oils, but they can be harmful if consumed in large quantities and for extended periods of time. Being thin decreases the load on our hearts and improves our circulation. Exercise helps to maintain muscle tone and allows us to eat more food, therefore achieving adequate intake of all nutrients.

Follow this process: . Have a fatty acid blood analysis done. Achieve ideal weight. Start with vegetable oils high in ω3 and supplement with fish oils if you need to reduce immediately the risk of dangerous clotting. This applies when you already have cardiovascular disease and are at significant risk for forming unneeded clots. Use blood tests to arrive at desirable clotting levels. Take more ω3's (fish oils, flax seeds, or soybean oil) if you clot too quickly; reduce your intake if you don't clot quickly enough.

Start with a mixture of ω3 and ω6 designed to shift your blood levels of EFAs closer to the ideal levels found in healthy people. Eventually you will be taking one to two tablespoons of soybean and safflower oil per day, mixed with flax seed oil if your blood levels of ω3 are very low. If necessary, take more ω6 (safflower oil) to lower blood fats and hypertension, or more ω3 to lower triglycerides or blood clotting.

Basic diet

Oil Source	Fish Oil	Soybean	Safflower
Treatment objectives	Fatty Acids to take		
	ω3 Derivatives	ω3 + ω6 EFA	ω6 EFA
Reduce Blood pressure	Increase	Increase	Increase
Decrease Cholesterol	Same/Less	Increase	Increase
Decrease Triglycerides	Increase	Try: varies	Same/less
Diabetic taking insulin	Increase	Increase	Increase

This chapter presents information to assist you in reviewing your treatment with your doctor. You should read it several times and then discuss these treatment strategies with your doctor or nutritionist.

There are several approaches to the correction of EFA abnormalities. The **preventive approach** uses small amounts of EFAs to maintain existing good health, mostly by eating natural foods (**physiological dose**). **Treatment** requires larger amounts of EFAs obtained from oils and oil extracts (**physiological to pharmacological dose**). **Some diseases** require far larger amounts of oils. Still others require oils obtained from exotic sources or oil mixtures which are being developed currently (**pharmacological dose**). Those who cannot absorb the fat require **intravenous feedings**. All patients require a balance of ω3 and ω6 appropriate for each condition. Because each person is

Putting it all together

different, the ideal mixture varies from one person to another. See the tables in this chapter for summaries of major changes in behavior depending on whether you are healthy and want to prevent disease, or are already ill with heart disease.

Most people who need treatment for cardiovascular disease are overweight. We suggest you start with our **Boston Egg White Diet for weight loss** or with any other weight loss program you like. Your objective is to lose at least one to two pounds per week and be as thin as possible without becoming ill. Being thin will clean your arteries of hard fat and give your heart, lungs and kidneys a break.

Prevention (Healthy) vs. Treatment (ill with heart disease)

Action	Prevention	Treat Heart disease	Severe Disease
Weight	Average-low	Low	Very low
Better underweight	Maybe?	Yes	Yes
Calories	As needed	Reduce	Few
Balanced Diet	Yes	Yes	Yes
Exercise	Yes	If safe	Careful
No smoking	Yes	Yes	Yes
Reduce stress	Perhaps	Yes	Yes

When to use fish and vegetable oils

Research has shown that most Americans are deficient in the essential fats because they eat a diet high in saturated fat and calories and low in essential fats. Excess calories are then converted to even more saturated fat. Excess saturated fat makes it difficult for the body to utilize the essential fats it has.

Eating more ω3 and ω6 fats and fewer calories allows the body to slowly substitute soft essential fat for hard saturated fat in arteries and other cells. Although this replacement also occurs when people substitute

Putting it all together

natural vegetables for animal fat, it happens too slowly for people who are already ill. Eating fish and vegetable oils speeds up the process.

General rules about fatty acid treatment

The EFA derivatives have a stronger and faster effect than the EFAs, but the body does not store them and their effects do not last as long. Gram for gram, an EFA derivative has a stronger effect than the EFA precursor which must be converted to derivatives before it exerts its effects. Eating EFAs allows the body to regulate and produce the EFA derivatives it needs. This approach is often effective in prevention, but may not work to treat and correct for years of neglect. For more immediate results, or when you need to eat large amounts of essential fats, eat EFA derivatives. For longer lasting and long term treatment, use EFAs. The plan proposed here starts you with a mixture of both,

Oil supplements vs. disease stage: rough guidelines

EFA Supplements	No Heart Disease	Heart Disease	Severe Disease
Increase PUFA?	Yes *if* EFA Insufficient	Almost always	Yes
More ω6?	Maybe	Yes	Yes, a lot
More ω3?	Maybe	Yes	Yes, a lot
Fish oils?	Rarely	Probably	Probably

and slowly weans you towards more EFAs and fewer EFA derivatives. EFAs are far cheaper and easier to take because they are found in common oils. EFA derivatives are far more expensive products.

The ω3s are more effective at lowering triglycerides than the ω6s, and far more effective at reducing platelet aggregation (clots). However, for optimal blood pressure and cholesterol levels you need a mixture of ω3s and ω6 which you can determine by trial and error (i.e., try a mixture for several months, see the effects on your clinical symptoms, have a fatty acid analysis, change one of the fatty acids, try again, and so on).

Always make one *small* change at a time, and wait at least three months to see the effects. Sometimes it may take six months before the effects are noticeable. Actual results depend on your body weight, how much oil you are taking, what other foods you eat, and your own unique metabolism. The tables in this chapter present general guidelines to remind you of possible action to take. When in doubt you should have your blood analyzed to find your fatty acid abnormalities and needs.

Soybean and walnut oil have similar ω3/ω6 ratios and amounts, and thus have similar effects. Safflower and sunflower oils are quite similar to one another, both being rich in ω6, and similar to corn oil (rich in ω6, but not as much as sunflower or safflower oil). These three oils contain almost no ω3s. Fish oils have ω3 derivatives.

Start with a mixture high in ω3

Because most people are more deficient in the ω3 than in the ω6 fats, the initial supplements must be high in ω3 compared to ω6 fatty acids. Eating soybean or walnut oil, rich in the ω3 linolenic acid, will usually provide all the ω3 most people need. The exception occurs when you are at high risk of developing a clot that could obstruct an artery (your doctor will know from your health condition and blood tests). In this case you want to start with fish oils to quickly reduce the tendency of the body to form clots. Fish oil supplementation is also useful in people who have reduced ability to convert the precursor linolenic acid to its derivative, **EPA**. This fatty acid is found in fish oil, and it reduces the tendency of the body to form clots. After replenishing your ω3 fatty acids, one tablespoon/day of a mixture of oils rich in ω3 and ω6 fats will replace your saturated fat with essential fats. You can continue with soybean oil, or take a mixture of safflower and soybean oil.

How long does it take to replace your saturated fat? The time it takes to replace the saturated fat stored in your body depends on how old you are, what you have been eating all your life, what else you eat, and what type of body you have. You can speed the process by losing weight (and burning saturated fat) and eating more oils. In general, after three to six months you should notice a significant decrease in your cholesterol and blood pressure. If you are taking drugs for your blood pressure, you will find that you need a smaller dose in order to maintain your current blood pressure. It is important that you revise your drug dosages if your blood pressure or cholesterol declines. Again, this requires medical supervision. Be persistent, but do not expect miracles. You cannot change 40 plus years of accumulated saturated fat in a few weeks.

Putting it all together

When do you need oil supplements?

The need for oil supplementation depends on the type of fat in your body, which in turn depends on the fat you have eaten all your life. Healthy people who have followed a prudent diet all their lives have accumulated plenty of essential fats (both the ω3 and ω6) in their body tissues. They are also lean and have little stored saturated fat. Because they do not need to replace tens of pounds of fat, they can

Meals to work towards different states of health

Action	Prevention	Treat Heart Disease	Severe Disease
Low cholesterol diet	May be	Yes	Yes
Low salt diet	Rarely	Yes	Yes
Low saturated fat	Yes	Yes	Yes
Low calorie meals	No	Yes	Yes
Strict diet adherence	Perhaps	Yes	Yes
Avoid sugar	No	May be	Yes
Avoid stimulants (coffee, tea, chocolate, etc.)	No	May be	Yes
Fish	Yes	Yes	Yes
Meat/Poultry	Yes	Some	Rarely
Egg yolks	Yes	Some	Rarely
Multiple vitamins/ minerals	Rarely	1-3/week	Daily (due to low calories)

obtain all their essential fats from vegetables. Fish and oil supplements are not needed, and may not even be healthy since excessive amounts of essential fats can be dangerous.

Unfortunately, most people have eaten too much saturated fat and not enough essential fats most of their lives. You may not feel sick, but you may have high blood pressure or elevated cholesterol and have a high risk of a heart attack. Drastic steps are thus required to substantially

Putting it all together

change the composition of your body fat and lower your cholesterol, clean your arteries, and soften your vessels (reduce your atherosclerosis and arteriosclerosis). Although the prevention diet could work for you, it may take too long, too many years. You need a shortcut. And consumption of oils provides that shortcut. The oils quickly change the fat composition of your body.

How much oil should you take? What type of diet should you follow?

People with "good genes" (a family history of longevity) do not need to be as careful as those whose family members have had a heart attack before age 70. Even without a family history, high cholesterol and blood pressure put you at risk: The higher your cholesterol and blood pressure, the more careful you have to be and the more you have to work at bringing them down. Only your doctor can tell you how to proceed and blood tests are important diagnostic criteria. In this book we provide the overall guidelines but you have to realize that it is impossible to give a specific program that works for everyone: Each person is unique and has different needs due to different human physiology, weight and metabolism of fatty acids.

ω3 vs. ω6: General guidelines

Oils can be taken any time of the day and mixed in any way as long as they are not cooked or heated. Try to keep approximately constant the amount of oil that you take every week. This will help you to maintain weight and to plan your meals. If you increase one oil, you should reduce the other. Each tablespoon of *any* oil contains about 130 calories. The oils can be taken once a day or distributed at each meal. You do not need to eat the same *exact* amount every day. You can eat more some days and less on other days or even skip some days.

To prescribe the exact amount and type of oil for each person, it is necessary to analyze your body fat. However, it is possible to provide practical guidelines without seeing blood test results. Although this approach may sound complicated, in fact it is quite simple because it does not need to be exact: What matters is the average food you eat over several months rather than the specific meals eaten each day.

Putting it all together

How to correct EFA abnormalities

A fatty acid profile determines your current fatty acid composition and compares your blood test results with those of a healthy person. Your goal is to achieve a fatty acid profile similar to one of a healthy person. In general, you start with a mixture of EFAs and then you either increase or decrease ω3 and ω6 intake until you reach your goals. There are two exceptions: 1) If you must rapidly decrease your clot formation, you must start with fish oils. However, as soon as possible you reduce your intake of fish oils because ultimately the ω3 from vegetable oils will be converted by your body to the same ω3 derivatives you have been getting from fish oil. 2) Another exception may occur if your fatty acid profile shows that your body lacks the ability to convert the EFAs to their derivatives. In this case, you will need to take the derivatives of both ω3 and ω6 until this changes.

General steps to correct EFA abnormalities

- 1.   Obtain a baseline fatty acid profile. The purpose of the fatty acid profile is fourfold: a) to determine your body' composition of EFAs, thus identifying any abnormalities; b) to determine if your body can make enough EFA derivatives; c) to determine whether you have too many TFAs stored in your body, and must cut down dramatically on food sources of TFAs; d) to determine whether you are a good candidate for fish oils. Eating fish oils quickly prevents dangerous clots. This is to be done when you are at immediate risk of death from clot formation because your blood forms clots too easily.

- 2.   Start with one to two tablespoons of a mixture of ω3 + ω6 EFAs; soybean and walnut oils contain a ratio of ω3:ω6 in an excellent proportion for humans.

- 3.   After 10-20 weeks, have another fatty acid profile and determine if your body is forming enough EFA derivatives. Also check whether your TFA levels have declined.

- 4.   If TFAs are still high, you must modify your diet to avoid most foods with hydrogenated oils and beef.

- 5..   If EFA derivatives are formed, and your **EPA/AA ratio** (eicosapentaenoic/arachidonic = 20:ω3/20:4ω6, see chapter I.3) is within desirable goals, continue with the existing diet.

Putting it all together

- 6.   If the ratio of EPA/AA is below your desirable goal, you will need to eat fish oils rich in EPA. It is impractical to attempt to increase the ratio by eating fewer ω6 fatty acids. When you reduce your intake of ω6s, the body frequently compensates by making more arachidonic acid. Patients with deficient or low levels of linoleic (ω6) fatty acid often have elevated levels of arachidonic acid. This is a common error overlooked in experiments where subjects eat different types of fatty acids.

  If the ratio is above your desirable goal, you may need to decrease your intake of ω3 fatty acids. However, if your total amount of arachidonic acid is low, you may need to eat more ω6s to produce more arachidonic acid. Some people cannot make enough arachidonic acid (an ω6, linoleic acid, derivative) because of age, disease or other nutritional deficiency.[1]

- Once you have reached your goals, continue with one to two tablespoons per day of a 50-50 mixture of soybean + safflower oil.

If you must reduce clot formation immediately, during the first 4 weeks you eat the equivalent of one teaspoon of fish oil per day, either as oil or in capsules, and additional oils up to 1-2 tablespoons per day. If you gain weight, eat less of other foods. If you have severe cardiovascular disease, try to eat more oils as long as you continue to lose weight. The fish oils are reduced in later weeks because you will begin to make ω3 derivatives from the vegetable oils high in ω3.

During the first three to six months eat 50% to 100% of your vegetable oil supplement as soybean or walnut oil. Afterwards eat 50% soybean or walnut, and 50% other oils such as safflower oil. These are approximate numbers. What matters is that first you eat more of the ω3 oils and later more of the ω6 oils. That is all. Modifications for specific diseases are discussed in later chapters.

Fish and vegetable oil therapy: More is not better

We know that too much fish oil is not healthy, and we suspect that too much of the other oils may also not be healthy. Therefore, you should eat enough oil to reach or continue to move towards your goals, but not any more. For example, once your blood is more fluid and less likely to form clots, you should reduce or stop taking fish oils. Otherwise, you may end up bleeding too much.

Putting it all together

Fish oil extracts promptly reduce the likelihood that a clot will obstruct an artery, often in less than one week.[2] Soybean oil, on the other hand, may take 10 or 20 weeks to take effect.[3] Fish oils are eaten in relatively small quantities and are not stored by the body. If you stop eating fish oils, they disappear from the blood within a few weeks and your body returns to your previous levels. Linolenic acid (ω3), the precursor of the fatty acids in fish oils, is found in many vegetables and vegetable oils. The body does store the linolenic acid you do not use (as well as linoleic acid, the other EFA precursor). These stores serve as reserves to make the ω3 derivatives. I have fed subjects special diets that consist of intravenous lipids (and practically nothing else by mouth) and I found that even ill patients can make enough derivatives from linolenic acid. However, some patients need fish oils to promptly decrease platelet coagulation or treat other conditions because they need the ω3 derivatives in quantities above those normally produced by their bodies.

Suggested schedule for ω3 deficient patients

Weeks	Fish Oil	Flax Oil	Soybean Oil
	ω3 Derivative	ω3 EFA	ω3 + ω6 EFA
1 to 4 weeks	One teaspoon	1/2 Tbl spoon	1-2 Tbl spoon
4 to 10 weeks	Reduce	Same	Increase
10 to 20	Reduce	Same	Same/less
Over 20	Same/Less	Less; more if ω3 deficient	Same/less

When to change oils

A patient taking fish oils who has an ulcer or diverticulitis could bleed internally and develop anemia. A minor bruise could become a major bruise. For these reasons we do not recommend that large amounts of fish oil be taken for many months unless other alternatives, such as vegetable oils, do not work. Vegetable oils are less likely to cause bleeding.

Your bleeding time should increase to approximately 8 to 10 minutes. It usually takes two weeks to three months for this to occur, depending on how much oil you use. At that point you should reduce the dose of fish oils to about 1/5 of the initial amount and continue with soybean oil. Between 10 and 20 weeks after you start the soybean oil, it will

Putting it all together

begin to produce an effect similar to the fish oil. Unfortunately, this does not happen with all people. If soybean oil alone or soybean together with less fish oil does not maintain your clotting factors at the desirable level, you can increase the amount of fish oil again. The variables to follow include: (1) your ability to form clots (measured by the tests called bleeding time or platelet aggregation); (2) the ratio of **eicosapentaenoic/Arachidonic Acid (EPA/AA** = 20:5ω3/20:4ω6). The blood test **EFA-SR** calculates these ratios and provides ranges for people with different conditions. These results assist your doctor or nutritionist in providing you with the best mixture of ω3 and ω6 fatty acids to eat.

Fish oil and soybean oil should increase your bleeding time, and decrease your triglycerides, cholesterol and blood pressure. If soybean oil and safflower oil continue to improve your well being, eliminate the fish oils. If you reduce the amount of fish oil you take and your progress is reduced (i.e. your bleeding time decreases substantially, your blood pressure goes up, or your cholesterol or triglycerides are elevated) then you may need to continue taking fish oil. If, after several months on fish oils (ω3s) you reach a plateau, a situation where you do not see further improvement, it is time to change the oil mixture.

Because the fish oil fatty acids EPA and DHA are not stored in the body, if you stop taking them your blood levels decrease within a few weeks. However, if you replace them with linolenic acid, most of the time your body can make enough EPA and DHA. If in doubt you can have your blood tested for ω3 composition.

If you have a deficiency of ω6 in the blood, you can use safflower or sunflower oils to increase the amounts of ω6 EFAs. Also, after a period of taking oils rich in ω3 there may be a need for additional ω6, particularly if there is a deficiency of ω6 and the ratio of EPA/AA is too high compared to your goal.

To decrease the ratio EPA/AA when the body has sufficient amounts of ω6 and ω3, decrease the intake of ω3. To decrease the EPA/AA ratio when you also have a superimposed ω6 deficiency (but plenty of ω3), decrease the intake of ω3 and increase the intake of ω6. To decrease the EPA/AA ratio when you have an ω6 deficiency as well as insufficient ω3s, maintain or increase the intake of ω3s but increase significantly the intake of ω6s.

Putting it all together

Fatty Acid changes to modify specific disorders

Disorder	Fish Oil	Flax Oil	Soybean Oil
	ω3 Derivative	ω3 EFA	ω3 + ω6 EFA
EPA/AA ratio*			
To increase	More	More	**Varies**
To decrease	Less	Less	
Bleeding Time**			
To increase	Increase	Increase	**Varies**
To decrease	Reduce	Reduce	**Varies**
IF: Blood pressure does not decrease			
	Increase a little	Increase	Increase ω6***
IF: Cholesterol does not decrease			
	Increase a little	Increase	Increase ω6***
IF: Triglycerides do not decrease			
	Increase	Increase	Increase

This table presents various options you have to accomplish the stated goal. Try each one until you find the best one for your condition. Selecting the optimal mixture of fatty acids is a matter of trial and error because of huge individual differences in metabolism.

* The EPA/AA ratio is the ratio of EPA to arachidonic acid (20:5ω3/20:4ω6). This ratio is used to monitor the body's ability to form clots quickly.

** Optimizing Blood Clotting. You want to change your fatty acid ratios so that you neither clot too quickly nor to slowly. There are many tests to monitor the body's ability to form clots. Here we use as an example the test called Bleeding Time.

*** Use any oil high in ω6. You may continue to use soybean oil as your source of ω6, as it has both ω3 and ω6 fatty acids. You may also change to an oil such as safflower if you need to eat fewer ω3s.

Putting it all together

Who needs fish oils?

Given enough time, most people will improve with vegetables and vegetable oils. However, some people cannot make the derivatives of the essential fats or need huge quantities of fish oil essential fats. If vegetable oils are not sufficient to improve your health, you may need constant fish oil supplements for years. Examples of people who may need fish oils for most of their lives are:

- **Individuals with genetic abnormalities.** Some people have a genetic system that does not work properly. They have too much cholesterol and too many triglycerides in their blood. An indication of such abnormality is having an unusual disease for your age or sex. For example, most people over 60 have heart disease, arthritis and high cholesterol. If you are under 40 and have such conditions, you may have "bad genes." Such people may benefit from consumption of fish oils. If your condition does not improve after taking vegetable oils for 6 months, you may have a disorder that makes you a reasonable candidate for fish oils.

- **People who have a tendency to form clots (hypercoagulable blood).** Fish oils quickly reduce the tendency of the blood to clot and can prevent clot formation that obstructs arteries and leads to heart attacks. For example, many people who need bypass surgery have hypercoagulable blood. After you recover from bypass surgery, it may be a good idea to start with fish oils.

- **Individuals who take drugs that inhibit the formation of ω3 derivatives from their precursor, linolenic acid.** In a healthy state, humans can make ω3 derivatives from linolenic acid. We suspect that insulin and TFAs interfere with this process. Diabetic patients who must take insulin may benefit from taking fish oils.

- **Elderly people.** Aging may decrease the ability of the body to form ω3 derivatives from their linolenic parent.

- **Immune disorders**. Fish oils have been found to reduce the inflammation associated with immune disorders or arthritis. Taken under careful supervision, the side effects are insignificant. The side effects of oil therapy are often far milder than the side effects of drugs.

Putting it all together

Most people also need more ω6 fatty acids

People who have a dietary history of foods low in ω6 need to supplement their meals with ω6 rich vegetable oils. At present we do not know whether excessive ω6s are dangerous. However, we do know that hypertension, elevated cholesterol, and triglycerides in the blood lead to premature death. Therefore, you should continue to take vegetable oils until your risk of heart disease is substantially decreased. If you need fish oils (with ω3 derivatives), you may also need a new type of ω6 derivatives which will become available in the near future. These extracts are to linoleic acid what fish oils are to linolenic acid.

Other conditions that respond to fatty acid mixtures

In addition to modifying your blood fluidity or coagulability, you may want to reduce your blood levels of cholesterol and triglycerides. The general rule is that ω3 fatty acids have a greater effect on triglycerides than on cholesterol, while ω6 fatty acids have a greater effect on cholesterol than triglycerides. However, the research supporting these findings is not convincing: There are far too many individual differences. My research has shown that we need to achieve optimal body levels of ω3 and ω6 to decrease total cholesterol and triglycerides. For many people this means eating large amounts of EFAs. Individuals with highly elevated blood lipids (mostly due to a genetic disorder) should try large doses of both ω3 derivatives and ω6 derivatives (such as borage oil, or new oils containing ω6 derivatives that will soon become available). By large dose I mean several tablespoons per day. You will need to try different mixtures to obtain the best effect which is unique for each person. In my clinical experience, ω6 derivatives can be highly effective in lowering very high cholesterol levels.[4]

If you have claudication (leg pain due to arteriosclerosis) or other kind of circulatory problem related to fat, the treatment is the same. Cold hands and cold feet are signs of poor circulation, and often improve after treatment with vegetable oils. The reason for this is the oils soften your arteries, allowing more blood to your extremities; this keeps you warm. Oils also prevent your skin from getting dry and cracking in the winter. Improved circulation keeps your skin soft and moist. The proper balance of skin fat retains and seals moisture into the skin.

In general, hypertension responds better to ω6 than ω3 fats. Diabetics on insulin may need fish oils and oils containing ω6 derivatives (such as GLA) because insulin may interfere with the mechanism by which the body makes derivatives from EFAs.

General comments about oil use

- You can use soybean or walnut oil interchangeably, and safflower or sunflower oil interchangeably.

- You can use seeds instead of the oil: tofu instead of soybean oil, fresh walnuts instead of walnut oil, etc.

- You can use any of the fish oils available on the market, or cold water fish instead of fish oil.

- Try to keep approximately constant the total amount of oil that you take in a given week. This will help you to maintain weight and plan your meals. Therefore, if you increase one oil you have to reduce another. Constant oil intake is a convenience, not a requirement, but maintaining ideal weight is essential.

- We do not know the possible long term consequences of eating fish oil extracts everyday. To be on the safe side, as soon as possible replace fish oils with cold water fish and vegetable oils.

Since oils have many calories and can impede weight loss, you may be restricted to one tablespoon of oil per day; otherwise you will gain weight. You also need additional vitamins and minerals. For each tablespoon per day of oil, take 50-100 I.U. of Vitamin E, and perhaps Selenium (this is difficult to tell and a blood test is the best solution).

Supplement your meals with uncooked oils; they can be very pleasant on foods such as salads or potatoes. Use the mixture appropriate for your condition, containing one of each group of oils high in ω3 and ω6.

Most people like to eat a lot of food. Oils are very high in calories and not very tasty. Therefore, if a patient is slim, has heart disease, and wants to prevent further disease without weight gain, his/her meals should be planned using foods high in ω3 and ω6 fats. This patient should eat large amounts of those foods rather than just oil supplements.

Putting it all together

Case study: A 71 year old with heart disease

Mr G, a 71 year old man, had cholesterol over 250. His blood pressure was over 160/90 after large doses of medication, and he had suffered one heart attack. He began his treatment with two teaspoons of cod liver oil and 1 ½ tablespoons of soybean oil per day. After three months he continued with one teaspoon of cod liver oil. After one year he reduced it to ½ teaspoon. He then shifted to a fish oil extract and took less than ½ a teaspoon because the extract is more potent than cod liver oil, and reduced the soybean oil from 1 ½ tablespoons per day to less than one tablespoon per day. Eventually his bleeding time (indicator of ability to clot) was over 12 minutes. He then stopped taking fish oil. He now takes less than one tablespoon of soybean oil per day, combined with sunflower oils and seeds, to prevent excessive blood clotting. He makes up the difference in total oil consumption with fish and green vegetables. Because he lost weight, and is taking little oil, he can now eat more food. After two years he reduced both his blood pressure medication and his blood pressure. His cholesterol is about 180.

Radical Nutritional Therapy

For people with advanced cardiovascular disease, strict fasting followed by great weight loss may be effective in cleaning out and opening their arteries. It has been reported that due to starvation during World War II, people were found to have cleaner arteries; deaths due to heart disease dropped significantly. Fasting burns fat and releases your body's stores of essential fats. However, fasting must be done under the supervision of a physician with expertise in fasting. The rationale behind fasting derives from the resilient nature of the fat that accumulates in the arteries. Hardening of the arteries may have resulted in so much fat in the arteries that even the loss of a lot of weight may not be enough to clean the arteries. However, the extreme weight loss caused by fasting or very low calorie diets may cause the body to burn the fat in the arteries. Then the body can replace the hard fat with the soft fat formed from liquid oils.

Instead of fasting, you may use a diet high in PUFA and very low in calories. Very low calorie diets can soften your arteries because they eliminate saturated fat, release the essential fats and lower high blood pressure and cholesterol. These diets require medical supervision; they may cause lethal abnormalities of potassium and other key substances.

Putting it all together

How to lower *trans* fatty acid levels

Many people have abnormally high levels of *trans* fatty acids (**TFAs**) found in processed fat (i.e., hydrogenated oils), margarines and beef. The profile **EFA-SR** will tell you whether or not your levels are so high that you need to drastically change your diet to lower them. You probably remember hearing about the dangers of TFAs during 1993 and 1994. Many scientists reported that TFAs contribute to heart disease. Dr. Lerman and I wrote a paper in 1993 which showed that TFAs are associated with coronary artery disease, and with increased levels of Total/ HDL cholesterol.[5] We recommended that people with elevated TFAs in their blood change their diet to reduce TFAs. Fortunately, my research indicates that it is not difficult to reduce your blood levels of TFAs. If you drastically cut your intake of TFAs from hydrogenated fats, processed fats, beef and margarines, you can reduce the TFAs in your blood by more than 20% in a few weeks, sometimes even faster. However, it requires a strong will to drastically change your diet and reduce TFAs. If you do not have too many TFAs in your blood it may not be worth the effort. Increasing your plasma levels of EFAs provides some protection against high levels of TFAs.[6]

Follow your progress

Periodic visits to your physician, and diagnostic blood tests will help you to monitor your progress. Two simple tests you can do yourself:

- Weigh yourself every morning after you wake up.
- Take your blood pressure every day at the same time.

To weigh yourself, use a good scale: Scales under $5 usually have an error of several pounds, not very important but something to consider. Changes from one day to another are not important: Sometimes you may go up or down a few pounds due to changes in the amount of water in your body. But if each day you are a pound heavier than each day of the previous week, your weight has gone up. You should expect to maintain your weight with variations of no more than 3 pounds.

Similarly, you can monitor your blood pressure. Sit for at least five minutes (preferably 15 minutes) before taking your blood pressure. You will notice large fluctuations from one day to another. This is normal. The important thing is that, over time, your blood pressure declines. If

Putting it all together

you are on high blood pressure medications, with continuous evidence of decline, your physician should reduce your dose.

Help your body regulate itself

Patients have a very important ally --- their bodies. Your body helps to regulate the effects of the oils, especially the effects of the vegetable oils. This is why for long term treatment we recommend vegetable oils rather than fish oils, unless the vegetable oils cannot bring about the desired therapeutic results. Because your body can regulate and monitor oils in the body, it is less important to eat the same amount of oil every day than to make certain that the amount averages out over several weeks. If the results you get with vegetable oils are not enough, or if you are severely ill, you may need to take more oil, change the oil type, or take fish oils.

Take control of your life

New knowledge of nutrition provides the means to control our lives. Changing our diets will lead to healthier and longer lives. So? Let's DO IT!. LET'S TAKE CONTROL OF OUR LIVES. (And let's celebrate our victory by running away from, not towards, the refrigerator.)

References and Notes

[1] This is not inconsistent. What happens is that it is very difficult to predict whether eating more linoleic acid (ω6) will increase or decrease your levels of arachidonic acid.

[2] Because they contain daughter ω3 fatty acids such as EPA and DHA.

[3] Because it contains parent ω3, linolenic acid, which the body must convert to EPA and DHA. It takes longer to act, but it is safer in the long run.

[4] It is unlikely that the federal government will approve the use of ω6 derivatives for the treatment of medical disorders. The FDA will most likely consider them a "drug" and require many years of testing before they are allowed. The cost would be prohibitive for the most likely sellers, health foods stores and supermarkets. And, if approved, it would be sold at pharmacies at prices probably 10 times higher. However, you could buy and use them as a food. Although a doctor may be reluctant to prescribe a medication not approved by the FDA, he or she can tell you to eat healthy foods, especially those low in cholesterol and high in ω6s.

[5] Siguel EN, Lerman, RH. *Trans* fatty acid patterns in patients with Angiographically documented coronary artery disease. *Am. J. Cardiology* 1993; 71:916-920.

[6] Based on research by Dr. Siguel.

Putting it all together

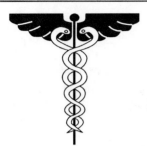

IV.5

DIETS FOR SPECIFIC DISEASES

"Aim treatment to the problem"

Topics: *Treatment approaches. Disease-specific combinations of essential fats. Heart disease. Hypertension. Stroke. Hyperlipidemia. Diabetes Mellitus. Poor blood circulation. Arthritis. Allergies. Dry and itchy skin. Cancer. Neurological disease. Inflammatory Bowel Disease. Short Bowel Syndrome. Cystic Fibrosis. AIDS.*

Summary

Cardiovascular disease requires a higher intake of ω3 and ω6 fats and reduced intake of other fats. The first goal is to prevent clot formation which leads to prompt death. Start with fish oils to promptly decrease clot formation, and replace them later with soybean oil to maintain optimal clot formation. Add ω6 fats (corn, safflower, sunflower oils) to soften the vessels. Hypertension improves with ω6 fats and small supplements of ω3 fats. Diabetes may require a reduction of carbohydrate and protein intake and replacement with essential fats, both precursors and derivatives (because insulin may inhibit the formation of derivatives). Therefore eat fish, lean animal fat and oils. Inflammatory bowel disease and Cystic Fibrosis require substantial amounts of vitamins, minerals and EFAs (due to poor absorption), so much that some patients require intravenous feeding. Arthritis and allergies improve with fish and vegetable oils which act as anti-inflammatory agents. Dry skin improves with topical applications of ω6 fats and vitamin E, and a diet high in essential fats. Most studies show that low calorie meals high in essential fats and low in saturated fat prevent cardiovascular disease and several types of cancer. Lowering cholesterol may also prevent colon cancer.

Treatment approaches

A wide range of medical problems improve with diets low in saturated fat and calories and high in essential fats. Here we explain which diseases require $\omega 3$ or $\omega 6$ fats, precursors or derivatives. The overall approach is to bring the patient's fatty acid profile closer to the profile of a healthy person by eating different mixtures of EFAs.

Most individuals have cardiovascular disease, manifested as either heart disease, hypertension, diabetes mellitus, elevated blood lipids (cholesterol and triglycerides) or a high risk for a stroke. Many of these conditions, when mild and incipient (i.e., just beginning to appear) have no obvious symptoms. That is the reason they are called "silent killers," and to diagnose them we must rely on blood and other tests. Because most people have cardiovascular disease, almost everyone could benefit from treatment of this problem in addition to any other medical problem they have. Fortunately, treatment of any disease with essential fats will have a beneficial side effect: an improvement in your cardiovascular status.

Mild conditions need to be treated as seriously as severe conditions. Mild cardiovascular disease does not go away: It merely gets progressively worse until you stop it. The key difference is that a severe medical condition requires a more drastic treatment and more stringent adherence to the rules indicated in this book. To obtain a good reference for future studies and treatment, it is very important that you have your blood tests done **BEFORE** you start eating more essential fats.

The tables in the appendix present the results of the test **EFA-SR** for patients with heart disease, obesity, Crohn's disease and other conditions. The treatment of each patient is described below. All cases are composites and do not describe any one specific individual. Obviously, your own condition is likely to be different from these composites and your doctor would help you apply these general guidelines to your own case.

Severe Heart disease; bypass surgery

This section applies to people who have severe heart disease, those who plan to have bypass surgery or already have had bypass surgery, and people who have had a heart attack (myocardial infarct).

Diets for Specific Diseases

Clot obstruction is the final event

Heart disease not due to an accident, infection, or congenital defect has three components: hardening and thickening of the arterial wall, narrowing of the arterial canal, and an increased tendency of the blood to form clots. The most immediate danger is posed by increased clot formation and narrowing of the arteries: One large clot could obstruct an artery in the heart, causing an infarct, or in the brain, causing a stroke.

In fact, the most common cause of death in the US is an obstruction in the vascular system due to a clot. If an artery is narrow, a small clot can obstruct it; if it is wide, a small clot is unlikely to obstruct it. Therefore, in cardiovascular disease the immediate danger to be prevented is unnecessary clot formation. Obviously, we need clots to prevent excessive bleeding. Thus, when we speak about prevention of clot formation we talk about a careful and difficult balance between forming clots to prevent excessive bleeding and close holes in vessels, but not forming clots which obstruct the flow of blood inside the vessel.

How to achieve proper clot formation

Studies have shown that most people with cardiovascular disease are in a **hyperaggregatory** state; that is, they form clots too easily. This is probably due to the excessive saturated fat and cholesterol in their vessels. Therefore, the first line of treatment is to use fish oils in modest amounts to decrease clot formation. You will remember that fish oils decrease clot formation because they interfere with platelet aggregation.[1]

Fish oils rapidly decrease clot formation

Most fish oils contain EPA and DHA (eicosapentaenoic acid, 20:5ω3, and docosahexaenoic acid, 22:6ω3). These oils are available in bottles (such as cod liver oil) or in capsules. Eating several capsules per day, in the range of 1 to 3 grams per day [you should check these numbers with your doctor] or about one teaspoon of most oils per day, will increase your blood levels of EPA and DHA within a few days and drastically increase the ratio EPA/AA. (Remember, AA refers to Arachidonic acid, an ω6 derivative, and EPA is an ω3 derivative.) The relative amounts of EPA vs. AA in your blood determine the formation of hormones that affect the ability of platelets to form clots. When the EPA/AA ratio increases, platelets aggregate less easily and clots are less likely to

Diets for Specific Diseases

form. Most people can increase their EPA/AA ratio by increasing their intake of linolenic acid (the ω3 precursor). Large amounts of linolenic acid are found in flaxseeds and flaxseed oil, but it takes several weeks (between 2 and 20) before the body starts to actively convert the linolenic acid to EPA. Thus fish oils must be used to address the problem immediately, until your body's own mechanisms kick in.

Eating the precursor, linolenic acid, allows your body to make as much EPA as it needs. However, if you learn that your body is unable to make as much EPA as it needs, or if you want to decrease your tendency to form clots immediately, EPA or fish oils may be your best choice. In any case, *be very careful about mixing ω3 fatty acids with other anticoagulants* such as aspirin. This is an area where a fatty acid profile is essential to determine whether or not you have desirable or undesirable EPA/AA ratios in your blood.

The proper amount of fish oils depends on the brand of oil used and your medical problem. A bleeding time test and a fatty acid profile (see Part II, blood tests) will help to determine how much ω3 fat you need. You can eat these ω3 fats from any of a variety of fish oils.

Less oil with bleeding, more with narrow vessels

After approximately three weeks of eating fish oils, your bleeding time likely will have increased dramatically, to around 10 minutes. Proper levels are between 8 and 12 minutes, again, depending on your medical condition. If you have any disease associated with increased bleeding (such as an ulcer or diverticulitis), you should keep your bleeding time below 10 minutes; if you have particularly narrow vessels it may be desirable to go over 12 minutes to prevent formation of even small clots which could obstruct your narrow arteries.

Other ω3 fats

Concurrently with fish oils you should start eating the precursor ω3 fat found in soybean or walnut oil (linolenic acid). Begin with about one tablespoon per day. (More for people with severe disease, less for a milder condition.) Keep in mind that fats increase your weight and weight reduction is the most important factor; hence you must reduce your total food intake or exercise more.

After three weeks on fish oils you should decrease them until you reach a level appropriate to your medical problem. Healthy people most

Diets for Specific Diseases

likely do not need to eat fish oils (see previous chapters). Individuals with heart disease will most likely have to eat fish oils for the rest of their lives to prevent risky clot formation. Over time, a combination of fish and vegetable oils will provide the optimal mixture of ω3 precursors and derivatives. The ω6 fats to be used are discussed under hypertension.

Poor circulation

Two factors will improve blood circulation: softer vessels, achieved by eating more ω6s (see below) and decreased platelet aggregation, achieved by eating more ω3 fatty acids. The recommendations outlined above for heart disease will also improve blood circulation. Over time your vessels will become softer and less narrow, and you will become less affected by the problems of poor blood circulation, such as cold hands and feet. Losing weight also helps because your heart can work more effectively, pumping more blood to your hands and feet.

Case Study: Coronary Artery Disease with hyperlipidemia and high *trans* plasma levels

42 year old male with elevated cholesterol, angina, 15% overweight, elevated 20:3ω9 /20:4ω6 and 16:1ω7 (indicators of EFA insufficiency), increased *trans*, reduced ω3/ω6. Recommendations: reduce weight; avoid processed food, beef and hydrogenated oils. Because plasma *concentrations* of all fats are elevated, a consequence of hyperlipidemia, weight loss and a slight increase of PUFA intake will reduce plasma concentrations of SFA and MUFA. Take 10 ml (about 2/3 of a tablespoon) per day of soybean oil plus 100 I.U. Vit. E per day. This plan aims to decrease the ratio of Total Cholesterol/HDL cholesterol, lower total cholesterol and triglycerides, shift towards reduced platelet aggregation, and reduce the risk of cardiovascular disease. A diet very low in TFAs is needed to give the body time to burn the excessive amounts of blood TFAs. If the patient did not have such high TFAs in his blood, we would not enforce a diet severely restricted in TFAs. After the TFAs return to more reasonable levels, the patient can continue to eat foods with some TFAs, such as beef or baked foods made with hydrogenated oils. Also notice that we primarily restrict beef rather than fish, poultry, turkey or pork. Beef is usually higher in TFAs than other animal products, but there are huge variations from one brand to

Diets for Specific Diseases

another. ***Livestock fed foods high in TFAs would themselves contain large amounts of TFAs.***

What causes hypertension?

Despite years and millions spent on research, little is known about the most common cause of hypertension. Conflicting theories abound. Some researchers attribute it to too much salt (Sodium Chloride); others to insufficient Calcium, Potassium, or even Magnesium. I believe that researchers will soon find Manganese deficiency in patients with high blood pressure and heart disease caused by hardening of the arteries.

Understanding basic biochemistry and physiology will allow you to make some sense out of the many conflicting theories. The cells have highly specialized "*pumps*" that control which substances leave and enter the cell, allowing wanted substances to enter or leave the cell, and not allowing unwanted substances either to enter or leave. These pumps regulate the composition of the cell. Many studies have shown that high blood pressure is associated with defective or poorly working pumps, but the cause is unknown. My research has led me to propose that the most common cause of hypertension is hardening of the arteries and inefficient function and fluidity of the arterial cell membranes. Cells with an imbalance of EFAs, with too much saturated fat and not enough PUFAs, function poorly. The pumps which push substances in and out of the cell to maintain its nutritional needs work poorly. Things from outside the cell leak in, and things inside leak out towards the blood plasma. The reason for the leak is simple: The leak occurs following the direction of pressure. Substances that exist in higher amounts inside the cell leak out; those that exist in higher amounts outside the cell leak in. In humans, most potassium, magnesium, manganese and calcium are inside the cells and most sodium and chloride are outside the cell, in the blood plasma. According to my research, most high blood pressure is due to abnormal EFA balance. Cells that contain too much saturated fat and not enough essential fats become hard and brittle, accumulate cholesterol and have membranes that do not work well and leak. With defective pumps and membranes, potassium, calcium and magnesium leak out of the cell and are eventually lost in the urine. This produces body deficiencies of these minerals. Sodium and chloride leak into the cell, leading to excessive accumulation.

Diets for Specific Diseases

Thus, according to my research, sodium and potassium imbalances are a consequence of the EFA abnormalities which cause high blood pressure. They are not a principal cause of high blood pressure. Understanding how cell membranes work helps us to develop the appropriate therapy. Ideally, we want to correct abnormal high blood pressure by treating the abnormal composition of cell membranes. This can be accomplished through an optimal diet. In the meantime, for hypertensives, deterioration can be prevented by eating less salt and more calcium, potassium, and magnesium. Individuals with hypertension should eat less sodium (found in common salt) because their bodies cannot cope with large amounts of sodium.[2] They should eat more potassium, magnesium and calcium because their bodies lose them in higher quantities. Most salt substitutes contain potassium and calcium instead of sodium and are excellent for hypertensive people. BUT beware: IF you have kidney problems, excessive intake of potassium, magnesium and calcium is dangerous. If you need additional potassium, magnesium and calcium to correct for body losses, you probably need larger quantities than those found in foods. You should obtain a prescription and monitor your treatment with periodic blood tests. This is not a do-it-yourself-treatment. You must have professional supervision.

This explanation of the cause of high blood pressure reaches the same treatment conclusions as the one proposed by other authors, but it is more exhaustive. Moreover, it points to the basic source of the problem: excessive saturated fat and not enough PUFAs. The ideal treatment, therefore, is not merely salt restriction, but eating more PUFAs and less saturated fat. This will in turn improve the function of cell membranes and pumps, and lead to more optimal use of the minerals sodium, chloride, potassium, magnesium and calcium. A healthy person does not need to worry about eating too much or too little of these minerals: Together, a balanced diet and the regulatory powers of the healthy body take care of preserving scarce minerals and disposing of excessive amounts.

About blood pressure

Hardening of the arteries makes it difficult for the blood to flow. It is like trying to water plants with an old and hard hose: Due to increased resistance, water flows slowly. To assure that enough blood reaches parts of the body that are far away, such as legs and the outer portions

Diets for Specific Diseases

of the kidney and the brain, the heart pumps harder. The result is higher blood pressure.

Unfortunately, while some vessels can resist the higher pressure, others cannot. Sometimes, a small vessel breaks in the brain, causing a stroke. Other times small vessels break in other parts of the body causing tiny damage which is not obvious or painful. Over time, this "tiny" damage accumulates and leads to reduced function of the kidneys, liver, stomach and brain.

Although the exact numbers are not known, based on current research and clinical experience I estimate that the average organ "dies" or loses about 0.5% of its function from natural wear and tear each year. Over 100 years we lose about 50% of the function. Because most people can live with about 30%, we easily should live to more than 100 years of age. However, because of pollution, environmental toxins, disease, etc., some organs deteriorate faster than 0.5%/year. When our organ cells die at the rate of 1% per year, which is about what happens to many people in America, our life expectancy is about 70 years, the time it takes to lose 70% of our cells. Of course, these are rough numbers. Usually one organ will die much faster than the others. The brain is one of the most resilient organs. Cell death in the brain doesn't kill us; it only makes us dumb. The liver, too, is fairly strong, but as it dies, it fails to eliminate toxic chemicals. When these chemicals accumulate in the body, they increase the rate of death of the kidney and the heart. Because there is only one heart, it is usually the first organ to go. But with some people, both kidneys die before the heart dies.

Treating high blood pressure with drugs usually means that we make the heart pump less hard. As a result, many organs do not get enough blood and they die a little bit faster than usual. Of course, others live longer because they are not killed by the high blood pressure. For some people, one organ (like the kidney or brain) may lose as much as 1% of its function every year. By the time the person is 70 years old most of the organ function has been lost and the person will die. Treatment of high blood pressure is a delicate balance between preventing the immediate danger caused by the high blood pressure while avoiding the side effects of the drug, including slow organ death (particularly brain death) and less effective supplying of the body with nutrients and oxygen. I believe that drug treatment of high blood pressure prevents early deaths due to stroke and heart attacks, but accelerates the rate of cell death and the deterioration of the brain and body. Ideally, the best

Diets for Specific Diseases

treatment for high blood pressure is to eliminate the cause, which often is hardening of the arteries.

Treatment for the most common condition

The most common cause of hypertension is hardening of the arteries. Eating more ω6 and ω3 fatty acids will soften the vessels. The amount of ω6 required depends on the severity of your hypertension. Of course, another essential step is to become thin. Practically every study has found that losing weight lowers high blood pressure,[3] and also lowers high glucose levels (helps to normalize hyperglycemia). You should supplement your diet with one teaspoon to two tablespoons of vegetable oil high in ω6 fatty acids (safflower, sunflower or corn oil). **Note**: There are *some types of hypertension that are not caused by improper nutrition*. These types may be caused by excessive hormone production, cancer, unusual genetic factors and other severe medical conditions. Failure to treat the underlying medical condition can be fatal.

After three months on a high EFA diet you should notice a reduction in your blood pressure. Remember that blood pressure undergoes significant changes from one day to another and during the day. It is common for a person to have a blood pressure of 130/80 one day, and 120/65 the next day. Therefore you should not worry over minor fluctuations. Measure your blood pressure every day at the same time after sitting for 15 minutes. If you do not see any reduction in either of the numbers (systolic = top number; diastolic = bottom number), it is time to either increase ω6 oils or **add** ω3 oils. If weight reduction and two tablespoons of ω6 vegetable oil per day do not lower your blood pressure after six months, you need to eat more oils rich in ω3s (but no more than one tablespoon per day). Hypertension has multiple causes and each patient requires different treatment. Plan your treatment in conjunction with your doctor and nutritionist to get the best benefits from nutrition and drugs when needed.

Stroke

People who have an increased tendency to form clots (your doctor can determine this from blood tests) should follow the same treatment indicated for heart disease. Fish oils are uniquely useful in reducing the tendency to form clots.

Diets for Specific Diseases

Individuals who have brittle vessels, which leak easily, must monitor their blood to insure that it clots properly. Fish oils, which increase bleeding, may not be an appropriate treatment for them, and if chosen should be used under medical supervision. Otherwise, a small leak could lead to a large loss of blood which can cause high pressure inside the brain and consequent brain destruction and paralysis. For such patients, a rough guide is to maintain the bleeding time between 5 and 8 minutes. This is one instance where blood tests are essential. Most other people can eat fish oils without having to worry too much about excessive bleeding. Obviously, this is a complex subject that requires medical evaluation by a qualified health provider. Achieving EFA balance will often strengthen brittle and weakened vessels.

Hyperlipidemia and dyslipidemia

This section applies to the approximately 5% to 15% of the population who have *very high* cholesterol or *very high* triglycerides (called "severe hyperlipidemia"). It also applies to another unusual lipid or lipoprotein disorder called "**dyslipidemia**" or "**dyslipoproteinemia**," a disease most likely caused by a genetic defect compounded by a bad diet. As a general rule, if your cholesterol is over 400 mg/dl or your triglycerides are over 300 mg/dl, you probably have an unusual genetic condition that increases your cholesterol or triglycerides. Another type of dyslipidemia is very low HDL, which significantly increases risk of heart disease.

Introduction to Lipid Metabolism

The fat in the blood is carried inside particles manufactured by the liver, called "lipoproteins". Researchers have found that some lipoproteins are heavier than others, thus all lipoproteins have been classified according to density. The particles are named "**VLDL**" (very low density lipoproteins), "**LDL**" (low density lipoproteins), "**HDL**" (high density lipoproteins), and "**IDL**" (intermediate density lipoproteins). When more sophisticated instruments have been used, researchers have found even more lipoproteins of differing densities: Now we have HDL1, HDL2, HDL3, LDL I-IV, and many more. Regardless of density, each lipoprotein contains some cholesterol, cholesterol attached to fatty acids ("cholesterol esters"), triglycerides, phospholipids, vitamins and apoproteins.

Diets for Specific Diseases

The cells in the body have receptor mechanisms to catch lipoproteins from the blood, absorb the vitamins and essential fats needed from them, and throw them out again into the blood. Many hormones regulate the way the body uses these lipoproteins. In women, huge changes occur at menopause, which apparently contributes to women's higher likelihood of heart disease after menopause. People with abnormal genes have abnormal metabolism of the lipoproteins and this defect is frequently associated with cardiovascular disease or stroke. A few people have genes that protects them against heart disease, but we do not know how.

Lipid disorders

Genetic lipid disorders are also known as "**familial diseases**" because usually more than one family member has the disease, which is transmitted through the genes. In these diseases, one or more genes are "different" or "defective". As a result, an enzyme which is important to the metabolism of lipoproteins is not made properly, and thus a small part of the body fails to work. Because the human body is an extraordinarily complex machine, even if 1/1,000,000 works poorly, the body dies.

There are physicians who specialize in the treatment of patients with severely abnormal lipids. Research studies have shown that "familiar hypercholesterolemia" (highly elevated cholesterol) occurs in about one in 500 persons. A specific defect in Apoprotein B, a protein that helps to make lipoproteins, occurs in about one in 700. A familiar defect that causes both elevated triglycerides and cholesterol, "combined hyperlipidemia", occurs in about one in 100.

Humans have two copies of every gene. When only one gene is defective, we say it is a heterozygous defect. When both genes are defective, we say it is a homozygous defect. People who have one defective gene have a mild form of the disease. People with both genes defective have a severe form of the disease.

About 15% of people with hyperlipidemia have at least one defective gene that regulates Apoprotein E4. This protein regulates the operation of the cell's receptor for low density lipoprotein. With a bad receptor, these lipoproteins accumulate in the body. High LDL cholesterol in the blood is strongly correlated with heart disease.

About 7% of people with hyperlipidemia have at least one defective gene that regulates Aproprotein E2. This protein regulates the update

Diets for Specific Diseases

of leftover lipoproteins, called "remnants" in the blood, and also the formation of LDL. Paradoxically, some of these people may have low cholesterol because they have low LDL cholesterol. However, they often have high triglycerides.

Hyperlipidemia

The word, "hyperlipidemia" literally means high levels of lipids (fats) in the blood. As a general descriptor, it can mean either an inflated number of lipoproteins, or an inflated number of the fats themselves, in the lipoproteins. In medicine, this term traditionally has been used for elevated total cholesterol or total triglycerides. However, modern research has shown that hyperlipidemia is more complex because there are many different types of lipoproteins; some may be present in higher than normal amounts, and others actually may be present in lower than normal amounts.

Most people who have abnormally elevated cholesterol and triglycerides have acquired disease, that is, one caused primarily by diet. When we say that a disease is "acquired" rather than genetic, we mean that our behavior plays a role far more important than our genes. Some people have abnormal lipids caused primarily by very unusual genes. In these situations the levels of different fats in the blood are very different from those of other humans who eat the same diets. However, because each human has unique genes, genetics always plays a role.

Treatment

When you are diagnosed with a genetic disorder of lipid metabolism you will need to follow a very strict and complex diet, and you may also have to take drugs. This is a situation where you must be seen by a specialist on lipids rather than a regular physician. Because each of these disorders is fairly unique and manifests itself differently in different patients, you need to work with your health provider to develop the optimal plan.

Based on my conversations with many physicians, my research and my clinical experience, I have found that many abnormalities of lipids improve when treated with *large amounts* of EFAs and EFA derivatives. You may need to take several tablespoons of oil per day, while reducing your intake of other foods (otherwise you will become obese). If you have severe hyperlipidemia you should follow the diet recommended for severe heart disease but eat more fish oil

Diets for Specific Diseases

supplements. Vegetable oils alone are usually not sufficient to bring very high blood lipids to normal levels. Fish oils (with ω3 derivatives), and, when they become available, ω6 derivative fatty acids, are recommended for most of your life.

As a general rule, ω3 fatty acids lower triglycerides. This effect is most notable for ω3 derivatives rather than the ω3 precursor, linolenic acid. Thus, fish oils are more effective than flax seeds. However, it is possible to take larger amounts of flax seed than fish oils, so a combination is always desirable. The ω3s also lower LDL-cholesterol and may increase HDL-cholesterol.

The ω6 fatty acids also lower triglycerides. This effect is most notable for ω6 derivatives, particularly arachidonic acid. However, in 1994 it was not possible to purchase oils with large amounts of arachidonic acid. The next best available ω6 derivative is GLA, found in borage, primrose and other unusual oils.

For hyperlipidemia, a general rule is that the amounts needed to be effective are large, often at least 2 tablespoons per day, but more likely to be several tablespoons per day. Each tablespoon of oil has approximately 130 calories. If you take 3 tablespoons a day every day, and do not reduce other calories or increase your exercise (often difficult for sick people), you will gain more than two pounds each month. This is not desirable because the most common disorder associated with abnormal lipids is heart disease; obesity could make this condition worse. Therefore, you must drastically reduce other things in your diet to make room for the oils. Because you are eating large amounts of oil, you also need to take more antioxidants. Approximately 200 I.U. of vitamin E every day is reasonable, as is about double the usual amounts of other antioxidants. Your doctor can advise you as more research is published regarding optimal dosage of antioxidants.

A few people cannot tolerate fat. They lack the enzymes to digest blood fat and get ill when they eat fat. A partial solution for this problem is to eat extremely low fat diets supplemented with essential fats. One tablespoon per day of a mixture of oils will provide the required essential fats. The purpose of this mixture is to maximize the amount of EFA and EFA derivatives while minimizing oil intake.

Diets for Specific Diseases

Diabetes Mellitus

My research has shown that patients with diabetes have EFA abnormalities. I believe that future research will show that most of the complications of diabetics are caused by abnormal EFA metabolism. Diabetic treatment has traditionally emphasized the proper use of carbohydrates. Unfortunately, a consequence of the diets followed by many diabetic patients is that they eat many carbohydrates and saturated fat. This diet, together with abnormalities in insulin metabolism typical of diabetics, worsens the cardiovascular diseases associated with diets low in essential fats. Insulin is needed for the proper use of essential fats, and insulin abnormalities found in diabetes cause abnormalities in the body's use of its essential fats. It is unfortunate that this topic has been overlooked by the vast majority of publications aimed at patients with diabetes. Both types of diabetic patients, those who use insulin and those who do not, will benefit from corrections of EFA abnormalities diagnosed by the test **EFA-SR.**

Diabetics should behave as if they are at very high risk for cardiovascular disease, which they usually are. They should follow the same diet recommended for the treatment of cardiovascular disease, but with greater care. In particular, they should eat ω3 fatty acids to decrease their tendency to form clots. This is recommended because diabetics are at higher risk of developing disease due to abnormalities of blood clotting, including loss of vision. Research on fatty acids indicates that loss of vision in diabetic patients can be prevented by a diet high in essential fats. This should be carefully monitored by blood tests for fatty acids.

A consensus panel of government scientists has agreed that weight loss is a proven treatment for diabetics who do not require insulin.[4] However, most government panels fail to state the importance of a proper balance of essential fats.

There is an additional problem in diabetes which complicates its treatment, and is probably a major factor in the eye and cardiovascular disease associated with diabetes. Published research and my own studies indicate that insulin interferes with the production of the derivatives of EFAs. Therefore, patients who require insulin or those who overproduce insulin because of abnormal glucose metabolism (often found in adult onset diabetes) should eat fish or fish oils for a source of ω3 derivatives.

Diets for Specific Diseases

Derivatives of the ω6 fats are currently found in primrose and borage oil and some other commercial products currently under development. Unfortunately, there is as yet no commercial equivalent of fish oils for ω6 fatty acids. Sources of very long chain ω6 fatty acids, such as arachidonic acid, will soon become available and they may also be quite helpful to diabetic patients. The fatty acid profile **EFA-SR** determines whether or not a diabetic needs to eat EFA derivatives and how much of each one.

A final advantage to including more EFAs in the diet of the diabetic patient is that fat slows the digestion process and increases the time that food spends in the stomach. For this reason, foods with fat are given to patients with diabetes to slow down the rate of absorption of glucose, lessening the amount which rapidly enters the blood.

Kidney Disease

Kidney disease caused by hardening and obstruction of the arteries is to be treated in the same way as other similar *severe* cardiovascular diseases. After an evaluation of fatty acid patterns in the blood, the patient should eat a diet very high in EFAs to quickly bring the patterns toward normal levels, while at the same time minimizing the likelihood that a clot will obstruct a kidney artery. For many people this means eating fish oils high in ω3s.

For many years physicians have prescribed diets restricted in protein. Because the kidney excretes byproducts of protein metabolism, eating a protein-restricted diet has been thought to correct or prevent kidney disease. Although animal studies have shown that restricting dietary protein protects the diseased kidney, similar results have not been obtained with humans. In a study comparing different protein restricted diets, none seemed to make a significant difference in preventing kidney disease.[5] Current research suggests that the key to preventing and treating kidney disease is to correct EFA abnormalities.[6]

Arthritis

Research suggests that arthritis occurs because the body produces antibodies against itself. There is an increased immune-inflammatory response that, instead of protecting the body, attacks the body.

Diets for Specific Diseases

Antibodies are molecules produced by the body to attack and destroy foreign agents that enter the blood. Arthritis is due, in part, to an incorrect or overactive defense system, or a confused response to a virus which triggers an inflammatory/immune defense. What happens is that the body mistakes itself for the foreign particle, so attacks itself.

Therefore, to treat arthritis, we need to alter the immune response and make it less active. Traditionally, this has been accomplished with antiinflammatory agents such as steroids, non steroidal drugs and aspirin. Diets low in saturated and high in essential fats also alter the immune system and may produce a favorable response in patients with arthritis. Fish oils decrease the inflammatory response and they usually have fewer side effects than drugs used in arthritis (however, *beware* that aspirin and fish oils both decrease clot formation and can produce bleeding). Some, but not all, experimental trials with fish oils have shown that they can be effective for some patients with arthritis. The trials that failed to show improvement may not have used a proper balance of EFAs or enough antioxidants. Under proper medical supervision to ensure that fish oils do not cause any complication (primarily excessive bleeding and anemia), fish and fish oils may be tried by most arthritic patients.[7] In addition, ω6 derivatives found in evening primrose or borage oil could also improve arthritis. All these essential fats act by modifying the activity of the hormones which regulate inflammation. However, substantial amounts of these oils may be required to have an effect. Please be aware that eating several tablespoons of oil per day would make you gain weight unless you cut other foods.

I have spoken with many arthritic patients who have been treated with essential fats without any knowledge about their initial fatty acid composition. In many cases they get disappointing results. Quite often, the dose and types of oils used are incorrect. Furthermore, they are used without appropriate antioxidant supplements and for an inadequate period of time. No blood tests are done to monitor the blood levels of essential fats and determine what changes are needed either before or during treatment. Additionally, overweight patients are not encouraged to lose weight, one of the most significant factors in minimizing the effects of arthritis. Regardless of the cause and treatment of arthritis, there is a simple factor upon which every scientist agrees: If you take an injured joint or bone, and place it under severe stress due to increased weight, you are likely to worsen the

Diets for Specific Diseases

damage. Therefore, people with arthritis should be extremely thin to minimize wear and tear on their bones.

Allergies and Asthma

Research indicates that allergies, like arthritis, are the result of an altered immune or inflammatory process. An allergy occurs because a person is oversensitive to a particular agent. Whenever faced with something foreign to our body, such as a bacteria, food, insect sting, or pollen, our body "attacks" it, thus producing an immune and/or inflammatory response. Such a response is a way to contain the foreign agent. But sometimes the body overreacts. Although the causes of overreaction are not well understood, research suggests that altered production of hormones known as eicosanoids[8] contributes to the allergic response.

Because essential fats modify the production of eicosanoids, scientists have experimented with foods high in different essential fats. They have found that some people with allergies may not be able to produce enough derivatives of the essential fats. This means that these people need to eat more essential fats found in fish oils (ω3's) and in fats derived from linoleic acid (ω6's).

To prevent or treat an allergy, several steps are indicated. You should try each one independently. Then try various combinations (up to three combinations). Of course, if you know the agent that causes your allergy, you should try to avoid it. But often people do not know what causes their allergy.

Basic step: Lose weight if you are overweight; regardless of your weight, eat less saturated fat. This is required to improve the function of your immune system. A low fat vegetarian diet usually decreases the allergic response. If the Basic treatment is not enough, move to Step 1.

- **STEP 1: Eat fish oils**. After a baseline fatty acid profile, start with fish oil capsules. Try them for at least three months. Repeat blood tests to see if you have changed your blood levels sufficiently. Many times the treatment fails because the patient is not eating enough ω3s. However, some patients actually manage to eat too many oil capsules. The only way to make certain of how your body uses the fatty acids in the oils is with a blood test. This is important because too much fish oil may cause you to bleed. If you notice improvements in your allergies after about three months, continue.

Diets for Specific Diseases

If you do not feel better and your blood tests indicate that you have taken adequate amounts, move to Step 2.

- **STEP 2: Eat evening primrose or borage oil** (or other ω6 derivatives when they become available).[9] Try them for three months. Again, measure the levels in your blood to see that you are taking enough. If no improvement is seen even with adequate levels for several months, move to Step 3.

- **STEP 3: Eat a mixture of ω3 derivatives (fish oils) and ω6 derivatives.** Continue for several months unless you feel worse. If you do, reduce the amount of oils. If your blood levels indicate that you are eating adequate amounts, and there are no side effects, continue even if there is no obvious improvement. Sometimes it takes months for the effects to be seen. Other times, the only effect is that your condition will remain stable. It may not improve, but it probably will not get worse.

The combined effects of the basic program (less saturated fat) plus the additional oils may require months before they take effect. Do not feel discouraged. If you do not get worse, these oils will help your cardiovascular system and you should try them for several years. You may feel an improvement the following year. Because you are eating large amounts of oils you will need to take antioxidants such as vitamin E, C and selenium. However, there is no need to take large quantities of these vitamins and minerals. I rarely suggest more than 100 I.U. of vitamin E per day, or more than 200 mg of vitamin C per day from all sources combined (i.e., including what you get from your food).

Dry and itchy skin

Deficiency of ω6 fatty acids cause a dry, scaly dermatitis, known as Seborrheic dermatitis. You will notice something like dandruff and redness around the nose, behind the ears or in the eyebrows, on a man's chest (if hairy) or under a woman's breast, or on other parts of the body where the skin is folded. Many people think that oily skin is due to excessive oils in the body, or that dry skin is caused by eating too much oil or not drinking enough water. In fact, oily skin may be caused by excessive levels of saturated fat, which alters the fat composition of the skin and makes the body produce excessive oil-like substances.

Insufficient levels of the essential fats produce ineffective skin cells. Without sufficient essential fats the skin loses water, producing a dry

Diets for Specific Diseases

and itchy skin. Drinking water and humidifying the environment may temporarily relieve the problem. However, eventually the defective skin will allow the water to evaporate. Usually this problem gets worse in the winter when the environment is dry, or in the summer when the environment is hot and water evaporates from the skin. A solution to the problem of dry skin may be to eat a diet rich in green vegetables and vegetable oils, but low in animal fat. Take vitamin E (about 100 IU/day) to prevent deterioration of the essential fats you are eating.

A temporary solution to dry, itchy skin, while waiting for dietary changes to have an impact, is to rub safflower oil (high in ω6) on your skin a few times per day.[10] Safflower or sunflower oils are often equivalent. Experiment first with very small quantities and increase them only if you have no adverse reactions. Wash your hands and face carefully, dry them well, and apply substantial amounts of oils to the skin and rub them in. I suggest that you apply these ointments on weekends early in the morning and leave them on all day. Be careful: The oil can get on your clothes, bed, etc.

Some people develop an allergic reaction to some oils. Before you apply a large amount of oil, try a small amount on a small portion of your skin to insure that you do not have a bad reaction. If you have no bad reaction and decide to use the oil, first apply first a small amount to your skin, increasing the amount as needed over a period of several weeks. If you have an allergic response (redness and irritation) to one oil, try another type or another brand. Additional guidelines for healthy skin include:

- **Be thin:** Thin people usually have tighter and better skin. When you lose weight for the first time your skin may be too big for your body. Do not worry: After a while the skin will catch up and readapt. BUT be careful: If you gain and lose weight repeatedly, your skin may lose its ability to readapt (see below).

- **Remain at a stable, healthy weight:** Going up and down in your weight stretches your skin and over time it loses its ability to adapt, making you look older.

- **Eat ω6 fats:** If you have dry and itchy skin, eat more safflower or sunflower oil and vitamin E: These oils have fats that may help your skin. However, if you are allergic to vitamin E or oil, you must consult a physician.

Diets for Specific Diseases

- **Miscellaneous:** Avoid exposure to the sun (long exposure to
  the sun wrinkles the skin), do not smoke, wear rubber gloves
  when using strong cleaning agents, wear soft clothing, and
  avoid strong washing detergents. Moisturizers also help to
  relieve itching, but highly perfumed products should be
  avoided.[11]

Cholesterol and fat in Cancer

Cancer is primarily a process where certain body cells divide and
reproduce without control. Two main factors contribute to cancer: One
is a genetic change in a cell which makes the cell divide endlessly; the
other is a cell environment which facilitates this endless division. By a
cell environment we are referring to the molecules that surround the
cell inside the body, not the environment outside your body. The most
popular theory about cancer states that several factors cause the
genetic change that induces the cell to divide, and a multitude of factors
which allow the cell to continue dividing. Every day we eat and breathe
chemicals that can **mutate** the cell (change the genes), or we are
exposed to other substances which can mutate the cell. Nearly
everybody agrees that cigarette smoking is one of the strongest
mutagens available. (Mutagens are substances that cause changes in
genes.)

Another general theory about cancer states that any process which
drastically increases the rate of cell division is likely to increase the
probability of getting cancer. When cells divide far more rapidly than
usual, there is an increased chance that one of the cells will become
abnormal and cause cancer. Therefore, any process that increases the
exposure of cells to mutagens or forces the cells to divide more than
usual increases the chances of getting cancer.

What are these processes? Any disease, particularly infectious
diseases, forces the body to reproduce its cells and also release potent
agents to attack the invading bacteria. These foreign invaders, or the
body's own attacking agents, may cause some cells to mutate into
abnormal cancer cells. Chronic gastrointestinal disease that forces
intestinal cells to replicate faster than usual can lead to cancer. Any
irritating agent that forces cells to reproduce faster can lead to cancer.
Repeated sun burns, skin abrasion, and lung irritants are the types of
agents that cause cells to reproduce at a faster rate. Most foods contain

Diets for Specific Diseases

a huge number of chemicals, many of which are potential mutagens, while others have opposite effects.

Some researchers believe that increasing the body's metabolic rate increases the release of the byproducts of metabolism and oxidation called "free radicals." These radicals can cause changes in genes. Every day we probably make thousands of different types of radicals. They have an important purpose in the body, namely participation in the natural chemical reactions which sustain life. But when too many are produced, the excessive amounts can contribute to cancer. To protect us against excessive radicals, many foods, particularly fruits and vegetables, contain a huge number of antioxidants. We do not know the correct balance of each antioxidant or radical, thus supplementation by vitamin pills can be counterproductive. Eating natural foods, especially many vegetables and fruits, appears to be the best way to protect ourselves.

Overeating, that is, eating too many calories, increases our metabolism and therefore our production of free radicals. This is one reason why being slim and eating few calories may protect us against cancer. Of course, if you become overweight you are less likely to die of cancer because you will die first of cardiovascular disease. Nevertheless, eating too many calories and too much total fat, particularly saturated fat, has been found to be associated with an increased incidence of cancer.

Nutrition researchers agree on several basic principles for cancer prevention:[12]

- **Eat less.** Animals who overeat are more prone to cancer and live shorter lives. Being thin, active, and eating little food usually prolongs life and prevents cancer.[13] Also, minimize alcohol consumption.

- **Avoid processed meats and saturated fat.** This includes: salt-cured, smoked or nitrite-cured foods like bacon, sausages, hams; charcoal grilled meats and other fat cooked at high temperatures (as in broiling or frying).

- **Eat well.** Eat foods high in fiber, vitamins A, C, and beta carotene, selenium and vitamin E. Vegetables provide these nutrients.[14] However, eating vitamin and mineral supplements alone may be counterproductive because you can cause a vitamin or mineral imbalance. Moreover, natural foods have hundreds of natural chemicals which current

Diets for Specific Diseases

research is finding to have protective effects against cancer.
Again, the goal is "balance": eating natural foods and
supplements only to correct deficiencies identified with
biochemical tests.

- **Eat more antioxidants if you eat more essential fats**.
  Most Americans, because of inappropriate diets, have
  insufficient levels of EFAs in their bodies and need to eat more
  EFAs. However, EFAs are highly susceptible to oxidation and
  may produce excessive free radicals. Thus, you must eat
  antioxidants when you eat more essential fats.

The same diet works for heart disease and cancer

Studies of different populations have shown that many people with
cancer have very low cholesterol. For a while, scientists did not know
whether the cancer reduced cholesterol in people or low cholesterol
induced cancer. Fortunately, recent studies have found that lowering
cholesterol prevents rather than causes cancer.[15]

Another area of concern has been the effect of fat on cancer. Most
studies have found that eating too much fat is associated with a higher
likelihood of developing cancer. These studies have shown that foods
high in saturated fat are associated with cancer, and eating large
amounts of polyunsaturated fat may help cancer cells to grow.
However, no one has shown that moderate amounts of polyunsaturated
fat, such as those indicated in this book, lead to cancer. There is
general agreement that the same foods which help to prevent heart
disease also prevent cancer, leading to healthier and longer lives.
These diets emphasize natural foods high in complex carbohydrates and
essential fats, and elimination of processed foods. Unfortunately, we all
die eventually. If we succeed in preventing death from cardiovascular
disease, then we are most likely to die from an infection, an accident or
cancer. Our objective is not to eliminate death, which is impossible, but
to prevent premature death.

Potential treatments

Many people with cancer lose their desire for food. We do not know
why this happens, but we do know the results. Eating a bad diet leads
to deterioration of the immune system, reducing the ability of the body
to fight cancer cells. Therefore, many scientists encourage cancer
patients to eat balanced meals regardless of whether they are hungry.

I wrote a paper[16] explaining why *some types* of cancer growth may slow down when the patient eats a low calorie, nutritionally balanced vegetarian diet. I suggested that patients who want to treat their cancer should eat little, and avoid all animal foods because they contain a type of fat that is necessary for cancer cell growth. Since I published that paper I have received numerous communications from patients and physicians, who told me that they followed my suggestions with good results.[17]

Neurological Disorders

Disorders such as Multiple Sclerosis and Alzheimer's disease lead to destruction of neurological tissue. Including more ω3's in the diet, particularly fish oil ω 3's, provides the body with critical raw materials to rebuild destroyed tissue. Even though the disease is not cured, its progress or deterioration may be slowed down. I have found, through blood testing, that many patients with neurological diseases such as Parkinson's disease, Huntington disease and multiple sclerosis have EFA abnormalities. Treating those abnormalities may not cure the disease, but it could slow down its progress. Without treatment, the brain is deprived of critical essential fats and probably deteriorates even faster.

Inflammatory Bowel Disease (Crohn's Disease and Ulcerative Colitis)

There are two major types of inflammatory bowel disease ("**IBD**"). Crohn's disease primarily affects the ileum, which is the terminal part of the small intestine. Ulcerative Colitis primarily attacks the large intestine. Both diseases cause damage to the cells that line the intestine. The damage makes it more difficult for the body to absorb food. Because the small intestine is one of the major organs involved in the absorption of EFAs and several vitamins (i.e., B_{12}) and minerals, deficiencies of these vitamins, minerals, and EFAs are quite common in Crohn's patients. The diarrhea caused by the malabsorption of food carries with it other minerals and nutrients, often making the disease much worse. In Ulcerative Colitis, the body primarily loses water and a few minerals, but these losses upset the balance of nutrients in the body, and can lead to malabsorption problems in other parts of the intestinal system. Such malabsorption, coupled with increased demand

Diets for Specific Diseases

for EFAs to repair the intestinal cells, results in deficiencies of EFAs in practically all patients. Besides increased losses and intestinal repair, the disease itself forces the rest of the body to use up more EFAs, thereby increasing the need for EFAs. It is common for patients with IBD to have wide fluctuations in their plasma EFA levels. Research has shown that EFA abnormalities contribute to the inflammatory process and further deterioration in IBD. My research is finding that EFA abnormalities are probably the most significant nutritional abnormality in Crohn's disease.[18]

When patients with IBD are relatively well fed or receive intravenous lipids, their EFA status improves. When the disease becomes more active, their EFA status gets worse, which in turn causes further damage to the intestine and makes the disease even worse. Most patients have a large whole body deficiency (that is, not enough EFAs in their bodies)[19] and it is difficult for them to eat enough EFAs by mouth to correct this deficiency. Treatment aims to prevent a rapid deterioration of the disease and prevent or correct many of the "systemic" complications (other severe problems that often affect patients with IBD).

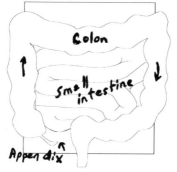

Based on my clinical experience, I have concluded that Crohn's disease is caused by an infectious agent. Some physicians think it is a "psychiatric" disorder; others call it an "immune" disorder (even though we do not know what causes immune disorders and many may be caused by infectious agents). I believe it is an infectious disease which is not very contagious, but, nevertheless, is worth taking care to avoid contact with. People with Crohn's disease and their family members should pay particular attention to bathroom use, being certain it is kept as clean and sanitary as possible. However, because the microorganism is primarily in the intestine, together with millions of other organisms, infection is rare. Because there is not enough money for research and, in my opinion, much of the current nutritional and drug research is misguided, the cause of Crohn's disease has not been found. The infectious agent may be found to be somewhat similar to the one that causes tuberculosis. Whatever it is, it is very difficult to identify because the intestine contains too many bacteria.

Diets for Specific Diseases

Crohn's disease produces a severe inflammatory response that in part obstructs the intestine and interferes with the absorption of food. This obstruction causes severe intestinal cramps, particularly after eating regular foods. Traditionally, some physicians and medical textbooks have recommended a diet low in fiber, referred to as a "low residue" diet. I have not found such diets useful. Low residue diets made with whole foods require digestion and still contain significant residue that irritates the cells lining the intestine. The exceptions are specially formulated diets that require practically no digestion and are very easy to absorb (see below). Our research has developed new approaches that could help when used under medical supervision.

Inflammatory bowel diseases, such as Crohn's Disease and Ulcerative Colitis, and short bowel syndrome often caused by surgical removal of a portion of the bowel, have several symptoms and problems that can be classified into major categories:

Diarrhea, due to poor absorption of fat and some other food nutrients , as well as to poor absorption of water and other body secretions such as bile.

Inflammation, because the intestinal cells react to the disease and become inflamed. An inflammatory response often spreads to other parts of the body.

Partial Obstruction of the intestine which interferes with movement of food and causes severe pain. It also causes increased bacterial growth that produces gas and interferes with food absorption.

Malabsorption and malnutrition, because some but not all nutrients are poorly absorbed.

Diarrhea

Diarrhea may improve with a diet high in fiber. Some leftovers from digestion, such as bile, produce diarrhea by irritating the intestine and acting as powerful laxatives. Some fibers, such as pectin and gum, may help to bind these food residues and reduce diarrhea.

Cholestyramine (sold under the name QUESTRAN™) has a similar effect when eaten 15 to 30 minutes before each fatty meal. Other types of fiber, such as cellulose, may prevent watery diarrhea by absorbing water in the colon. There are several bulk fiber chemicals that you can buy for similar purposes. A diet with a wide variety of vegetables and fruits, low in animal fat and high in fiber, may also prevent this type of

Diets for Specific Diseases

diarrhea. However, *caution* must be taken if the intestine is obstructed.

Inflammation

Increased intestinal inflammation is the most important characteristic of IBD. It is difficult to detect with conventional blood tests. Many physicians order a wide range of tests to detect or monitor inflammation. Unfortunately, most of those tests are practically useless. If you feel sick, you are sick even if the test is "normal". If you are sick and the test is abnormal, there is little the physician can do that he could not do without the test results. If you feel great, and the test is abnormal, then you may not want to do anything because the test may either be in error or does not reflect your current well-being. In IBD the most important test of the activity of the disease is how you feel. The next most important tests are the nutritional tests that help you to decide how to specifically change your diet to correct nutritional deficiencies or excesses. A fatty acid profile such as the **EFA-SR** is very important because it helps you to correct EFA abnormalities, prevent unusual clot formation (which is common in IBD, particularly in patients who require intravenous feeding), and helps your doctor to modify the inflammatory response. Because the balance of EFAs determines the nature and extent of the inflammatory response, your doctor may recommend that you eat more ω3 in the form of EPA or linolenic acid, or more ω6 in the form of linoleic or GLA, to drastically change the inflammatory response. This is one situation where EFA derivatives may be indicated and the test **EFA-SR should be repeated frequently**. With frequent monitoring you can plan your optimal diet. Because the cost of frequent hospitalization is extraordinarily high, fatty acid analysis is highly cost-effective even if it only saves you a few days of hospitalization every year. IBD is a very expensive disease to treat, and treatment is rarely effective. Patients and doctors should aim to minimize and prevent complications by correcting nutritional abnormalities.

There is one test which I recommend for most patients with IBD: protein electrophoresis (see section II). This test is inexpensive and uses tiny amounts of blood. With modern technology and the aid of a highly trained specialist, this test measures a wide range of inflammatory proteins and other indicators of health status. Very few physicians are aware of the wide range of applications of this test.[20]

Diets for Specific Diseases

Obstruction

A partial obstruction can get worse with a diet high in fiber. This effect is difficult to predict. However, a diet very low in fiber may actually produce a greater obstruction because when the intestine contracts, there is not enough food inside it to prevent the intestine from contracting so tightly that it obstructs itself. In fact, this is believed to lead to diverticulitis and other problems. Therefore, for each person there is a certain amount of fiber which will help to prevent the pain associated with obstruction and also decrease diarrhea, and a larger amount that will cause an obstruction. Only you can tell by trial and error, and the amount may vary according to the state of inflammation of your intestine.

A partial obstruction is caused by a combination of factors. With IBD, the skin-like tissue that lines the intestine becomes thicker and harder, and the intestine becomes narrow and less flexible. In addition, the cells become inflamed and swollen. Outside the intestine, and inside the abdomen, the intestine becomes twisted because of the force caused by food trying to get through. Twisting the intestine, like twisting a hose, causes a partial obstruction. In obstructed areas, water accumulates because it cannot move fast enough, and there is overgrowth of the bacteria which produce gas. Food cannot pass through quickly enough and keeps pushing against the wall of the intestine, causing pain. The pressure of the food causes the intestine to distend and touch other organs. In IBD, you will notice abdominal distention, an increased urge to urinate (because the bowel is pressing against the bladder), and leg and knee pain as the intestine presses against the sciatic nerve. Sometimes the only symptom of intestinal inflammation and partial obstruction is pain in the knee and diffused leg pain. Many physicians diagnose "arthritis" when the real problem is intestinal inflammation pressing against a nerve. A similar situation occurs with back pain. Severe back pain may indicate a large intestinal infection or inflammation. The treatment for intestinal inflammation consists of bowel rest (intravenous feeding or elemental diet) for several days to weeks until the inflammation subsides and antibiotics if the inflammation is severe. You may need a wide spectrum mixture of intravenous antibiotics, to prevent or treat a hidden abscess. There is a great danger in treating this "arthritis" with steroids, because many times the inflammation is associated with small abscesses. The inflammatory process used by the body to fight the abscess and prevent the bacteria from spreading to other parts of the body can be reduced by

Diets for Specific Diseases

steroids. Using steroids could cause a small infection to propagate to other parts of the body.

In treating IBD, we suggest that you start with a small amount of fiber. Try that amount for several weeks. Increase it slowly. If it causes you more pain, then decrease it. Allow time for the body to adapt to it. Modify the fiber composition by trying different foods, ONE AT A TIME so that you can identify any specific food which is not good for you.

Malabsorption

Inflammatory bowel disease, such as Crohn's disease, is characterized by diarrhea and malabsorption. Among the major nutrients, carbohydrates are the easiest to absorb, protein is next and fat is the most difficult to digest and absorb. Individuals with inflammatory bowel disease are prone to develop severe deficiency of essential fatty acids. Because fat usually increases diarrhea, the best diet is very low in fat supplemented with one to two tablespoons of a mixture of $\omega3$ and $\omega6$ oils, both precursors and derivatives.

Malnutrition

Malnutrition is a complicated problem. It refers to having adequate body weight and adequate amounts of some nutrients, but having an *imbalance* in your nutrients. You may have normal or increased weight and look fine, and still be malnourished. To detect imbalances in protein, fat, minerals and vitamins one needs sophisticated blood and urine tests which require a specialist to interpret. Once the imbalance is determined, proper therapy is provided. Malnutrition manifests itself through subtle symptoms, such as muscle weakness, cramps, impaired vision or decreased mental abilities.

Most people with inflammatory bowel disease have nutritional deficiencies caused by poor absorption of some nutrients.[21] (In contrast, most other Americans have nutritional excesses along with deficiencies.) They simply cannot absorb some nutrients. The most common deficiencies involve most vitamins and minerals, and can be corrected easily with oral supplements. Most of the common multivitamins are not appropriate because they do not have vitamins and minerals in the proportion these people need them. They often have too much Iodine and not enough calcium, potassium, B_{12}, Folate and Biotin. In particular, deficiencies of magnesium are quite common and very difficult to correct.

Diets for Specific Diseases

Very thin people with malabsorption diseases need to eat more food because they are not getting enough calories. However, most people do get enough calories, but develop deficiencies of selected vitamins and minerals. Our studies have shown that the most common types of nutritional deficiencies in patients with malabsorption diseases are:

- **Deficiency of EFAs.** This is probably the most significant deficiency, which is difficult to treat because patients have to take large quantities of oils. Treat by eating a mixture of ω3 and ω6 oils, similar to the one used for heart disease. Quite often the deficiency is severe and recurrent, and patients require periodic intravenous infusion of lipids to replenish the body with EFAs. Even when corrected with intravenous lipids, the deficiency recurs because of the disease. Fat malabsorption due to Crohn's disease or short bowel treatment leads to Absolute Essential Fatty Acid Deficiency and requires frequent monitoring with a fatty acid profile to determine when intravenous lipids are needed. This is one of the few conditions where intravenous supplements may be needed because the person cannot absorb enough EFAs.

- **Vitamin deficiencies.** The most likely deficiencies are of B_{12}, Biotin, A, D, E and K. You can easily supplement your diet with these vitamins and, if necessary, you can obtain a special formulation of these vitamins in a water soluble form that is easier to absorb. Vitamin K deficiency can occur because the bacterial combination in the gut is altered; sometimes too many important bacteria are killed by antibiotics and cannot produce enough vitamin K. A second cause for vitamin K deficiency is simply that there is not enough vitamin K in the diet, and whatever is in the gut is poorly absorbed. Most patients with a diseased ileum (terminal part of small intestine) require periodic vitamin B_{12} and Vitamin K injections. These injections can be replaced, in many cases, with large oral doses, but oral doses may not be enough for some patients. Even if they get absorbed, they are not properly used by the body. Subcutaneous injections should be used about once every 3 to 8 weeks.

- **Mineral deficiencies.** The most common deficiencies include potassium, magnesium, manganese, zinc, copper and calcium. Patients often need to take very large doses of these

Diets for Specific Diseases

supplements. They usually need to obtain a prescription and use specially prepared supplements. Cramps in the legs often indicate potassium deficiency; cramps in the hands may indicate magnesium deficiency. Zinc deficiency often produces a scaly dermatitis. Except for potassium deficiency, which is characterized by muscle pain (particularly cramps in the morning when you wake up and stretch your legs), most other deficiencies are difficult to diagnose through symptoms. instead, specialized tests are required.

- Some patients require periodic intravenous or submuscular magnesium, or a small dose of magnesium many times per day. The problem with magnesium is that a single large dose may produce diarrhea (magnesium is a good laxative) and could make the diarrhea worse).

- **Additional supplements**. Two additional supplements are sometimes required: carnitine and choline. Muscle weakness and tiredness after rapid exercise are symptoms of carnitine deficiency (but they can also indicate potassium, magnesium or manganese deficiency).

Be careful with supplements. This is not a do-it-yourself-job. If you eat the wrong mixture of supplements you can easily overdose on one. One easy mineral to overdose on is Iodine, which is easily absorbed and found in many foods, salt and vitamin supplements.

To correct existing EFA abnormalities and supply daily requirements, most patients with malabsorption disease would need to take between 1 and 3 tablespoons of oil per day. For some people, this is too much fat, and causes more diarrhea (which can be minimized using cholestyramine and eating 1/2 of the oil in the morning and the rest in small amounts). Do not expect quick results. It often takes years to correct severe EFA deficiency in IBD. People with coronary artery disease or abnormal cholesterol levels associated with excessive weight usually have enough EFAs. Their problem is too much saturated fat which interferes with the proper use of the EFAs. In IBD, most people are thin and do not have enough EFAs in their body. Because IBD patients have fat malabsorption, they cannot eat too much fat and therefore it takes a long time to correct EFA deficiency. Those who can eat and absorb large amounts of fat (i.e., 3 tablespoons per day), may gain quite a bit of weight and should reduce other sources of calories and increase exercise. In severe cases, intravenous feeding with fats is

recommended to correct severe absolute (whole body) EFA
deficiency (see chapter I.3).

Treatment of Crohn's disease

Treatment of Crohn's disease aims to correct the symptoms. Until we
identify the organism that causes the disease, we will not be able to
have antibiotics against it. Surgery is to be avoided as long as possible.
Even the worst cases, where patients have intestinal fistulas or "holes,"
or abscesses and infections, can often be treated with total parenteral
nutrition and bowel rest for several months, and also with intravenous
antibiotics for 10 days followed by oral antibiotics if needed. The
disease recurs after surgery practically every time, while the
nutritional deficiencies caused by removal of the bowel remain forever.

Treatment should diagnose and correct nutritional abnormalities that
are a major factor in premature death in Crohn's disease, as well as the
cause of many other health problems. Successful treatment should
relieve intestinal inflammation and obstruction, and reduce diarrhea.
There is an approach for each one of these problems (which will be
discussed at length in another book).

After many years of research, scientists now agree that the best
treatment for Crohn's disease is "complete bowel rest," meaning that
the bowel should not work digesting food. There are two "foods"
available which I consider best for the treatment of Crohn's disease:
Vivonex™ and Tolerex™. These are powder formulas composed
primarily of simple amino acids, small carbohydrates, vitamins and
minerals. For this reason they are called "elemental diets" (meaning
very simple in chemical composition). They require practically no
digestion and are absorbed almost immediately, without requiring
much involvement from the intestine. After a period of 2 to 4 weeks on
this formula, practically all patients improve drastically. Their
nutrition improves because the formula is nutritionally balanced and
contains all essential vitamins, minerals and amino acids.
(Unfortunately, the exceptions are EFAs; see below.) In addition, the
intestinal inflammation subsides. An even better treatment would be
exclusive intravenous feeding, known as Total Parenteral Nutrition.
However, this treatment is expensive (as much as $30,000 per month),
and dangerous because the intravenous lines can get obstructed or
infected.

Diets for Specific Diseases

Most people cannot tolerate Vivonex™ and Tolerex™ by mouth. They must drink it using a tube inserted through the nose into the stomach. The tube is connected to a pump that feeds the solution continuously for 15 to 24 hours per day. Sometimes people drink it slowly with a straw all day long. Drinking it fast causes diarrhea.

To reduce diarrhea, I recommend the use of a product like "Questran™" or a similar resin. This type of product binds to bile (one of the substances made by the body which helps with digestion) and prevents it from reaching the large colon where it becomes an irritant that causes diarrhea. "Questran™" is also effective in lowering cholesterol (rarely a problem in patients with Crohn's disease) and has been shown to have very few side effects. I suggest you use 1/3 or more of the usual envelopes of "Questran™" about 10 minutes before you start to eat any meal that contains fat. You can also add one envelope of "Questran™" for each 3 envelopes of Vivonex™ or Tolerex™.

Many times in Crohn's disease, the intestinal obstruction gets substantially worse, because of increased inflammation and/or because of "bacterial overgrowth". Bacterial overgrowth means that the bacteria which normally live in the intestine have grown too much. Once out of balance, they cause gas and other problems. There is also a high probability that small abscesses (sores with pus) or tiny infections develop within the intestine. My clinical experience has shown the best treatment to be significant doses of a mixture of antibiotics targeted to the common bacteria found in the intestine. Treatment for about 10 days resolves the problem. This matter must be discussed with your physicians because many doctors refuse to believe that antibiotics work in Crohn's disease, in part because they often use the wrong mixture of antibiotics.

The elemental diets given to Crohn's patients have practically no fat in them. This is done intentionally to facilitate absorption and prevent complications. Because many people must drink the elemental diet with a tube while they are sleeping, it is important that the food leave the stomach very promptly. Otherwise there is danger that it could be regurgitated and enter the lungs. Fat slows the digestion process and increases the time that a food spends in the stomach.

Because elemental diets contain practically no EFAs, and usually zero ω-3s, you must supplement your diet with soybean oil. Because patients with Crohn's disease develop severe EFA deficiencies, they must be monitored regularly and eat as much oil as they can tolerate.

Diets for Specific Diseases

If possible, I suggest two tablespoons per day of soybean oil, one first thing in the morning and one late in the afternoon. Take the oil at least 2 hours before going to bed to prevent food from staying in the stomach too long and regurgitating into the lungs. In the morning the body may produce the largest amount of bile and this could make it the easiest time to absorb the EFAs. Always precede a dose of oil with about 1/3 envelope of Questran™. If oral EFAs are not enough, a patient may need to receive periodic Intravenouos lipids.

Many patients will find that a diet very low in fat along with EFA supplements is best for them. Very low, particularly zero fat foods are easy to digest and minimize diarrhea. Oils high in EFAs provide the required essential fats with a minimum of fat intake. Vegetables often decrease diarrhea, but you must be careful not to eat too many vegetables at a time if you have a partial intestinal obstruction. Vegetables are high in fiber and indigestible matter that can worsen an obstruction. If you develop the symptoms of a complete obstruction, which include feelings of nausea, vomiting, and severe, continuous abdominal cramps that seem to occur in cycles (on for a few minutes, off, and then on again), you should be seen immediately by a physician. The on-off-on pain cycle occurs as the intestine tries to push the food through the obstruction.

Short bowel syndrome

Some people have "short bowel syndrome,", meaning that their bowel (intestine) is shorter than normal. Quite often this occurs as a result of an accident or a disease. For example, a person may have had a cancer that required removal of part of the intestine. Or s/he was involved in an accident or shooting which caused him/her to lose part of the intestine. The nutritional deficiencies in short bowel syndrome resemble those of patients with Crohn's disease or Ulcerative Colitis. The type and extent of the deficiency depends on how much of the intestine is missing. Fortunately, the remaining parts of the intestine are not diseased in these patients; consequently, they rarely suffer from obstructions or massive malabsorption in the remaining parts. On the other hand, some patients have lost huge sections of the intestine and have similar symptoms and deficiencies as patients with severe Crohn's disease. In other words, they appear to have severely dysfunctional intestines.

Diets for Specific Diseases

Cystic Fibrosis (CF)

The nutritional problems pertaining to EFA abnormalities in cystic fibrosis (CF) are similar to those in Crohn's disease. "The basic defect in cystic fibrosis increases the metabolism of EFAs and thereby gradually gives rise to EFA deficiency, which is a well documented finding in most cases with this disease." EFA abnormalities and their metabolic products, i.e., different eicosanoids, and *EFA deficiency ". . .will cause gastrointestinal symptoms and the sequence of this development will mirror the natural history of the disease"*.[22] Often, a decrease in total fat, and probably EFA abnormalities, are the first detectable signs of the deterioration characteristic of cystic fibrosis.[23] There is evidence that in CF there is an impairment in the conversion of EFA precursors to their derivatives, as well as biochemical evidence of EFA deficiency.[24] It is recommended ". . .that close monitoring of plasma EFAs be carried out in CF, because of the high incidence of EFA deficiency despite efforts to improve and liberalize fat intake."[25] These authors recommend the analyses of plasma for the detection of EFA abnormalities and cite my research to describe their findings. The authors suggest that correction of EFA abnormalities will assist with easier ". . .control of chest infections, marginally better respiratory function, and perhaps extended survival." These results, together with those of numerous other published articles, provide compelling evidence that the treatment of CF prior to 1994 has ignored fundamental effects of EFA abnormalities on CF.

- EFA abnormalities and EFA deficiencies are highly common in CF and probably affect most or all patients. These deficiencies are highly complex and vary from one patient to another. Individualized diagnosis and treatment is necessary.

- EFA abnormalities contribute to impaired function of all organs, including lung function and gastrointestinal disease, and are likely to be a major factor in premature death.

- EFA abnormalities and deficiencies can be corrected with appropriate oral or intravenous supplements.

- Correction of EFA abnormalities provides significant improvement to patients with CF.

Correction of EFA abnormalities may require large amounts of oil and could take years unless intravenous lipids are used. Intravenous lipids may be required because of fat malabsorption. These issues also occur in Crohn's disease.

Diets for Specific Diseases

Case study: Cystic Fibrosis and Crohn's disease with EFA Deficiency

35 year old woman with Crohn's disease for over 5 years, partial intestinal resection. She has elevated $20:3\omega9$ /$20:4\omega6$ (See chapter I.3), and significantly decreased levels of EFAs and derivatives. Both the percent and the absolute quantities of EFAs are decreased, a condition we call Absolute EFA Insufficiency. The purpose of therapy is to achieve normal results as measured by the test **EFA-SR**. Because EFAs are essential for the intestine to repair itself and make more cells, correcting abnormalities of EFAs will minimize complications of the disease and increase bowel healing.

Recommended treatment: Oral soybean oil supplements (15-30 ml/day) plus 200 I.U. Vit. E/day, plus cholestyramine to minimize diarrhea. (Large vitamin E doses are needed due to malabsorption.) A repeat of the fatty acid profile after three months found that EFA levels increased significantly and derivatives were formed. Although there was a marked increase in the percent of PUFAs, due to the severe extent of the deficiency, the patient was still very deficient. We estimated that it would take many years to correct the deficiency using only oral supplements. The patient was then hospitalized for one week to receive a "loading" dose of EFAs with intravenous lipids and extra supplements of trace minerals, vitamins and other minerals. Now at home, she continues on a diet which includes a mixture of regular foods, an elemental diet, and EFA oral supplements. Repeated analyses have shown significant normalization of the fatty acid profile **EFA-SR:** The $\omega3$s have returned to normal but $\omega6$s are still deficient. Her oral dose of oils was then changed to 1/2 safflower and 1/2 soybean mixture, to increase the $\omega6/\omega3$ ratio.

Infection - AIDS

Some infectious agents alter the metabolism of fatty acids and make it more difficult for some parts of the body to get enough essential fats. Many AIDS patients lack essential fats. It appears that the AIDS virus alters the utilization of essential fats and deprives the body of EFAs. The disease also causes malabsorption and losses of EFAs from the intestine. A surgeon I know treats patients with AIDS using intravenous infusions of EFAs. The reason for using intravenous fats is that severely ill AIDS patients have difficulties absorbing fats. He has

Diets for Specific Diseases

found that the patients' immune systems improve and the progression of the disease is stopped. This work may provide a scientific basis for the observation that diets low in fat and high in essential fats help some patients with AIDS, and improve the immune system. A proper balance of EFAs is essential for the immune system to work. When the balance is upset, the body cannot fight infection. I recommend that every patient with AIDS be evaluated for abnormalities of EFAs, and correct any discovered abnormalities with oral or intravenous oil supplements.[26]

Adrenoleukodystrophy (ALD) and related disorders

Most people with ALD have seen the movie "Lorenzo's oil." The movie describes the story of a child with a disease that makes it difficult for his body to eliminate long chain fatty acids. There are several genetic disorders where humans lack enzymes to properly use fatty acids. In many of these conditions, long chain SFAs (C22 to C28, that is, molecules with 22 to 28 carbons) accumulate in the blood and tissues. [For comparison purposes, the EFAs have 18 carbons, their common derivatives have 20 to 22 carbons, but some new derivatives found in the eye and brain appear to have 24, 26 and even more carbons.] It is hypothesized that the accumulation of these long chain SFAs damages the myelin (the white matter which serves as a protection cover) of nerves, causing severe disease and eventual death at an early age. Based on the fact that in *humans*, elongation and desaturation fatty acid enzymes have preference for unsaturated over saturated fatty acids (which I have shown in a study published many years ago[27]), researchers proposed the use of MUFAs to stop the formation of long chain SFAs. With the aid of chemists, researchers developed a mixture of MUFAs which were used to treat people with ALD. Feeding the MUFAs indeed causes a shift in fatty acid production and reduction in blood levels of long chain SFAs. Instead of making long chain saturated fatty acids, the body makes very long chain monounsaturated fatty acids. Unfortunately, MUFAs cause problems perhaps as severe as the original problem. Feeding large quantities of MUFAs to a patient causes severe EFA deficiency, a problem which I pointed out several years ago and have since identified in the leftover blood sent to me by physicians treating patients with ALD.

I have proposed that a better treatment for ALD would be to use long chain EFA derivatives. I have shown that in humans the elongation and desaturation enzymes follow this **preference:** ω3 > ω6 > ω9 > ω7 > **SFAs**. Therefore, a mixture of ω3 and ω6 fatty acids would be far more effective than MUFAs (which are a mixture of ω9 and ω7 fatty acids) in the prevention of long chain SFAs, while at the same time preventing EFA deficiency. In this situation, unfortunately, correction of the fatty acid abnormality is unlikely to prevent premature death in individuals who have a severe genetic defect. However, there are many people with mild forms of the disease. In these cases, I recommend a blood analysis for all types of fatty acids, and subsequent therapy based on increased levels of long chain EFA derivatives. These derivatives may monopolize the enzymes that produce undesirable levels of SFAs and MUFAs, in a sense, "turning them off." These long chain EFA derivatives are now commercially available from specialized chemical companies. In treating ADL, it is important that the fatty acid profile used be similar to the **EFA-SR** test and measure concurrently the percent and concentration of key fatty acids. This will determine whether the deficiency is absolute or relative (see chapter I.3).[28]

Sickle Cell disease

One of the major causes of sickle cell disease is the death of red cells. Improving the EFA composition of red cells through better diet makes the cells more resistant and flexible. I have proposed that EFA supplements may improve the survival of patients with this condition.

References and Notes

[1] ω3 fatty acids found in fish oils modify the production of a type of hormone known as eicosanoids, and this alteration decreases platelet aggregation.

[2] As not all people with hypertension are "salt sensitive", the amount of salt you may eat safely depends on your unique responsiveness. Furthemore, if you are on a medication that leads to an increase in blood potassium levels, consult with your doctor before using salt substitutes or potassium supplements. Many salt substitutes replace sodium with potassium.

[3] Buddhist Monks and Nuns on vegetarian diets have fewer retinal abnormalities and less hypertension than Chinese non-vegetarians of a similar age. *Medical Tribune*, page 3, Nov. 19, 1986.

[4] Research News, *Science*, Vol. 235, Page 163, January 9, 1987.

[5] Klabr S et al. The effects of dietary protein restriction and blood pressure control on the progression of chronic renal disease. *N. Engl. J. Med.* 1994; 330:877-84.

Narins RG, Corters P. The role of dietary protein restriction in progressive azotemia. *N. Engl J. Med* 1994; 330:929-30.

[6] Dasgupta A, Kenny MA, Ahmad S. Abnormal fatty acid profile in chronic hemodialysis patients: possible deficiency of EFAs. *Clinical Physiol & Biochem*, 1990; 8:238-43. This study shows that EFA deficiencies are associated with kidney disease, and treating them could prevent or correct kidney disease.

[7] Kremer J M et al. Fish-Oil Fatty Acid Supplementation in Active Rheumatoid Arthritis. Annals of Internal Medicine, Vol. 106, pages 497-503, April, 1987.

[8] Eicosanoids (a type of hormone) such as prostaglandins and leukotrienes are involved in the regulation of the immune and inflammatory response.

[9] There are many similar oil capsules available at health food stores, by mail, or from a pharmacy or nutritionist. These capsules contain GLA or DGLA, a special type of ω-6 essential fat.

[10] Dr. Siguel has developed a cream that treats dry skin, dandruff and minimizes hair loss. While many products exist to remove dandruff, Dr. Siguel's cream aims to correct the biochemical abnormalities that cause dry skin, dandruff and hair loss. The cream is based on Dr. Siguel's research. At the time of this writing it is not available for sale, while he is waiting to develop marketing agreements.

[11] Skin: getting the wrinkles out of aging. National Institute on Aging, US DHHS, March, 1981.

[12] Nutrition and Cancer: Cause and Prevention. American Cancer Society Special Report. *CA-A Cancer Journal for Clinicians*, Vol. 34, No 2, pages 121-126, March/April, 1984. Laboratory Management STATlines, pages 15-16, October 1986.

[13] Cancer lower among active men. *The Boston Globe*, June 28, 1987, report of American Cancer Society study .

[14] See: Colditz G, et al, Increased green and yellow vegetable intake and lowered cancer deaths in an elderly population. *The Am Journal of Clinical Nutrition*, vol. 41, page 32-36, January 1985. However, excessive vitamin A or C intake, or too much fiber, may also induce cancer as reported by Dr. Herbert, Science Vol. 233, Aug. 29, 1986 (letter: Diet and Cancer). The best way to avoid excesses is by eating foods rather than food extracts or supplements like vitamin pills.

[15] Many patients with cancer do not eat well. It is well known that cholesterol declines drastically when people stops eating. One of my duties in the hospital was to review and interpret all the cholesterol tests of patients with heart disease. I noticed that patients admitted to the Coronary Intensive Care Unit often had very low total cholesterol, and even an excellent ratio of Total/HDL cholesterol because they were not eating. Similarly patients with cancer often have low cholesterol values because these patients frequently eat few calories.

[16] Siguel EN. Cancerostatic effect of vegetable diets. *Nutrition and Cancer*, 4:285-289, 1983.

[17] It is now possible to analyze your cancer cells to determine whether they require EFA derivatives to survive, and whether a low calorie, no EFA derivatives diet would help. In addition, one can test if the cells reproduce more slowly in the presence of high levels of ω3s. Although these tests are not commercially available, they are not difficult to conduct. Of course, you would need quite a bit of money to have these tests done.

[18] In the appendix there are test results from a patient with Crohn's disease.

Diets for Specific Diseases

[19] Overweight patients may have plenty of EFAs in their body fat, but too much saturated fat. Patients with IBD are rarely overweight and do not have enough EFAs in their body fat.

[20] As part of my training in clinical pathology (laboratory medicine), it was my job to review the protein electrophoresis test results on most patients at a major university hospital in Boston. I learned that a huge amount of useful information could be obtained from the test. However, it takes more than 30 minutes to interpret the test results. Most insurance companies do not pay enough for test interpretation and therefore doctors rarely do it.

[21] Different parts of the intestine absorb different types of nutrients. The nature of the deficiency depends on the diseased part. In Crohn's disease, it is usually the terminal part of the small intestine, called the ileum, which is responsible for the absorption of EFAs, B12, vitamin K and several other nutrients.

[22] Strandvik B. Relation between essential fatty acid metabolism and gastrointestinal symptoms in Cystic Fibrosis. *Acta Paediatr. Scand. Suppl.*, 1989; 363:58-65.

[23] Tomezsko, JL, Scanlin, TF, Stallings VA. Body composition of children with cystic fibrosis with mild clinical manifestations compared with normal children. *Am J. Clin. Nutr.* 1994; 59:123-8.

[24] Lloyd-Still HD, Johnson SB, Holman RT. Essential fatty acid status in cystic fibrosis and the effects of safflower oil supplementation. *Am. J. Clin.Nutr.* 1981; 34:1-7.

[25] Lepage G, Levy E, Ronco N, Smith L, Galeano N, Roy CC. Direct transesterification of plasma fatty acids for the diagnosis of essential fatty acid deficiency in cystic fibrosis. *J. Lipid Res.* 1989; 30:1483-1490.

[26] It is important to perform a fatty acid analysis as I have described in my patent and it is done by the test **EFA-SR**. AIDS patients may have at least one of three different types of abnormalities: not enough EFAs in the body (absolute EFA deficiency), enough EFAs, but not enough in proportion to the total fat (relative EFA deficiency, often caused by excessive blood levels of saturated fatty acids), and a transport deficiency (also relative EFA deficiency) which makes it difficult for the EFAs to reach the cells that need them. This is not caused by excessive amounts of saturated fatty acids, but instead caused by the AIDS virus which interferes with the optimal use of EFAs by the body. A similar phenomenon has been found in other infectious diseases.

[27] Siguel, EN, Maclure, M. Relative enzyme activity of unsaturated fatty acid metabolic pathways in humans, *Metabolism* 1987; 36: 664-669. Read chapter I.3, where I explain why the enzymes have preferences as follows: $\omega 3 > \omega 6 > \omega 9 > \omega 7$.

[28] Many people still believe that Lorenzo's oil should be used to treat these patients. I disagree, unless the oil is supplemented with EFA derivatives. For a discussion on the current treatment, see Letters to the Editor, *New Engl. J. Medicine*, More on Lorenzo's Oil, 1994; 330:1904-5. By A Odone and M Odone, myelin project. P Aubourg, INSERM, WB Rizzo, Medical College of Virginia. Also see Aubourg P, Adamsbaum C, Lavallard-Rousseau M-C et al. A two-year trial of oleic and erucic acids ("Lorenzo's Oil") as treatment for adrenomyeloneuropathy. *N. Engl. J. Med.* 1993; 329:745-52.

Diets for Specific Diseases

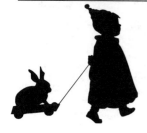

IV.6

THE EFFECT OF AGE, GENES AND TEMPERATURE

"We may all be created equal but we are physically different"

Topics: Food and age. Your genes. Do your ancestors come from a cold or a warm climate? Temperature and diet.

Summary

Children and adolescents require proportionately more calories than adults, which provide additional energy, vitamins, minerals and essential fats. Compared with adults, they need more nutrients because they are building more cells. Supplements may be required if their calories come primarily from foods with low nutrient value. Adults must eat only enough to maintain weight and replace dead cells. Sedentary individuals require vitamin, mineral and oil supplements because the smaller amount of food they need to maintain weight may not provide enough necessary nutrients. Some elderly individuals may need to eat EFA derivatives because the ability to form derivatives of the essential fats may be impaired as one becomes older. Eat more essential fats in cold climates or during the winter because essential fats protect against the cold. Supplement the essential fats with vitamin E and other antioxidants to prevent oxidation of the essential fats.

Introduction

In previous chapters we introduced general principles for food selection. Healthy people should eat a balanced mixture of many different foods, primarily natural foods in their natural state. Individuals with cardiovascular disease need to quickly and drastically modify their body composition. Just eating natural foods may take too long. Therefore we indicated oil supplements, which help to replace saturated with essential fats.

In this chapter we explain what foods and supplements are appropriate for specific population groups. No two humans are alike (except for identical twins). It is impossible in one book to prescribe individual diets for each person in the country. Instead, we have grouped people into broad categories of specific nutritional need. Much of the information presented here is controversial and being investigated. Therefore, you may find researchers who disagree with my advice. I think I am right, but only time will tell.

Children

Growing children require nutrients to create new cells. Therefore, children should eat a large number of foods, in greater variety than adults and in greater quantity. It is important to concentrate on vegetables and fish in order to insure an adequate supply of essential fats, which are needed for optimal body and brain growth.

Most children in the USA follow a diet very high in sugar, processed carbohydrates, saturated fat and processed oils, which are the main ingredients in most cookies, candy bars, and other foods provided in fast food restaurants and school cafeterias. Many food bars appeal to people because they are made with "natural foods". Some parents think their children are eating the "right way" because they eat organically grown processed foods, unbleached flour, and products made with whole wheat flour. Unfortunately, these "natural" foods are mainly food extracts high in carbohydrates, sugar, corn syrup and processed oils. These foods are transformed by the body into saturated fat, and may also contain other undesirable ingredients such as *trans* fatty acids. Remember, "natural" does not necessarily means healthy. Many food bars contain processed oils and pure carbohydrates which the body sees biochemically as being similar to those in chocolate brownies or cookies. Furthermore, most processed foods have been deprived of their EFAs.

Age, Genes and Temperature

Because many foods are vitamin fortified, children may eat too much of some vitamins and minerals and not enough of others. Variation in the composition of processed foods (such as cereals) makes it impossible to predict whether a child is eating too little or too much of a particular vitamin and mineral. I find it impossible to scan the food labels and calculate my daily nutritional intake to verify that I am eating the proper amounts of vitamins and minerals. I cannot remember all the food labels and correctly multiply their food composition by the amount I eat every day.

Food labels are practically useless for me because they do not tell me the important things I want to know: the amounts and types of essential fats, TFAs, and levels of toxic contaminants, antibiotics, or other undesirable additives in the food in question.

Ideally, you would like your child to eat natural foods. Sometimes this is impossible. Therefore, an alternative approach involves guesswork and compensation for current bad dietary habits. If your child follows a bad diet, you could try a multiple vitamin with minerals two to four times per week. A multivitamin once every day is very rarely needed and may lead to a vitamin overdose. Select one pill with the RDA (as explained in other chapters).

Encourage your child to take vegetables and fruits to school. Eat a fruit as dessert instead of a cookie or ice cream. Instead of ice cream buy sherbet or very low fat ice cream. Add one tablespoon per day of soybean and corn oil (half and half) uncooked to meals (adding these oils to mashed potatoes or salads is a good choice).

Children should be slim. If your child is not slim the primary reasons are that he/she is not exercising enough and he/she eats too many sweets and processed foods. Do not be confused with theories about fat cells, hormones and enzymes. Those theories make fascinating discussion at scientific meetings and may explain overweight in a few exotic cases reported in scientific journals. Most overweight children are overweight because they eat too much of the wrong foods. You rarely see overweight children in countries where people are dying of starvation.

It is preferable that children exercise in order to eat more foods and consequently obtain a proper balance of nutrients. Food deprivation in children, that is, eating foods low in calories, may lead to nutritional

Age, Genes and Temperature

deficiencies. Children should lead an active physical life and eat foods naturally low in saturated fat and calories and high in nutrients.

Infants and very young children

Infants and very young children require a large proportion of their fat as EFAs. Both ω3 and ω6s are needed by all cells to grow and reproduce. The ω3s are used to create new brain cells and make connections among cells. Infants and young children deprived of ω6s develop skin disorders. A skin dermatitis in newborn children is often due to ω6 deficiency. Well-trained intensive care and newborn units are aware of this ω6 deficiency and treat it with topical applications of safflower oil (or similar treatment) and, when needed, oil provided intravenously. Unfortunately, few provide extra ω3 because decreased mental ability is not obvious in infants. EFA deficiency is also a contributory factor in reduced cell life, including reduced red cell life and increase in bilirubin in the blood. I recommend that all infants born from mothers with suspected nutritional deficiencies be tested for EFA abnormalities using the blood test **EFA-SR**. A deficiency of ω3s leads to impaired brain growth, behavior abnormalities and reduced brain function. Children fed diets deficient in ω3s are likely to grow up to be less smart than they could have been.

Women's milk contains a more balanced amount of EFAs than cow's milk or most formulas. However, women who are EFA deficient cannot produce milk with enough EFAs to meet the needs of their children. Some infant and children's formulas on the market contain small amounts of the EFAs linoleic and linolenic acid. They contain practically no EFA derivatives. The reason for this is that EFAs, particularly the derivatives, are very unstable and deteriorate rather quickly. Children would not eat formulas that taste "fishy" or "rancid." Furthermore, fat in a meal delays the emptying of the stomach. Putting fat in infant formulas will mean that the food will stay longer in the stomach. Because many infants and children eat lying down or go to bed shortly after a meal, the food in the stomach may regurgitate back up into the lungs. Foods without fat are rapidly digested and leave the stomach sooner.

Although many companies plan to add more EFAs to their formulas starting late in 1994 and 1995, this change could cause additional problems. If you feed your child foods high in fat, you want to wait for at least 30 minutes (maybe longer with a large meal) before putting

Age, Genes and Temperature

your child to lie down in bed. This is necessary to allow time for the food to leave the stomach. I know that many parents feed a bottle to their child while the child lies in bed. This procedure could be dangerous when the food contains a lot of fat. The food could be regurgitated and damage the lungs. In addition, formulas with EFAs need additional antioxidants or special protection against deterioration. Of course, the best approach is to breast feed. Children get fresh EFAs right from the original source. ***Women's milk is high not only in EFAs, but also in EFA derivatives.*** This is very important for infants and young children who may not have the enzymes to make EFA derivatives. These EFA derivatives are freshly made by the women's bodies. Furthermore, most babies are breast fed somewhat vertically (nobody breast-feeds a baby with his or her feet up), which means that the food is unlikely to back-up into the lung. But I have seen babies drink from a bottle while putting their feet and stomach up against the bed. When your child starts to eat foods, you can feed him/her foods rich in EFAs, particularly ω3s needed for brain development. Foods high in TFAs may interfere with the body's ability to make EFA derivatives, so it is wise not to feed any of these foods to infants and very young children.

I strongly recommend that children who may not have obtained enough EFAs at some point in their lives have a blood test to determine if they have enough EFAs now. Although some of the damage done may not be reversible, you can prevent further brain deterioration by supplementing their diets with a proper mixture of EFAs and EFA derivatives. It is highly unfortunate that most parents and many physicians are not aware of the need for EFA supplements. This issue was raised at several US and World nutrition conferences during 1994, and I and other scientists, particularly in Europe and Canada, have been lecturing about it for more than 15 years.[1]

The best approach to insure that children get enough EFAs is to be certain that pregnant women have enough EFAs for their babies. I believe that the vast majority of women do not have enough EFAs in their blood to feed their babies before or after they are born. This is an unfortunate nutritional problem which I believe is a major contributory factor to decreased mental ability.[2] In addition to impaired brain function, EFA abnormalities are a major factor in the elevated cholesterol and blood pressure that now affect a significant number of children raised in America.

Age, Genes and Temperature

Late adolescents and adults

While children and early adolescents need foods to grow organs, late adolescents and adults need foods to preserve their bodies. Their requirements for vitamins and minerals are smaller, and they have vast stores which allow them to tolerate longer periods of excesses or deprivation. Therefore, nutritional deficiencies are less likely in adults than children. Adults who are usually less active than children should eat less food proportionate to their body size, or they will become overweight. Adolescents should eat enough EFAs to prevent EFA insufficiency when they become older.

Middle age

Most Americans who have reached middle age have accumulated over 40 years of bad nutrition. It is impossible to change the foods you have accumulated in your body during 40 years in one week or even one month. However, it is possible to change them slowly, over time, while preventing further deterioration.

For most people, the most likely problem is an excess of saturated fat and insufficient essential fats in their bodies. This can be compensated for by eating oil supplements as previously described.

Elderly

Elderly people and those with sedentary jobs need to follow a careful diet to prevent nutritional deficiencies. They usually do not eat enough food to get all necessary nutrients, and if they do eat enough food, they gain weight.

Most elderly people exercise very little. An active child may eat 4,000 calories per day and rarely become obese. An active adult may eat 2,000 calories per day and maintain his weight. An elderly person may eat 1,500 calories per day and gain weight. In fact, many overweight elderly people move so little that 1,000 calories per day provide all the energy they need.

If you eat few calories per day (under 1500), you may need vitamin and mineral supplements

It is difficult to obtain an adequate supply of vitamins and minerals on less than 2,000 calories per day. Therefore, many elderly individuals need to take one multiple vitamin plus mineral supplements three to six times per week. In addition, they must take at least one tablespoon of oil, the combination of which depends on the diseases they want to treat or prevent. If they have a significant deficiency of essential fats, they must take EFA derivatives to correct it quickly. An elderly person cannot afford to wait 10 years to correct a deficiency of EFAs. Elderly persons should be particularly aware of imbalances of EPA/AA (see previous chapters) that leads to increased formation of clots. They should also be concerned about ω3 deficiency because it will lead to decreased mental ability.

Our research suggests that many healthy elderly individuals can survive eating only precursor EFAs (vegetables and vegetable oils). However, a very small amount of fish or fish oil is not likely to hurt and may help. Fish is preferable, but overweight individuals on low calorie diets can supplement their meals with 1 to 3 grams of ω3 oils per day (about 2 to 6 oil capsules or a small teaspoon).

Some research suggests that elderly people may not be able to form enough derivatives of the essential fats and therefore should eat fish oils to obtain ω3 derivatives. How can you tell what you need? The fatty acid profile will indicate whether or not a person can form EFA derivatives from precursors. If the test shows that you cannot form enough EFA derivatives, you should eat more fish oil and ω6 derivatives. If you are quite healthy by merely eating vegetables and fish, please continue. However, if you have any of the conditions that may be improved by EFA derivatives, try them.

Aging reduces the capacity of our organs (heart, lungs, kidneys). Therefore, elderly people must have smaller bodies to function well; in other words, they must be thin. Most physicians agree that the most significant factor in ill health and "being tired" among the elderly is overweight. Remember, what may be average weight for a young adult is overweight for an elderly person who has a smaller heart and lungs barely able to supply the needs of an average body.

Age, Genes and Temperature

Your ancestry or genes

We know that some people live to 100 and others die of a heart attack at age 35. We rarely know why, but it is clear that some people have genes which determine their better body chemistry, protecting them from disease, and deterioration in old age. Some may have genes that help to destroy harmful chemicals. Others may have genes that protect their essential fats from oxidation (destruction). Whatever it is, some people have it, some do not. However, good or bad genes are not the determining factor in good health. Some people are born wealthy and squander their money; others are born poor and achieve great wealth.

Eating a healthy diet will help your body, whether you have good or bad genes. Individuals with bad genes, usually indicated by a family history of death at a young age, need to be more careful in their food selection and stick more consistently to healthy foods.

Ancestry

My research suggests that individuals who originated in warm climates, characterized by dark skin and eyes, have been optimally designed to exist in these warm climates. For example, these individuals are less likely to be burned by the sun. When these people move to a cold environment their requirements for essential fats increase. If you have dark skin and eyes I suggest that you eat more green vegetables and oils, and more fish. (But first test your blood to see whether or not you have enough EFAs). Dark-skinned people living in cold climates, particularly blacks (either from Africa or Latin America), should be tested for EFA abnormalities. People from India living in cold climates usually eat quite a few vegetable oils in their traditional meals, and are less likely to have EFA abnormalities.

Your environment: cold or warm climate

Research has shown that plants and animals adapt to cold weather by eating and manufacturing more essential fats. Fish who migrate from warm to cold areas produce more essential fats. This is one reason why cold water fish are rich in $\omega 3$ fats: They produce them as a protection against the cold because essential fats do not solidify in cold temperatures, while non essential fats do solidify. If a fish were made up of SFAs and moved to the Arctic, it would freeze solid, and die.

Age, Genes and Temperature

Humans are similar, except that we have modified our environment with artificial heat and air conditioning. These artificial modifications change our nutritional requirements in unpredictable ways. However, as a general rule, you can do the following:

- Eat foods natural to your environment.
- Eat warm area foods in the summer, cold area foods in the winter.
- Eat more essential fats and fish oils in the winter.

References and Notes

[1] The International Society for the Study of Fatty Acids and Lipids, together with major European health organizations, are recommending that infant food formulas contain ω3 and ω6 precursors and derivatives. Unfortunately, medical and nutrition groups in the USA have not paid enough attention to this major health problem. Instead, we find that government groups provide mothers, infants and children with foods high in saturated fats and low in EFAs.

[2] I have brought this matter to the attention of the US Department of Health and Human Services, the National Institutes of Health ("**NIH**"), the Food and Drug Administration and the USDA. None of these agencies have cared. I proposed that they fund surveys of pregnant women, children and adolescents to determine the extent of EFA abnormalities. They refused. The NIH has reviewed many of my research proposals and the review panels have repeatedly stated that my methods to measure fatty acids are *"state of the art"* and that I *"have considerable expertise in the area of fatty acid metabolism"* (4/07/94) and that I have *"clearly labored with the difficult identification of EFAs in human plasma through the development of sophisticated GLC techniques, meticulous preparation of serum samples for analysis, and activities related to the management and analysis of data obtained from improved GLC separation of plasma into various fatty acid profiles."* Unfortunately, it seems that the government prefers to spend hundreds of millions of dollars to test exotic drugs and to investigate complex and expensive invasive diagnostic procedures, while it fails to identify a problem that affects most of the children and adolescents in America. Ironically, President Clinton is trying to encourage more preventive medicine and improve children's opportunities while lower level government employees defeat his proposals by failing to identify and correct the most significant nutritional abnormality of children.

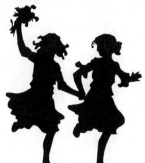

IV.7

OTHER POPULATION GROUPS

"Women require different mixtures of EFAs than Men"

Topics: *Modifications for men and women. Pregnant women. Active and inactive people. Executives. Athletes.*

Summary

During pregnancy, women often need to eat more essential fats from vegetables and fish, but they should avoid fish oils unless their blood tests show excessive tendency to clot. Very active individuals may eat more calories from animal fat because they will burn the saturated fat and store the essential fats. More sedentary individuals should eat fewer calories, and should eat proportionately more essential fats by eating more vegetables and oil supplements.

Men and women

It is amazing how little we know about the differing fatty acid needs of men and women. It is clear that women have a significantly different metabolism than men. Yet, how these differences translate into different nutritional needs remains to be determined. Because researchers have been concerned mostly with SFAs and cholesterol, they have overlooked research on EFA needs in women and men. My research aims to find the factors associated with heart disease, and the types of fatty acids that prevent heart disease and stroke. I have studied about 250 men and 250 women who participated in the world-famous Framingham Heart Study. I found significant EFA abnormalities in more than 25% of the subjects. I evaluated these patients using the blood test **EFA-SR**, which I developed. I use these methods to diagnose EFA abnormalities in men and women, and study how these abnormalities relate to abnormal cholesterol levels, high blood pressure, heart disease and diabetes. I have found that, on average, women have different EFA abnormalities than men. There is great variability in EFA patterns for both sexes. For that reason, a particular diet may work for one person and not for another.

Calories

Most women have a smaller body size than men do, and therefore require fewer calories. In other words, women need to eat less than men do. Moreover, in the USA, women tend to perform tasks that require less physical strength and therefore they consume fewer calories. Of course, if a women works performing constant and strenuous physical activity, her caloric requirements are increased. But most work does not require large amounts of calories. Similarly, a man with sedentary work does not burn many calories.

Even positions considered quite active, such as that of a police-man or woman, involve relatively minor exercise unless most time is spent chasing criminals by foot. Pressing the accelerator pedal in the car requires very few calories. Active strenuous exercise means the equivalent of running continuously for over 2 hours per day. Lumberjacks, athletes and those in similar professions consume large quantities of calories. Almost everyone else has, in comparison, a sedentary job.

Weight and weight loss

A healthy weight for a woman is less than the weight for a man of similar height. Because women have less body mass, usually less protein and bone, and smaller body organs, they require fewer calories to maintain their bodies.

The response to the same diet by two apparently similar people could be quite different depending on their body amounts of essential fats. I have found that some overweight people have large amounts of EFAs in their body, while others have very little. When a person with large amounts of EFAs in his/her body fat loses weight, the body primarily retains the EFAs and burns mostly saturated fat. As this person

---

Other Population Groups

becomes more lean, the ratio of PUFA/NoPUFA (NoPUFA = SFA+MUFA) (the amount of PUFA in proportion to other fats in the body) increases and may reach optimal levels. A person with large amounts of essential fats in his/her body may follow a very low calorie, low fat diet without EFA supplements and actually increase the amount of EFAs in his/her body, even after considering the need for daily EFA to repair the usual wear and tear of the body. This person will also see deep declines in total cholesterol and blood pressure.

A person who has little PUFA in the body and follows a very low calorie diet will lose weight, but will not get enough EFAs. As a result, although it is possible that the PUFA/NoPUFA ratio will increase, it will still remain abnormal. Practically everyone who goes on a very low calorie diet sees a drastic decline in cholesterol and blood pressure. However, when a PUFA deficient person starts eating again, cholesterol and blood pressure increase because the fundamental reason for the condition, low levels of EFAs in the body, has not changed.

Premenstrual syndrome

The activities of a group of hormones called "eicosanoids," which includes the prostaglandins, play a major role in menstruation and may account for the intensity of the premenstrual syndrome. Alterations in the relative amounts of various hormones affect the length and intensity of the menses. Because essential fats are the substances from which these hormones originate, modifying the relative amounts of $\omega3$ vs. $\omega6$ fatty acids may modify the intensity of the premenstrual syndrome. However, little is known that works for all women. The best policy is to try a therapy that, even if it does not help, will not hurt.

The following suggestions are likely to help without introducing additional complications. When you anticipate having premenstrual syndrome, change your diet as follows:

- Eat more green vegetables, and foods high in fiber to prevent constipation.
- Take fewer stimulants like coffee, tea and chocolate
- Eat several small meals rather than one large one. Eating frequent meals often provides psychological relief and may keep your body occupied with digestion, as well as prevent low blood sugar levels (hypoglycemia).

Other Population Groups

- Eat an ω6 rich oil such as safflower, or one with ω6 plus ω3 such as soybean. Experiment with both, using one for several months then shifting to the other, or to a mixture of the two. Trial and error will help determine which works best.. Remember, you need to try one oil at a time for several months and determine whether or not the pain associated with menstruation declines or remains the same.

Because each woman reacts differently to the prostaglandins, experiment with oils which have different effects to determine which one is better for you. Fish oils or flax seeds will have a similar but stronger effect than soybean oil, and you can use them instead of or in addition to soybean oil. The oils may be particularly useful for people who have a diet relatively low in the essential fats contained in these oils, that is, women who eat the standard American diet of animal food, sweets and processed food rather than the diet suggested in this book.

Pregnant women

Pregnant women have increased nutritional requirements. Because a child is growing inside of them, they need more of almost everything. But they need more of some nutrients than others. Pregnant women should take a multivitamin designed for pregnant women, or the one their physician prescribes after blood tests. A healthy pregnant woman does not need and probably should not take the multivitamin every day, but rather only a few times per week. Pregnant women are likely to require more Iron, Magnesium, Potassium, Vitamin B_{12} and folate. These nutrients are needed to produce cells and they are usually stored in relatively small quantities in the body.

One very important nutrient too often overlooked by most physicians is the increased need for essential fats. Pregnant women should increase their intake of vegetables and vegetable oils, with emphasis on soybean oil which provides both the ω3 fatty acids needed by brain tissue and the ω6 fatty acids needed by other cells. All cells need a mixture of these fatty acids, but brain tissue requires more ω3 fatty acids. In fact, current research suggests that some complications of pregnancy, such as diabetes, increased blood pressure, preeclampsia, and delayed or complicated delivery may be due to alterations in the structure of cells and hormones (prostaglandins); these changes are induced by insufficient intake of essential fats. If fish oils are used during

Other Population Groups

pregnancy, they should be used with great caution and perhaps should be stopped several weeks prior to delivery. Since fish oils decrease clotting, they could lead to increased bleeding after delivery.

Active vs. passive physical activity

Athletes and active individuals burn many calories and therefore eat more foods. Very active individuals can easily consume 4000 calories per day without gaining weight. Because they burn primarily saturated fat, even those who follow a relatively bad diet are able to accumulate essential fats and obtain required nutrients. Athletes therefore eat meals which behave as if they were low in saturated fat and high in essential fats. These facts may account for the finding of increased HDL and decreased cholesterol in active athletes.

Individuals who primarily have desk jobs, such as "Executives," tend to exercise rarely and thus burn few calories. Inactive individuals who eat more than 2000 calories per day usually gain weight. Because inactive people eat fewer foods, they must watch their meals and eat balanced foods to assure a proper supply of nutrients and essential fats. They must also be careful to eat foods low in saturated fats.

Anemia, bleeding, burns, disease

Any disorder that requires that the body make more cells increases the demand for EFAs. Burns, depending on the extent, requires that the body form a huge number of skin cells. Disease usually increases the metabolic rate and the demand for EFAs (which are used to form hormones and replace diseased tissue). Menstruating women may lose a significant amount of blood every month. Because the blood is lost to the body, the body cannot recover the nutrients in the blood. In contrast, when blood is lost through internal bleeding, such as from an ulcer in the stomach, the body often recovers many of the nutrients in the lost blood. The result is that women often need to take higher quantities of some vitamins and minerals than men do. They also need to replenish EFAs in their bodies with a balanced diet and/or oil supplements. Women who eat too much ω3, could have excessive menstrual bleeding.

Women who follow a vegetarian diet should supplement their diet with iron (about 4 mg per day is enough; most multivitamin pills contain 18

Other Population Groups

mg) and vitamin B_{12}. A multivitamin with iron containing 100 % of the RDA (as indicated on the label), once or twice per week, is usually enough. Occasionally, supplements of the vitamin folic acid (folate) are necessary, particularly during pregnancy if the diet is not balanced. People who have lost quite a bit of blood or other cells due to disease, burns, or a similar health problem need to eat more EFAs to replenish those lost. The blood lost and the cells lost carry EFAs with them.

Other Population Groups

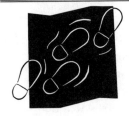

V.1

HOW TO EVALUATE A DIET

"To eat or not to eat is not the issue; the question is what to eat."

Topics: Types of diets. Which diets to select and why. How to evaluate a diet. Typical American diets. USDA recommended diet. American Heart Association diet. Vegetarian diets. Benefits and disadvantages.

Summary

There are two basic kinds of diets: diets aimed at weight loss and diets aimed at changing your nutritional status. Most weight loss diets are quite restrictive: They usually leave you hungry and may in fact lead to nutritional deficiencies if followed for long periods of time. A balanced diet will not leave you hungry and will provide a wide variety of appetizing foods. It will maintain or reduce your weight while improving your overall health.

Most diets do not require absolute adherence, but you cannot deviate often if they are to work for you. Occasional deviations are not likely to cause you any problem. But if the exception becomes the rule, if the occasional beer becomes a once a day drink and the monthly pizza, pastry, or heavy fatty meal becomes a weekly treat, then you are likely to counteract some beneficial effects of the diet.

The key is quite simple: Eat more green vegetables, legumes, seeds, nuts, fruits and cereals; avoid animal fat products and processed foods. Among the best decisions you could make is to shift towards more natural foods. A more vegetarian diet allows you to eat a great variety of foods, and you will rarely be hungry if you eat such a balanced diet. Because your nutritional status will improve, you will find that your energy level and your ability to do things are greatly improved.

Types of diets

A "diet" is a combination of specific meals and foods. There are three basic kinds of diets: (1) day-to-day diets that most people should use to maintain good health and prevent disease, (2) diets that help you lose weight, to be used for a short period of time, and (3) diets that improve your overall health and are used to correct existing disease, without necessarily causing weight loss.

Which diets to select and why

If you are overweight, you should start improving your health by losing weight, since eliminating excess pounds is probably the most important thing you can do to prevent heart disease.

A problem with most diets

No matter how good the intentions of the authors and how nutritionally sound a diet is (that is, how good the diet is from a scientific point of view), it is one thing to read about dietary recommendations and quite another thing to eat what they prescribe. Most Americans like prepared foods: pizza, cookies, cakes, soft drinks and beer. Given the choice between a hamburger with French fries or rice with green beans, most people will not have a hard time making a selection.

We suggest that you follow the diet that you like; then you will be more likely to stick to it. It is impossible to review all the available books and we have therefore selected a few examples from each category. You can pick out any cookbook at the library and make your own diet as long as you eat enough essential fats, and other basic nutrients.

Most common diets produce only mild improvements

Many diets are easy to follow but have the disadvantage of producing only mild improvements in your health. If you are young and healthy, following these diets may prevent cardiovascular disease. But if you are middle aged and already sick, these diets may be too mild, and the results they produce too negligible to make a major difference in your health. But they cannot be discounted out of hand. Even a small improvement in your health may extend your life, and that is certainly not something to be taken lightly. Some diets may actually be counterproductive, depending on how you implement them. Mostly

How to evaluate a Diet

vegetarian diets such as the ones we propose are likely to produce major improvements in your health.

The following diets recommend eating less saturated fat and refined sugars, and reducing salt (sodium) intake while at the same time eating more complex carbohydrates. The differences lie in the level of detail presented and the specific approach that they suggest. Some diets are quite specific and include many recipes, which you may or may not like.

The American Heart Association diet

I do not consider the American Heart Association (**AHA**) diets useful to treat heart disease because they fail to emphasize the role of ω3 vs. ω6 fatty acids. The AHA diet is easy to follow. Most nutritionists and physicians are familiar with it. The Heart Associations (local and national) provide a multitude of brochures that describe the diets, present recipes and give other recommendations for improving one's cardiovascular health. It is easy to call these associations and ask questions of their staff. You may purchase a brochure from them and use it as a guide for planning your meals. The AHA tells you the nutritional benefits of each food group, and within each group it tells you what foods are all right to eat and which foods to avoid.[1]

Research on the benefits of this diet is still in progress. The AHA diet is likely to prevent heart disease when compared with the traditional American diet. However, I doubt that the diet will have a significant effect as a treatment program for people who already have cardiovascular disease (or elevated blood pressure). The dietary changes may not be substantial enough to correct the effects of many years (30 or more, for most adults) of bad eating habits.

I do not recommend some of the approved foods which have been listed in the past in AHA brochures. Among the fats and oils, the AHA used to state that partially hydrogenated soybean oil is an acceptable food. I disagree: Partial hydrogenation destroys the beneficial ω3 fatty acids. Similarly, I suggest you avoid margarine, another food that was formerly recommended by the AHA, because it is made with partially hydrogenated oil. Aside from its saturated fat content, I am not against the sparing use of chocolate. Although chocolate may not be altogether advisable, cocoa can be used safely in your meals.

For treatment purposes (i.e., to lower your cholesterol, high blood pressure and reduce your risk of heart disease), please read my

How to evaluate a Diet

chapters on the use of vegetable and fish oils. Treatment requires drastic changes in your body chemistry. I recommend that more emphasis be placed on eating vegetables and vegetable oils (for treatment) and less emphasis on animal food products: You should eat less of the animal and dairy products approved by the AHA.

The main criticism I have of the AHA diet is its position on fat. The AHA does not incorporate the effects of EFAs on health and disease as described in this book. I have been writing to them for some time, to suggest that they ought to emphasize essential fats rather than saturated fats, and they ought to recommend avoiding *trans* fatty acids, but they have not been interested. I submitted abstracts for presentation at the 1993 annual meeting of the AHA describing the role of essential fats in health and disease and the extent of essential fatty acid abnormalities in the US. The AHA review committees told me that they were not interested in these topics. This astonished me, as one of my proposed research posters explained that I had identified one of the most significant nutritional factors associated with Total cholesterol/HDL cholesterol, a topic often discussed in AHA literature. My research had found that calories from essential fats were the most significant issue in creating healthy cholesterol levels and ratios.[2]

In contrast, the American College of Cardiology (**ACC**) accepted my research for presentation at their annual meeting in March, 1994. Furthermore, it considered my research so significant that it called a press conference (3/14/94) to announce my results. This situation illustrates the inconsistency of the many scientific review committees and may explain the often contradicting recommendations made by nutrition researchers.

The US Department of Agriculture recommendations for a "healthy diet".

It is my position that the USDA diet would cause more heart disease than it would prevent. Most processed foods such as pasta, breads, and cereals, placed by the USDA at the base of their pyramid, to be eaten in the largest amounts, have virtually no EFAs. Moreover, some of the carbohydrates in these foods are converted to SFAs when eaten in excess, and these fats can upset the balance of EFAs in the body. The USDA claims that fats and oils "provide calories and little else nutritionally." I consider this statement, made in "The Food Guide

---

How to evaluate a Diet

Pyramid" on p.5, to be incorrect. Although some fats provide calories without any other nutrients, many oils contain EFAs which are essential to human life. **Grouping oils with EFAs in the same category as candies, soft drinks and butter misrepresents what is necessary and what is irrelevant in nutrition.**

The USDA publishes several brochures with Dietary Guidelines for Americans.[3] You can obtain a copy of one of them for free or purchase one of several books that contain detailed information about the nutrients in each food. These recommendations were recently changed and now are represented by a pyramid of foods, with the foods to be eaten in the largest quantities placed at the bottom of the pyramid.[4] A copy of the pyramid is included in the Appendix.

The USDA recommendations are similar to what many Americans concerned about their health do now: Eat a variety of foods; maintain desirable weight; avoid too much fat, saturated fat, and cholesterol; eat foods with adequate starch and fiber; avoid too much sugar; avoid too much sodium; if you drink alcoholic beverages, do so in moderation. Because the USDA guidelines (like those of the AHA) overlook the differences between the ω3 and ω6 fatty acids which are the keys to good health, you may expect to obtain only slight improvements in your health. Worse, you may find that your chances of getting a heart attack increase if you eat a diet very low in EFAs.

The USDA tells you that oils have little value and encourages you to use them "sparingly" (p. 5 of The Food Guide Pyramid). The USDA and most other government agencies encourage a low fat diet. Most of the foods recommended by the USDA to be eaten in large amounts have very few EFAs. If you follow the USDA guidelines, your intake of EFAs would be quite small. If you also follow a low fat, low calorie diet, your intake of EFAs would be practically zero. Furthermore, even if you avoid saturated fats, my research indicates that if you follow the USDA diet high in carbohydrates, your body will convert them to saturated fats. This problem is further compounded by the recent decision by the Food and Drug Administration (FDA), which requires that foods labels indicate the amount of saturated fats but not the amount of PUFAs or TFAs, as I have been requesting from the FDA for many years. Without information about the PUFA content of foods, it is impossible to determine which foods are good or bad for your fatty acid balance. Labeling the saturated fat content of foods is, according to my research, practically useless and a waste of government and private money.

How to evaluate a Diet

Failure to eat EFAs for prolonged periods of time would make you EFA deficient. An EFA deficiency will put you at higher risk for cardiovascular disease, stroke, and numerous other health problems. The truth is that many people do not have enough EFAs and need to eat more of them. In an article published by the journal *Metabolism* in 1994, I provided the scientific basis that explains why essential fats are critical to human health, and why the current emphasis on saturated and monounsaturated fatty acids is misguided. In an article accepted in June, 1994, for publication by *the American Journal of Clinical Nutrition*, I explain why the USDA pyramid and the emphasis on low fat diets can cause more heart disease than they can prevent. It is time that the Secretary of the USDA and the President bring some common sense to nutrition. I believe that they ought to shift back towards the private sector (and the unemployment lines) a huge number of the bureaucrats involved in nutrition research and regulations. Let them read labels and eat pasta and bread.[5]

Diets that are quite different from the typical American diet

These diets require a substantial modification in the way you are accustomed to shop for food and in the way you prepare and eat your meals. You must be ready to introduce drastic changes in the types of foods you usually eat. The rewards of these diets are dramatic reductions in cholesterol and blood pressure, and the likelihood of a significant positive impact on your health and your life expectancy.

If you have cardiovascular disease you may find that the previous diets are likely to produce only minor, if any, noticeable improvements (and could even make you worse). The more radical diets, in contrast, would significantly improve your condition no matter how sick you are. In fact, if you are scheduled to have heart bypass surgery in two weeks, and you are willing to change your life style, you could try these diets for two weeks and perhaps avoid surgery. Even if you have your operation, a drastic program of diet modification will significantly improve the chances that you will live for a long time.

Vegetarian Diets

Vegetarian diets have been used for many years. They are classified into four major groups, beginning with the most radical.

How to evaluate a Diet

Vegetarian (vegans): Includes vegetables, legumes, grains, cereals, seeds and fruits. No meat or dairy products.

Ovo vegetarian: Includes eggs in addition to the vegan diet.

Lactoovovegetarian: Includes dairy products in addition to the ovo-vegetarian diet.

Mixed: Allows occasional animal foods or fish in addition to foods of the first three groups.

While the typical American diet contains 30% to 45% of its calories as fat, most of it saturated and partially hydrogenated fat (processed fat), vegetarians eat 15% to 30% of calories as fat, mostly natural polyunsaturated fat in their foods. While most Americans eat processed carbohydrates in the form of sugars and syrups, vegetarians usually eat natural complex carbohydrates in cereals, legumes and vegetables which contain many nutrients and essential fats.

Features

Research has shown that vegetarian diets produce remarkable results in reducing the risk or severity of cardiovascular disease. For many years scientists regarded vegetarians as adherents of a strange religion or as faddists or fanatics. However, during the 70's and 80's extensive research was done in the USA and Europe by many reputable and well known scientists, using groups that were known to follow vegetarian practices, such as the Seventh Day Adventists, macrobiotic followers, and individuals who volunteered to follow controlled and observed vegetarian diets. The results of the studies showed that vegetarians have the following positive features in their health profiles:

- Among the lowest cholesterol levels in the USA. Their values are usually around 130 mg/dl (while most Americans have values well over 200 mg/dl).
- Among the lowest blood pressure levels, around 110/70.
- Very low incidence of cardiovascular disease and of several types of cancer, particularly colon cancer.
- Among the highest longevity, and most disease-free lives.

When vegetarians shift to a diet containing large amounts of animal fat, after even four weeks, their cholesterol levels and blood pressure increase dramatically. When people on a regular American diet shift to

How to evaluate a Diet

a vegetarian diet, the opposite results are found: Cholesterol and blood pressure decline dramatically.

What causes these effects is not fully known. Studies have shown that the effects are not only due to the type of protein vegetarians eat, but also due to the type of fat that vegetarians eat. The vegetarian diet is very high in essential fats and low in total calories. A diet high in legumes, nuts and green vegetables is also a diet very high in fiber, and in ω6 and ω3 essential fats. You will recall that diets high in fiber and essential fats and low in calories prevent cardiovascular disease and other health problems.

Vegetarian diets do have some problems. Vegetarian diets require that you eat large amounts of natural foods and then exercise to burn excess calories, to allow your body to retain the nutrients it needs. Most people do not exercise enough and therefore may not eat enough foods to get all the nutrients they need. However, vegetarians may develop deficiencies of calcium, iron, riboflavin (a vitamin), vitamin B_{12} and possibly of vitamin D as well (unless they get adequate sun: Sunlight helps the body make vitamin D). These deficiencies may be corrected by appropriate vitamin and mineral supplements or by eating foods, particularly nuts, legumes and green vegetables, which are rich in these nutrients. Expert advice is required to plan a lifetime vegetarian diet. In particular, pregnant women and children have increased requirements for nutrients which make them more likely to develop deficiencies.

Comments

Vegetarian diets are recommended for almost everyone. You do not need to follow a strict vegetarian diet. In any case, the best policy is to improve your diet by eating more vegetables and less animal food products, emphasizing unprocessed natural foods, preferably eaten uncooked. Vegetarians, particularly strict vegans and those eating similarly restricted diets such as macrobiotic followers, should obtain expert nutritional advice during pregnancy and on how to feed their children adequately.

Macrobiotic Diets

Macrobiotics is a special type of vegetarian diet that emphasizes whole cereals and grains. The diet is part of a philosophical outlook towards life. Overall, the macrobiotic diet delivers results similar to those

How to evaluate a Diet

reported above for the vegetarian diets and, if followed with caution, it is likely to substantially improve the health of most Americans.

Follow a macrobiotic diet as often as you can, supplemented by vegetable oils as indicated in other chapters

The macrobiotic diet has slowly evolved over the years. You may soon find that some of the macrobiotic supporters have modified their diets to reflect modern nutrition and the need for EFAs.[6] The macrobiotic diet is a diet very high in complex carbohydrates and very low in saturated fat. When supplemented with seeds and vegetables it has adequate amounts of essential fats. Moreover, one can eat a lot of this sort of food and still lose weight.

It is difficult for any reader of macrobiotic books to determine what makes sense and what does not because of their mixture of science with philosophy. For instance, a main component of their program is the balancing of foods eaten, using their philosophy of food's energetic properties, described in terms of yin and yang. This is interesting enough but entirely unscientific. For those intent on trying macrobiotic foods, their recipes and exercises may be useful. The standard macrobiotic diet usually consists of about 15% fat (2% saturated, 8% monounsaturated and 5% polyunsaturated), 12% protein and 73% complex carbohydrates. Saturated oils such as palm and coconut oil, and hydrogenated oils (found in margarines) are to be minimized or avoided. Some macrobiotic diets recommend fish oil supplements to obtain ω3 fatty acids. However, vegetarian diets are high in ω3 fatty acids found in plants, and therefore fish may not be necessary for most vegetarians.

Scientific studies and results using macrobiotic diets are similar to those using vegetarian diets. Basically, these diets have the potential for drastic health improvements. My main concern is the confusion between nutrition, science, religion and philosophy.

However, a **word of caution** is required here. Strict adherence to a macrobiotic eating program could lead to a deficiency of EFAs, since an overemphasis of cereals and grains and an underemphasis of vegetables or vegetable oils leads to insufficient consumption of EFAs. In addition, too much emphasis on rice leads to an imbalanced diet with possible vitamin and mineral deficiencies.

How to evaluate a Diet

The Living Foods Diet

Ann Wigmore in Boston developed a nutritional program primarily based on the use of uncooked vegetables, which she named "living foods." This is a special type of vegetarian diet. While macrobiotic followers emphasize cereals and grains, including almost entirely cooked foods, and de-emphasize vegetables (at least in earlier versions of their program), Ms. Wigmore's program emphasizes raw foods and vegetables and de-emphasizes the more concentrated grains, nuts, and legumes.

But these statements, alone, are misleading. A major characteristic of her program is the way foods are prepared. Foods are not cooked, and instead are prepared using "natural" means, that is, with no artificial ingredients or heat above 115 degrees Fahrenheit. Ms Wigmore's diet is low in calories, fairly well balanced in protein, high in essential fats, particularly high in ω3 fatty acids, and high in most vitamins and minerals because some of the recommended foods are specially grown using a soil enriched with vitamins and minerals. Foods are eaten uncooked, and consist primarily of green vegetables, sprouts, and juices made from vegetables and seeds.

The staple of the diet, greens, are grown indoors using composted soil. Leftover food is used to make compost for growing greens and wheat grass. She recommends that other fruits and vegetables be organically grown. Seeds and legumes are grown to sprouts or fermented in water. Foods are eaten in special combinations as many times per day as is necessary. In fact, her diet advocates eating quite a bit of food and people rarely go hungry (this is similar to other vegetarian diets). But because the foods are extremely low in fat, particularly saturated fat, and very high in fiber, the caloric intake of the diet is low and most people lose weight when they follow her diet.

This is a comprehensive program for growing and preparing food suitable even for apartment dwellers living in cities. It emphasizes self-sufficiency. The diet is very low in saturated fat and high in EFAs and complex carbohydrates. You can eat a lot of food and still lose weight.

There are very few available scientific studies of the Living Foods program which, unfortunately, has not attracted enough medical attention. Because the program emphasizes organically grown foods which are eaten uncooked, and a wide variety of foods is emphasized, it is likely that the diet is fairly well balanced.

How to evaluate a Diet

Yet many issues remain: What is the long term effect of a lower-than-average protein diet? In what vitamins and minerals is the diet deficient, if any? Unfortunately, these questions will have to await further research. It is difficult for many people to get accustomed to growing their own foods and to preparing them the way Ms. Wigmore recommends. Still, one does not need to follow everything she says: Whatever aspects of her diet that you incorporate into your nutritional habits are likely to help your overall health.

Although most of her food recommendations and instructions for food preparation are probably correct, the theoretical explanations of why her diet work contain scientific errors, which I have discussed with her many times.[7] She attributes the benefits of her diet to effects of enzymes on the blood. This reflects an incorrect belief about enzymes: The enzymes that we eat are destroyed in the gastrointestinal system and never reach the blood, unless we have a disease that allows large molecules to leak inside the body. And if the enzymes in food were to reach the blood they would most likely produce a severe immune response because the body would consider these enzymes to be a foreign virus. All organisms, including humans, manufacture the enzymes they need from protein; they cannot directly use the enzymes they find in food. However, food enzymes can assist with digestion. The beneficial effects of the living foods diet are probably due to improved digestion, optimal mixture of vitamins and minerals found in foods grown according to her recommendations, and in the high level of EFAs in many versions of the diet. Unfortunately, not everybody who follows her diet eats enough EFAs!. While she was alive, I analyzed the fatty acid composition Ms. Wigmore's blood , as well as the blood of another person which she considered a "model" for following the living foods program. Ms. Wigmore had significant vitamin B_{12} deficiency. Both blood samples also had significant EFA deficiencies, particularly $\omega 3$ fatty acids.[8] I also analyzed the blood of a third volunteer who followed the living foods diet for about 3 years, but ate considerable amounts of flax seeds and other seeds. This person's blood had large amounts of $\omega 3$ fatty acids, moderate amounts of $\omega 6$ fatty acids, but other blood abnormalities which were perhaps not due to the diet but caused by other factors.

The living foods nutritional program, with modifications to reflect modern nutrition, is likely to be among the best diets that one can follow. Raw foods are more natural than cooked foods and more likely to preserve vitamins, minerals and essential fats. The emphasis on

How to evaluate a Diet

vegetables is consistent with our views that a diet high in essential fats (found in green vegetables) is the best overall diet. However, living foods must be followed with care because it suffers from some of the same difficulties found in all vegetarian diets. Protein balance can be a difficult goal for the follower of the living foods diet, and vitamin and mineral deficiencies may develop unless one has access to top quality soil and grows one's own food carefully. One possible way to insure against the possible harmful effects of this regimen is to follow the diet with occasional protein, vitamin and mineral supplements.

References and notes

1   American Heart Association, National Center, 7320 Greenville Ave., Dallas, TX 75231. Brochure 7-86-750M. The American Heart Association Diet: An Eating Plan for Healthy Americans.

2   It is my position that the current (pre-1994) emphasis on saturated and monounsaturated fatty acids is misplaced.

3   Dietary Guidelines for Americans. US Department of Agriculture,, Human Nutrition Information Service, Federal Building, Hyattsville, MD 20782.

4   The Food Guide Pyramid. USDA Home and Garden Bulletin 252, August, 1992 (I requested the latest available by June, 1994, and this is the one I received from the USDA).

5   Perhaps we should have a "nutrition" test before we allow people to provide advice. If they cannot provide evidence that they eat a healthy diet and follow the regulations that they sponsor, they ought to be excluded from making food regulations.

6   See *Diet for a Strong Heart* by Michio Kushi with Alex Jack; St. Martin's Press, New York. I understand that researchers familiar with my work on essential fatty acids have been recommending changes to the typical macrobiotic diet. The book describes Michio Kushi's Macrobiotic dietary guidelines for the prevention of high blood pressure, heart attack and stroke. Unfortunately, the authors mix valid statements about the relationship between diet and disease with other statements which derive more from philosophy than from science. I believe that concepts such as a Yin/Yang classification of cardiovascular disease (p 137 of their 1985 edition) have no proven medical validity.

7   I spent quite a bit of time explaining to her staff the pros and cons of her diet, and the need for balanced nutrition and essential fats. I found that there was a huge turnover in staff at her "nutrition center" in Boston, which made it very difficult for me to provide meaningful advice. Unfortunately she died in 1994 as a result of an accidental fire at her home.

8   Most people think that diets without fish do not have *omega*-3 fatty acids. This, as explained before, is a mistake. Most green vegetables are rich in *omega*-3 fatty acids, and the vegetables Ms Wigmore uses are particularly rich in *omega*-3 fatty acids.

How to evaluate a Diet

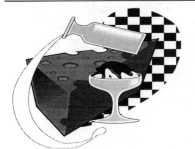

V.2

MORE DIETS

"Watch your diet: Choose a good one"

Topics. *Weight Watchers diet. The New American Diet. Pritikin Diet. Scarsdale die. Other diets.*

Summary

Diet and nutrition books can be classified into three major groups: a) nutrition books; b) weight loss books; c) cookbooks. Choose a good nutrition book to learn how to select foods and plan your meals.

To eat well and remain healthy you must combine a program of balanced meals with exercise. The key is to modify your habits so that you avoid sweets, and also foods high in calories and low in EFAs. The diets in this chapter are aimed at weight loss or overall well-being. For your information we describe the best features of each diet. Notice also that even if the nutritional advice provided by a particular diet is only partially correct, their recipes may provide you with increased variety in your meals.

Losing weight and being thin is the cornerstone of disease prevention. Weight loss is essential even though weight loss alone is not sufficient. Statistics do show, however, that thin people are less likely to develop cardiovascular disease and cancer. If you are thin, you are placing less weight on your bones and joints. Thus, they do not wear rapidly. If you have arthritis or almost any bone or joint disease, placing less weight on your body will decrease pain and prevent further complications. Moreover, a smaller body requires less work by the heart. And a heart that works less is less likely to die prematurely. Therefore, any diet that helps you lose weight without causing complications is a helpful diet.

There are no magic foods that make you lose weight. Weight control is achieved with a reduction in calories, especially by eating meals with less fat and less carbohydrates, sugars and sweet syrups.

The Weight Watchers diet is perhaps the most popular and successful weight reduction diet. The New American Diet improves upon the diets recommended by the American Heart Association and the USDA. The Pritikin Diet is usually very low fat and aimed at prevention and treatment of cardiovascular disease. It appears to be effective. However, over the long term I believe people should eat more EFAs.

Types of Diets

My main objection to most existing diets is that they do not provide a proper balance of essential fats. Many diets, even if partially deficient in essential fats, can be improved as I indicate or used to prepare interesting meals from the foods I have recommended before. The books described here have been widely read by the American public. Keep in mind that there is no secret formula for losing weight and eating well. To lose weight you must simply consume fewer calories. Low calorie diets followed for over one month require vitamin and mineral supplements as indicated in Section III, chapter 7.

Weight Watchers (WW)

This is one of the best established plans for weight reduction. The program uses traditional meals prepared with an emphasis on low calories. It is well organized and balanced. There are many ready-made foods that meet the requirements of this diet. Groups all over the country meet to help people plan and remain on the diet. The Weight Watchers' Diet has had success; many people have lost weight and kept it off with this diet.

In my opinion, the Weight Watchers' diet has shortcomings as a diet for treatment of high cholesterol and high blood pressure because it does not significantly change the fat composition of your body. It is generally more expensive than diets that are built around natural food products since many prepared meals are sold at relatively high prices. The diet primarily addresses the problem of weight loss rather than treatment of specific medical conditions or reduction of cholesterol or high blood pressure. This is a good diet to follow, but first measure any EFA abnormalities you may have using the test **EFA SR** and then supplement the diet with oils as indicated in Section IV to correct existing abnormalities.

More Diets

The New American Diet

The authors of this diet are nutrition researchers with extensive practical experience.[1] The program incorporates several phases to slowly move from the current American diet high in saturated fat and simple carbohydrates and low in complex carbohydrates to a diet low in saturated fat and high in complex carbohydrates. Meals are planned to slowly substitute better foods for less healthy ones. The diet is similar to the ones sponsored by the American Heart Association and the USDA.

The New American Diet is an easy one to follow. It is flexible and balanced and provides the proper nutrients. It has been developed as a result of several years of research and experimentation with human subjects, and incorporates modern concepts in nutrition. The authors have used fish and fish oils with their subjects, and they make specific recommendations for the use of these oils. Research suggests that using this diet improves cardiovascular disease. One may expect results similar to or better than those obtained from following the American Heart Association Diet or the USDA diet.

However, little is said about the uses and differences of vegetable and fish oils. The authors review neither the differences between ω3 and ω6 fatty acids presented in this book, nor the need to have individual diets for each adult based on the current composition of EFAs in their blood. My research indicates that this diet may be too mild for people with advanced cardiovascular disease or cholesterol over 240. Individuals with heart disease, high blood pressure, or abnormal cholesterol levels usually need to eat far greater quantities of EFAs than those indicated in this diet.

This book contains many useful and specific hints about which foods to eat and which to avoid, such as a table indicating what cheeses are recommended and which are not. It is an excellent choice from a nutritional point of view. You can make your own recipes if you do not like the ones in the book, but you can use the ones recommended there as a starting point. However, if you are willing to change your eating habits to accomplish a significant improvement in your health, the vegetarian diets described in the previous chapter may produce better results. The New American Diet is certainly useful as a transitional path from the standard American diet to a vegetarian diet.

More Diets

The Scarsdale Diet

The Scarsdale diet[2] is basically a low calorie diet (under 1000 calories per day) designed primarily as a weight reduction diet. Because an average person needs 1500 to 2000 calories per day, he or she will have a deficit of 500 to 1000 calories per day. This translates into 3500 to 7000 calories per week, which is equivalent to 1 to 2 pounds (see Part I of this book). Any diet that provides only this number of calories will accomplish the same result. The major claim of this diet is that it "works": It is simple, balanced and curbs the appetite. People on the diet apparently do not go hungry.

Many people claim to have lost weight with this diet and it may work for you. The diet is recommended for 14 days, but it is supposed to encourage good eating habits that you can continue for the rest of your life. One point of contention I have is that the Scarsdale diet book (page 30) recommends that you eat your salads without oil. Instead, I suggest including oil with your meals. It is very important that you be tested for EFA abnormalities before you start and after you finish with this diet.

The Pritikin Program of Diet and Exercise

This is a high carbohydrate, low fat diet. The Pritikin program incorporates a Regression Diet (for treatment) and a Maintenance Diet (for follow-up). The "ideal diet" would appear to be a diet with almost no fat in it. Of course, this is almost impossible to achieve. Therefore, the Pritikin diet consists of typical American foods but avoids fats and oils and limits your intake of foods high in fat.[3]

The Pritikin Diet is a low calorie diet and many people lose weight following it. It has been developed through many years of extensive testing and it has been followed by thousands of people. It is practical and most people can follow it. Research studies have shown that the Pritikin diet can indeed lower cholesterol, triglycerides and decrease the risk of heart disease. However, these results were obtained using foods that contain sufficient quantities of essential fats and do not completely avoid fat. Strictly following a very low fat Pritikin diet would result in meals deficient in essential fats; however most practical implementations of the Pritikin program contain some fat, mostly essential fats, and the meals consist of vegetables supplemented with

More Diets

small quantities of low fat animal meat.[4] This could be a good diet to follow if you keep in mind these issues:

- This diet is particularly helpful for overweight people who usually have large amounts of essential fat stored in their body, and which is released when they lose weight.

- You should supplement the diet with soybean and other oils indicated in Section IV if you have average weight or suffer from one of the conditions described in Section IV.

- Follow this diet for a short period of time (under one year).

The Setpoint Diet

The premise of this diet is that everyone has a particular set point or weight which one tries to maintain.[5] For most people, that set point is too high. Lowering the set point means a decision to achieve and maintain a lower weight. The set point is thus a psychological weight that each person has accepted as "normal". Lowering this psychological weight leads to weight loss.

The diet is balanced and uses mostly natural foods. It reduces saturated fat and total caloric intake. It is an easy diet to follow and fairly flexible. Research is in progress, but apparently it has been used successfully by the employees of several US corporations. It contains specific guidelines to plan meals and it is primarily aimed at reducing weight rather than correcting medical problems due to past poor nutrition. Most food recommendations are similar to the AHA or USDA diet. In my opinion, the diet does not address the balance of essential fats in the body. I do believe that many people set a point for their own weight. Thus, if they substitute low fat for high fat foods, they will eat more of them to maintain what they see as their "acceptable" weight.

References and Notes

[1] Sonja L. Connor, William E. Connor. *The New American Diet*. Simon and Schuster, 1985.

[2] *The Scarsdale Diet* (The Complete Scarsdale Medical Diet by H. Tarnower and SS Baker; published by Rawson, Wade Publishers, Inc., N.Y., 1978).

[3] In a recent revision of the diet, the authors recommend that people eat more essential fats. See *Beyond Pritikin*, by Gittleman, AL. Bantam Books, N.Y. 1989. Throughout the book there are statements quite similar to things I have been

writing about for years, but there are many statements which I consider incorrect, among the following (see first page of their book):

". . .essential fat helps burn excess calories instead of depositing them as fatty tissue." I think this is nonsense. Essential fats are fats and do deposit as fatty tissue. This is good, because they replace saturated hard fat with PUFA, soft fat.

". . .essential fat inhibits cancer cell growth". This is true for some but not all cancers.

". . .essential fat functions as an antiinflammatory catalyst". There are many types of essential fats. It is the balance of ω3 and ω6 EFAs and derivatives that matter, not the total amount of essential fats. Furthermore, the inflammation response is very important. Without it, we would not be able to fight infection. Many authors mistakenly believe that we must fight inflammation.

On p. 157 the authors present their diet, "The New Nutrition Diet Prescription". They recommend two tablespoons of essential-fat oil, but omit the fact that different oils have different ω3 and ω6 composition and what may be good for one person may be bad for another. They recommend that people eat ω6 EFA derivatives, GLA, and ω3 EFA derivatives, EPA. These supplements should be taken only by people who cannot make them from EFAs. Those who take them without a need for them are drastically altering their body's ability to regulate EFA metabolism and can cause serious harm to themselves. The GLA and EPA inhibit the regulatory conversion of EFAs to derivatives and the function of EFAs in the body. I do not think that any human can regulate all the biochemical reactions of his/her body. Instead, we must assist the body but not force it to do something. If your body cannot form enough EFA derivatives, you may need GLA or EPA. The type and amount depends on each person.

4   I brought this matter to the attention of the Pritikin staff several years ago.

5   Gilbert A. Leveille. The Setpoint Diet. Ballantine Books, 1985.

More Diets

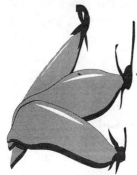

V.3

THE EFA DIET IN THIS BOOK

"Essential fats are an important determinant of good health"

Topics: *The unique features of my recommended diet. Similarities and differences with other diets. Prevention vs. Treatment.*

Summary

The key difference between my diets and those proposed by other authors lies in the emphasis placed on the essential fats ω3 and ω6. I utilize the different scientific and medical applications of the four groups of essential fats which I described in my publications, the ω3 and ω6 parents (precursors) and daughters (derivatives). Our programs explain which fats you need to eat, when, and how much of each one. We recommend the use of natural foods instead of food extracts or processed foods, and the avoidance of partially hydrogenated fats and processed fats.

All scientifically-accepted diets share a recognition for a balanced meal containing proteins, carbohydrates, vitamins, minerals and fiber. All agree that saturated fat should be avoided and should be replaced by polyunsaturated (essential) fat. My prevention diet emphasizes natural foods; the treatment diet uses oil supplements to speed up the process of replacing the body's saturated fat with essential fat.

The approach of this book

We emphasize the scientific and medical applications of the four groups of essential fats (PUFAs, or polyunsaturated fat): parents and daughters of the ω3 and ω6 fats. Some authors only speak about the ω3 derivatives found in fish and fish oils. We describe all of the essential fats and their role in good health and disease, and explain which fats you need to eat, when, and how much of each one.

Elements common to all diets

All scientifically accepted diets share a recognition for a balanced meal containing proteins, carbohydrates, vitamins, minerals, and fiber. Most agree that saturated fat should be avoided. Most nutritionists advise that simple carbohydrates (sugars and candy) and saturated fat should be replaced by complex carbohydrates. Most researchers agree that, as a general rule (exceptions do exist), thin people are likely to live longer than overweight people. I do not believe that we should replace most fat with carbohydrates. Instead, we should eat more essential fats and fewer total calories.

The role of the essential fats and natural, raw foods

I will share with you the results of my research that have led me to conclusions different from those held by many nutritionists.

- **Eat ω3 and ω6, not just ω3.** Many authors only mention the ω3 fats, and only those derived from fish and fish oils. I explain the need for a proper balance of ω3 and ω6 fats and the role of the precursor ω3 (linolenic acid) found in vegetables. While other researchers often recommend monounsaturated fatty acids (**MUFA**), such as olive oil, to lower high cholesterol, my research indicates that the essential fats are far more effective. I do not recommend that people eat more MUFAs. My research has shown that eating MUFAs is almost as bad as eating saturated fatty acids (**SFAs**).
- **Eat natural foods and avoid processed fats.** I recommend the use of natural foods in their native form, instead of food extracts or processed foods. I recommend that people avoid partially hydrogenated fats which include *trans* fatty acids (TFAs) and other isomers.

I did some of the pioneering work showing that *trans* fatty acids (**TFAs**) and other isomers in blood are associated with coronary heart disease and undesirable levels of cholesterol. However, while some researchers blame TFAs, I warned against the danger of other types of fatty acids,

The EFA Diet in this Book

called "isomers," which are not essential to the body and are
found in many processed foods. These isomers are not TFAs, and are
not essential fats. They are fats with different structures. I also warn
that beef and beef fat contains many isomers and TFAs, and thus
should be limited. I do not think that we must exclude them altogether
from our diets, but we should limit the amounts we eat. Cows have too
many TFAs and isomers. We should expand the use of other types of
animal food. Finally, I emphasize that the real issue is the balance of
EFAs. If we have plenty of EFAs, the impact of TFAs and isomers is
very small, as I have shown in my research. *People who have high
levels of TFAs and isomers and low levels of essential fats are at
the highest risk for premature death.*

- **Eat more raw foods.** I encourage you to eat more raw foods,
  for example, raw bean and seed sprouts (of course, you must be
  careful if the foods have toxic microorganisms or pesticides).

- **Eat foods in season.** I suggest that you eat foods in season
  and according to your climate: more fruits in the summer,
  more essential fats and fish in the winter. Your diet should
  change according to the temperature of your environment.

Role of Essential Fats

In a leading medical journal, I have described the classification of the
essential fats into the four groups repeated below (with examples in
parentheses). This classification is fundamental to our understanding
of the role of fat in health and disease. We explained before how much
you need to eat of each kind of fat, and how to use these various fats to
prevent and treat disease. People with a long history of foods low in
essential fats need to take supplemental oils to increase the storage of
these fats in their bodies. Younger individuals should eat foods that
contain little saturated fat and plenty of essential fats of the ω3 and ω6
families. Healthy individuals do not need to take oil supplements:
They will get their essential fats from vegetables and seeds.

Different diseases respond to different types of essential fats. However,
keep in mind that as far as we know now, people can live quite well
without eating animal fat. In fact, diets very low in animal fat may be
the best for the Western World.[1] However, you must eat more than 10
grams of essential fats (PUFA) each day. [2]

The EFA Diet in this Book

Most authors recommend an amount of essential fats (also known as polyunsaturated fat)[3] stated as a percent of total calories. They will say: Eat 10% of your total fat as polyunsaturated fat (suggested by the American Heart Association). I recommend that you eat a minimum amount of 10-20 grams of essential fat per day—the equivalent of one to two tablespoons of vegetable oil per day. About 50% to 70% of these essential fats should come from ω6 fats; the rest from ω3 fats. The specific amounts and proportion depend on your fatty acid profile, age, sex, weight and health status. Unless you are one of the few individuals who require the essential fats found in animal and fish foods (derivative fatty acids), you may get your essential fats from vegetables, seeds and vegetable oils. A small amount of animal food (preferably fish) high in protein --- such as one to two ounces each day or an equivalent quantity a few times per week--- will provide 1 to 3 grams of daughter fats.

If you eat very few calories per day because you are on a restricted diet,

Family	Parent	Daughters = Derivatives
ω3	Linolenic	EPA, DHA and others
ω6	Linoleic	GLA, DGLA, arachidonic
Found in	Vegetables	Animals (ω6), Fish (ω3)

do not exercise enough, or are old and require few calories, you should supplement your diet with oils. If you are a very active person who consumes over 3,000 calories per day, you may not need oil supplements. Instead, you may need to eat more animal products or nuts: It is difficult to get 3,000 calories per day eating only vegetables, grains and fruits. Adults with significant diseases must eat far larger amounts of EFAs to replace large amounts of saturated fat in their bodies with essential fats.

How to use other diets

Section V describes diets that are generally correct in most aspects except their scant discussion of fat. These diets were designed before recent research on oils had been published by myself and others. You can use these diets with the following modifications:

The EFA Diet in this Book

- **Eat less saturated fat and more polyunsaturated fat.**
Follow the guidelines described in this book, which mean fewer
animal fat products, more vegetable products, and oil
supplements for those who have a long history of a diet high in
saturated fat and low in essential fat. These recommendations
are generally in agreement with the ones stated by other authors.
The difference is quantitative: We recommend a greater
avoidance of saturated fat, fewer calories, increased amounts of
essential fat, avoidance of processed and hydrogenated fat, and
more green vegetables. Green vegetables are recommended
because they are high in essential fats.

- **Take vitamins and minerals while eating low calorie diets.**
If you are losing quite a bit of weight, you may become deficient
in some vitamins or minerals. This is one of the instances when a
multiple vitamin and mineral supplement is helpful. Eat a
vitamin plus mineral complex that contains the RDA
(recommended daily allowance) of each vitamin and mineral ---
read the label. One several times per week is usually sufficient.
There is no need to take one every day. In fact, one each day
could produce toxic effects after many years of continuous use. In
particular, eat more vitamin E to protect the essential fats.
About 100 IU should be adequate for most people.

- **Use fish extracts (oils) if you cannot make EFA derivatives
or you need to drastically reduce clot formation.** You
should eat more fish and less meat, and, as indicated before,
supplement the diet with a fish oil extract only in unusual
circumstances and under medical supervision. This is important
to prevent clot formation and avoid bleeding. While a decreased
tendency of the blood to clot may be beneficial for one person, it
may be dangerous for someone else. Some authors now writing
about ω3 and ω6 fats fail to indicate who can benefit from fish oils
and what risks are involved.

Prevention vs. Treatment

My research has led me to the conclusion that a book on the prevention
and treatment of cardiovascular disease must really propose three
different diets: one for weight loss, one for prevention, and one for
treatment for those readers who already have cardiovascular disease.
Thus, we present three diets:

The EFA Diet in this Book

- 1. The Boston Egg White Diet for weight loss.
- 2. The Modern Prevention Diet based on a program of balanced meals that emphasizes vegetables and fruits in their natural state, and encourages only occasional use of animal meat. This diet is to be used by individuals in good health to maintain their health, supplemented with a few essential fats if they do not eat enough calories to obtain the essential fats from natural foods.

3.   The Modern Treatment Diet, which goes beyond the prevention diet and indicates what oils to take to correct for years of neglect and bad eating habits. In this diet you will eat larger amounts of essential fats to replace the saturated fat in your body. Blood testing for fatty acids is essential for optimal treatment.

References and notes

[1] It is different if you live in the arctic, where a diet high in fish fat is probably essential to survival.

[2] Remember, technically the essential fatty acids are only Linoleic and Linolenic acid. These two fatty acids, together with all their derivatives (the sum of the ω3 and ω6) form the polyunsaturated (PUFA) fatty acids. To simplify, we refer to the PUFAs as the "essential fats".

[3] People who eat oils must take additional vitamin E to preserve the essential fats in their body. We do not know how much vitamin E is needed, but 100 IU appears to be a safe amount.

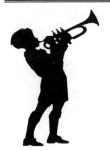

V.4

SHOPPING FOR THE RIGHT FOODS; RECIPES

"Desserts that lower your weight and your cholesterol"

Topics: *Where to buy: health food stores vs. supermarkets. Generic vs. brand name vitamins and minerals. Recipes. Desserts.*

Where to buy

Health food stores usually sell a wide variety of vegetable products. If we can believe what they are saying, some of them may have products which contain fewer pesticides than those sold at your local supermarket. The problem is that, unfortunately, there are no federal requirements on this matter. This is one area where the federal government should inspect and impose better labeling.

Organically grown foods may be superior to those grown with artificial fertilizers. However, that is often impossible to know. It is very difficult to agree on the appropriate criteria. Soil, water and air content has been altered so much in most places that the natural composition of the soil or water may contain more dangerous chemicals than artificial fertilizers.

Most health food stores have a wider selection of oils than supermarkets. Moreover, they are often fresher and may last longer than the supermarket variety. But some supermarkets sell top quality oils. Your best bet is to buy and try them (see the chapter on buying and storing oils). One of my favorite oils, walnut oil, is rarely available at Supermarkets. When you buy it, I suggest you purchase the one without strong flavor (which is also the cheaper kind) unless you particularly like a strongly flavored walnut oil.

Health food stores also sell more prepared foods made with grains, vegetables and soybeans. Even though expensive, these foods are often low fat products which provide variety and good taste. They are often the only source of meat imitators made with soy protein, flour and a variety of soy products. Soybeans are an excellent food: They have high quality protein and contain both ω3 and ω6 fats. Recently, many supermarkets have begun to carry soybean products such as Tofu, which I recommend.

Many stores also sell "ice-cream" like products very low in saturated fat, in which soy, rice, or skimmed milk replace the cream of conventional ice cream. Soybean based products are a good choice. When you buy processed foods, such as bread, buy products that contain very little fat. Processed fat, even if high in essential fats, may not be desirable because the chemical composition of the fat changes with cooking.

Fatty acid related products

There are a wide range of products available on the market. Because of differences in manufacturing and labeling, it is impossible for me to comment on all of them. As a general rule, I suggest that you use more conventional oils rather than exotic ones.

Lecithin is a type of fat usually extracted from soybeans, but found in all cells (vegetables and animals). It is rich in essential fats and choline. Unfortunately, the extraction process often alters a significant portion of the essential fats and creates artificial chemicals. Without sophisticated analysis it is impossible to tell whether the lecithin is OK. Vegetable oils provide similar ingredients and may be healthier. Lecithin can become rancid and you may not be able to tell.

GLA, usually sold as evening primrose oil or borage oil, is very useful for individuals who cannot convert the ω6 linoleic acid to its derivatives. If your blood test indicates a need for GLA, you ought to take it, probably in significant amounts. Otherwise, your deficiency may interfere with the normal and healthy metabolism of EFAs.

Flax seeds and flax seed oil are very high in the EFA ω3, linolenic acid. They are recommended for people who must increase their intake of ω3 fatty acids. I have analyzed several samples of both flax seeds and flax oil, and they seem to be fine and high in ω3 EFAs. However, ω3s are very unstable and thus you should try to obtain very fresh products. There are also a wide range of seaweed and algae on the market. Most of them are high in linolenic (ω3) fatty acids and also contain some ω3 derivatives, such as EPA. However, these fatty acids are very unstable. By the time they reach the stores, the important ω3 fats may have deteriorated.

Many companies sell "lipid formulas" with strange compositions. If you do not understand the label, these products are probably not for you. You may need to eat very large quantities of these "formulas" or capsules because the active ingredients are a very small percentage of each capsule. When you eat many capsules per day you are also eating the capsule and other materials put inside. You must verify that these substances are not harmful in large amounts. Unfortunately, you would probably need an advanced degree in chemistry and access to highly sophisticated equipment. Also, please write to your Congressman and the FDA to request that they establish industry standards and appropriate labeling.

As a general rule, you need to eat about 20 grams of EFAs or PUFA every day. If you take 5 capsules per day, each of which contains about 300 mg of the EFAs, you get less than 10% of your daily needs from the capsules (and pay a high price for it). Two tablespoons of soybean oil or equivalent amounts of Tofu give you most of your daily EFA requirements.

Fiber bars provide a mixture of different types of fiber. Most likely they are what they appear to be. However, it is more fun to obtain fiber while eating regular foods. If you eat healthy foods, you eat enough fiber. If you eat unhealthy foods, eating fiber supplements will not improve the quality of your food. One possible exception: Fiber sometimes improves constipation --- but too much fiber also may cause constipation. Therefore, each individual must determine his or her own optimal fiber intake.

Brown sugar is usually made with white sugar plus molasses. There is nothing particularly good about it.

Molasses, particularly black molasses, is very high in minerals. This is the product leftover after white sugar is extracted from sugar cane. You can use it for color and flavor and to make your own brown sugar at a lower cost.

Shopping for the Right Food

Artificial sweeteners are potentially dangerous because they may induce cancer, but there is no definite proof of this. If you are over 50, your chances of dying of heart disease are far greater than your chances of getting cancer. In this case, it is fair to use artificial sweeteners to lose weight, if they help you to eat fewer calories.

Fat replacements

These replacements may be useful if they help you lose weight. If you eat more food to compensate for the calories saved using low calorie fat replacements, you should not use them. The comments made about artificial sweeteners apply to fat replacements with one additional rule. Replacing fat with fat substitutes eliminates the essential fats. If you do not eat essential fats, you will remain hungry because your body sends you a signal that you need to eat essential fats. Remember to add essential fats (from vegetable oils, fish and vegetables) to your meals. Diseases such as cancer usually take 10 to 30 years to develop, and therefore the risk of dying of cardiovascular disease is probably much greater than potential risks of fat replacements eaten for 10-30 years if you start eating them after you are 50. I do not recommend fat replacements, artificial sweeteners, or any other artificial foods for children and adolescents, who could suffer ill effects from eating these artificial substances for periods greater than 30 years.

Incidentally, you can probably eat most natural herbs and spices in reasonable amounts: They contain very few calories and can make your meals more interesting. But remember that even a product made from ingredients found in nature also may be considered artificial, because the ingredients are in a concentration and mixture which is not natural to the human body. The only truly natural substances for humans to eat are foods found in nature, in their unadulterated and fresh form. Unfortunately, natural foods are hard to find without pesticides, added drugs such as hormones, and a variety of pollutants from the air, water and ground. If we don't already, soon we will have tens of thousands of dangerous chemicals in our body and it will be impossible for medicine to take them out.

How to prepare meals using oils.

Because cooking alters the chemical composition of polyunsaturated fat, do not cook with oils that are very high in polyunsaturated fat. The essential fats will be altered into potentially dangerous chemicals. Use

Shopping for the Right Food

corn oil in cooking, instead of safflower, soybean, sunflower or other highly polyunsaturated oils. In fact, cooking with butter may be preferable to cooking with oil. Scientists do not know. Use as little fat as possible when you cook at high temperatures for a long period of time. Using very small amounts of oil for frying and broiling protects you against the hazardous effects of saturated fat and cooked oils. Moreover, eating fewer greasy foods fried in oil decreases your total caloric intake. You can also use almost any edible raw oil, in small amounts, for flavor, with practically zero ill effects and many potentially good ones if it is high in EFAs.

Saturated fat made from vegetables, such as shortening, is not necessarily better than butter. It may contain artificial chemicals whose effects on the body are not known. It is possible that cooking with corn oil is better than cooking with butter, but we do not know.

Your best approach is to add oils to most of your meals, after they have been cooked or prepared: Make your own salad dressing with oil, vinegar, lemon and spices; add oils to noodles, salads, baked potatoes, mashed potatoes, apple pie (after it is cooked), bread, etc. Excellent dessert sauces can be made with oils and cocoa, maple syrup or honey. Obviously, you must decide how to balance the risks and benefits or pleasures of different oils. Knowing your blood fatty acid profile can help you know where you are and whether or not you must make drastic changes in your eating habits.

Food preparation

The general rules to follow are:

1. Process your foods as little as possible. The longer the cooking time and the higher the temperature, the more likely it is that you will destroy essential fats and vitamins and create toxic chemicals.

2. Eat more of your foods in their natural state. For example, fresh peas may be eaten raw. Frozen vegetables do not require cooking, merely defrosting which can be accomplished by leaving the foods at room temperature, washing them with hot water, or warming them up in a microwave oven. Eat more vegetable sprouts (grass, bean, seed sprouts).

Shopping for the Right Food

3. When you cook, do not overcook. Simple? Cook vegetables by steaming or microwaving them until barely done and still crisp.

4. Better broil or bake than fry. Microwaves most likely preserves the oils better than broiling or baking.

5. Freeze fat out. To delete saturated fat from foods such as gravies, first refrigerate or freeze the food (i.e., gravy) for a brief period to solidify the fat, and then remove it. To keep the gravy soft and add moisture to the meat, add water or oil to the gravy.

You can make your own mayonnaise

You may want to make your own mayonnaise to match your unique needs. Your own mayonnaise can include fresh ingredients and the types of oils whose taste you like and whose essential fat balance is best for your health. The following are suggested ingredients for mayonnaise:

Two egg yolks, one teaspoon salt, one tablespoon sugar, one teaspoon dry mustard, ¼ teaspoon paprika, ¼ cup vinegar, two cups corn oil.

Alternative ingredients include: two tablespoons of vinegar and two tablespoons of lemon juice instead of ¼ cup vinegar; safflower, soybean, walnut, or sunflower instead of corn oil; a little bit of olive oil in lieu of some of the other oil (for enhanced flavor). You may also wish to experiment with other ingredients.

There is a trick to making mayonnaise: The oil must be very gradually beaten into the egg yolks to form an emulsion. If the emulsion separates into two layers, slowly add another egg yolk while beating slowly.

Mix the egg yolk with all the ingredients except the vinegar and oil. Add ½ the vinegar and then ½ the oil slowly. Then add the other ½ vinegar and ½ oil. Using a blender, mix for about 2 seconds at a time.

Recipes for chocolate lovers

I must confess one weakness: I love chocolate. Chocolate has some "bad" things (such as caffeine-like chemicals) and a few good things (like potassium and magnesium). But many books state that chocolate is high in saturated fat. The truth is that cocoa, the active ingredient in chocolate, is a vegetable and has practically no fat (and, of course, no cholesterol as vegetables rarely have cholesterol). Chocolate is often prepared by combining cocoa with a saturated fat and sugar. You can make your own "healthier" chocolate desserts by using cocoa, and also pay substantially less than the market value of chocolate.

To prepare your own chocolate dessert you need several types of ingredients. Which ingredients you use and in what quantities depend on the use that will be made of the chocolate (for baking cakes, for flavoring foods, for puddings, "ice cream", sauces, etc.). The ingredients are:

1. Cocoa (pure cocoa, such as Hershey brand cocoa). Read the label: it should say 100% pure cocoa with nothing else.

2. Oil: any of the polyunsaturated oils discussed elsewhere in this book (walnut, soybean, safflower, corn). Some provide a better texture to food than others: Try them and select the one you like. Or you can use Tofu which is usually high in essential fats (read the label to see much how PUFA it contains).

3. Sweetener: sugar, honey, maple syrup, molasses. Sugar will often give a better consistency to most cooked products.

4. A protein source, such as low fat Tofu, or even regular Tofu (high in EFAs), skim milk, egg whites, even an egg yolk (excellent to blend things together).

Example of chocolate pie or mousse.

Purchase either the low fat Tofu or the regular kind. Whether to use the hard or soft type depends on your taste. For a mousse, use the softer kind; for a pudding-like texture, use the harder type. Take 8 ounces of tofu and whip it until smooth. In a separate container, take 1/4 cup of honey or syrup. If honey, melt it in the microwave for about 30-90 seconds. Add 1/6 cup of cocoa powder. Mix until smooth with a blender. Add 1 tsp of vanilla. Mix the chocolate mixture with the tofu. Pour it into a pie shell or into a cup. Obviously, you can vary the ingredients to make more or less. If you use regular rather than low fat tofu, you may need slightly more cocoa or vanilla or sweetener. You can also add a few drops of rum or some other liquor. For dark semisweet puddings use the regular firm tofu; for "creamier" mousse use the softer tofu and less cocoa. Top everything with a few slices of bananas and safflower or pumpkin seeds. The result is a highly nutritious dessert with essential fats, high quality protein, and a wide range of vitamins

Shopping for the Right Food

and minerals. This dessert will meet your protein needs with minimal amounts of fat, many of them essential fats. Try this and similar desserts and send me your results.

Have your toast and eat it too

Toasts seem to be part of the American way of life. Most breads are primarily carbohydrates, although some have added vitamins and minerals or may have natural fiber in them. They are not bad foods, but they can become dangerous foods when supplemented with foods high in saturated fat. There are new margarines in the market that are high in EFAs, contain only natural oils and no *trans* fatty acids. They are made solid through new processing that apparently does not alter the fatty acid composition of the original oil. I personally suggest you use soybean, walnut, or corn oil. Margarine made from oil tastes the same as the original oil and it just melts on the toast. So, why not use the original oil which is often cheaper and better? Just put a little bit of oil on your toast after it is toasted.

Food supplements to take

If you eat more foods high in EFAs, such as tofu or oils, you need to eat more antioxidants to protect them. However, you should not overdose or spend a fortune on them. Most people only need 50 to 100 I.U. of vitamin E per day. You can buy a 400 I.U. or 800 I.U. vitamin E capsule on sale at your local drugstore and take one a week. Vitamin E levels accumulate in the body and you do not need to take it every day. For Selenium, I recommend that you take about the average amount recommended by most nutritionists. Again, you do not need to take it every day. The 25 mcg found in most multivitamins is enough; one multivitamin 3 times per week is enough for most people. (Remember that you get vitamins and minerals from your meals.) Two exceptions listed in previous chapters include people on weight loss diets with severely restricted calories and patients with gastrointestinal disease who cannot absorb food.

Eating out

Many years ago, "health experts" recommended that fast-food restaurants replace their animal fat with vegetable oils. The reason was that animal fat was high in saturated fatty acids (**SFAs**) and also contained cholesterol. Pressed by public health interests, consumer groups and practically everybody, restaurants changed their fat from

Shopping for the Right Food

animal fat to vegetable oil.[1] To avoid further criticism, they sought to avoid tropical and other highly saturated oils. Instead, they chose partially hydrogenated oils. These oils are cheap and stable. The natural vegetable oil is high in EFAs and is very unstable when cooked at high temperatures. If fast-food stores used natural oils, they would have to throw them away frequently, increasing their costs and the hazards of disposing of very hot oil. Furthermore, highly unsaturated oils are unstable at high temperatures and may produce chemicals toxic to humans. Hydrogenated oils are far more stable, but contain *trans* fatty acids (**TFAs**). At the time the recommendations were made to shift to hydrogenated vegetable oils, scientists were aware that TFAs had undesirable health effects. However, I believe that there were significant political and economic factors that silenced those who opposed this change. I have attempted to speak against TFAs since before 1980, and particularly in the early 1980's. However, I was forced to stop. There has been evidence since the 70's that TFAs interfere with the metabolism of EFAs, and that saturated fats, in small amounts, are not dangerous. I believe a better solution would have been to encourage people to eat more EFAs and fewer calories. If you are slim and eat enough EFAs, and want to eat fried foods, it may be better for you to fry then in saturated fats. If you are overweight and have low EFA levels, then eating foods fried in hydrogenated oils can worsen your EFA deficiency. Of course, it is best to avoid fry foods, but we are free to drink and eat as much as we want. There are too many people anyway.

Cooking

As a general rule, microwave cooking is similar to boiling because microwaves cook by heating the water in the food. Microwave cooking is preferable to baking because it uses a lower temperature. Baking is preferable to broiling, because baking temperature is usually lower than broiling or frying temperature. Broiling may or may not be better than frying. It depends on how long you cook the food, and what its cooking temperature is. The higher the cooking temperature and the longer you cook something, the more likely it is that the oils will change to an unhealthy form. Incidentally, beware of oils that are used for prolonged periods, as is common in many fast food restaurants.

Preference order of cooking techniques:

Shopping for the Right Food

raw > microwave = boiling > baking > frying

Where there is a will, there is a way

This book tells you how to eat better. Now you must decide to do it.
Good will and good luck.

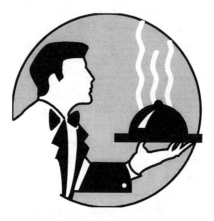

---

[1]   Letters to the Editor, *New Engl. J of Medicine,*. Health-related claims at fast-
food chains. 1994; 330:1908-1909. By DM Elston, MD (Major, M.C., USA); RM
Reeves, Institute of Shortening and Edible Oils, and M Kenkins, A.P.R., Wendy's
International. I wrote to several food chains to alert them about the nutritional
problems with their food preparation and the fact that they fail to tell customers
that the oils used contain TFAs and perhaps other undesirable chemicals.

Shopping for the Right Food

GLOSSARY

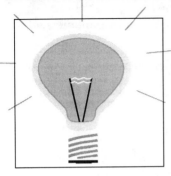

Absolute EFA Insufficiency. Insufficient levels of EFAs in the body. The cells do not get enough EFAs because the body does not have enough. The condition is found with fat malabsorption and in people who eat very few calories, such as anorexia nervosa.

Atherosclerosis. A type of hardening of the arteries in which cholesterol, fat, and other blood components build up on the inner lining of the arteries. Eventually the arteries may narrow so that oxygen and nutrients cannot reach important organs.

Arachidonic acid, AA. A polyunsaturated fatty acid derived from linoleic acid. The precursor to series 2 eicosanoids. Formula 20:4ω6.

Cholesterol. A soft, waxy substance. It is made in sufficient quantity by the body for normal body function, including the manufacture of hormones, bile acid, and vitamin D. It is like a fat and helps to maintain the optimal function and fluidity of membranes. In large amounts it forms crystals which harden the arteries.

Derivatives. Fatty acids derived from another fatty acid. Usually used to refer to derivatives of the two essential fatty acids.

Di- Homo Gamma Linolenic Acid, DGLA, 20:3w6, an ω6 derivative derived from 18:3ω6. Precursor of series 1 eicosanoids. Also called **Homo Gamma Linolenic Acid.**

Docosahexaenoic Acid, DHA. A PUFA derived from linolenic acid. Formula 22:6ω3. Found in fish, fish oils, mother's milk.

Eicosanoids. A group of hormones, which includes the prostaglandins, thromboxanes and leukotrienes. The regulate a huge number of physiological processes, including menstruation. They are formed in the body from PUFA in cells.

Eicosapentaenoic Acid, EPA. A polyunsaturated fatty acid derived from linolenic acid. The precursor to series 3 eicosanoids. Formula 20:5ω3. Found in fish, fish oils, mother's milk. Decreases platelet aggregation and clot formation.

Glossary

Essential Fatty Acid, EFA. Fatty acids that the body must obtain from the diet because it cannot make them. Linoleic and Linolenic acid are the EFAs.

EFA Insufficiency. Insufficient levels of EFAs in the body.

EPA/AA Ratio. The ratio of EPA to AA. The higher the ratio the less likely that platelets will form clots.

Gamma Linolenic Acid, GLA. A derivative of linoleic acid, $18:3\omega6$.

Fatty acids. One of the three nutrients that supply calories to the body. Fatty acids provide 9 calories per gram. Carbohydrates and protein supply 4 calories per gram. Fatty acids consists of three major types: saturated, monounsaturated and polyunsaturated. The natural form is called "*cis*". A form produced by processing is called "*trans*".

    Saturated Fatty Acids, SFA (also called saturated fat). It is formed by straight molecules. It is found primarily in animal fat. SFAs are solid at room temperature. Eating more SFAs increases total blood cholesterol, causes hardening of the arteries and increased clotting.

    Unsaturated Fatty Acids. It is formed by molecules that have one or more kinks or bends.

    Monounsaturated Fatty Acids, MUFA. It is formed by molecules that have one kink or bend. MUFAs are liquid at room temperature, solid in the refrigerator.

    Polyunsaturated Fatty Acids, PUFA. It is formed by molecules that have two or more kinks or bends. PUFAs are liquid at room temperature and remain liquid in the refrigerator. They are also called the essential fats, and consist of two families.

    Omega 6 ($\omega6$). One of the families of PUFAs. The precursor is linoleic acid. Derivatives include GLA, DGLA and arachidonic acid (AA).

    Omega 3 ($\omega3$). One of the families of PUFAs. The precursor is linolenic acid. Derivatives include EPA and DHA, found in cold water fish and fish oils.

Hydrogenation. A chemical process that changes liquid vegetable oils (unsaturated fatty acids) into a more solid saturated fat. This process improves the shelf life of the product, but in the process it creates *trans* fatty acids.

Glossary

Linoleic Acid, LA. An essential fatty acid, 18:2w6.

Linolenic Acid, ALA. An essential fatty acid, 18:3w3. Technically known as **Alpha Linolenic Acid,** to distinguish it from **Gamma Linolenic Acid,** 18:3w6, an ω6 derivative.

Lipoproteins. Protein-coated packages (particles) that carry fat and cholesterol through the blood. Lipoproteins are classified according to their density.

High density lipoprotein (HDL). Lipoproteins that contain a small amount of cholesterol and carry cholesterol away from body cells and tissues to the liver for excretion from the body.

Low density lipoprotein (LDL). Lipoproteins that contain a large amount of cholesterol. One possible role for LDL is to bring EFAs to the cells.

Membrane. The protective layer, like a skin, that surrounds a cell.

Precursor. One of the essential fatty acids or a fatty acid from which derivatives are formed.

Metabolism. The sum of all the biochemical processes in the body. The chemical reactions to make or change substances.

Plasma. The liquid part of the blood when the blood does not coagulate. It is obtained by precipitating the cells by centrifugation.

Platelets. Small cells in the blood that form clots.

Relative EFA Insufficiency. Insufficient levels of EFAs in the blood, primarily because there is too much saturated fat in the blood. The cells do not get enough EFA even though there may be enough EFAs in adipose tissue.

Serum. The liquid part of the blood when the blood coagulates. It is obtained by precipitating the cells by forming a big clot.

***Trans* Fatty Acid.** An unsaturated fatty acid that has no kinks at the position where the normal "cis" unsaturated fatty acid has a kink. It is produced by hydrogenation and by cows.

Trienoic to tetraenoic ratio, T/T ratio. The ratio of 20:3ω9/20:4ω6. This ratio increases with essential fatty acid insufficiency. It is a marker of EFA insufficiency.

Glossary

APPENDIX

This appendix contains tables and figures with test results from the analyses of fatty acids in humans, tables with the fatty acid composition of common foods, guidelines for blood and urine testing, and recent (revised 1993) government recommendation to lower cholesterol and prevent heart disease.

A. Tables and figures with test results from the analyses of fatty acids in humans.

B. Blood and urine tests. Different types of tests that assist to diagnose nutritional abnormalities. How to prepare to have a test.

C. Tables of Fatty Acid Composition of selected foods, with emphasis on ω3 fatty acids. Contains the amount of fat per 100 grams of edible food, raw.

These tables contain preliminary data prepared by the USDA. The headings in each column refer to fatty acids. Total saturated fat equals total SFA, total monounsaturated fat equals total MUFA, and total polyunsaturated fat equals total PUFA. The number 18:3 refers to 18:3ω3, linolenic acid. The number 20:5 refers to 20:5ω3, **EPA**. The number 22:6 refers to 22:6ω3, **DHA**. To calculate the total amount of ω6 fatty acids, use the following formula:

$$\text{Total } \omega6 = \text{PUFA} - 18\text{:}3\omega3 - 20\text{:}5\omega3 - 22\text{:}6\omega3$$

Although not stated, practically all of the ω6 listed in the table is linoleic acid. All the ω6 in vegetables is linoleic acid (with a few rare exceptions). Animal fat has, approximately, 90% linoleic and 10% arachidonic acid. This is a very rough approximation. For practical purposes, all you need to know is the total amount of ω6 and ω3. If you need to eat ω3 derivatives, you need foods high in EPA and DHA, mostly cold fish and fish oils.

The most important use of this table is the total amount of PUFA and linolenic acid. Look for foods that are high in PUFA and linolenic acid, as a proportion of total fat. For example, about 70% of the fat in wheat germ is PUFA. About 50% of the fat in broccoli is PUFA, with 25% being linolenic acid. Of course, you would need to eat a lot of broccoli to get enough EFAs. In 100 grams of broccoli we find 0.4 grams of fat, 0.2 grams of PUFA. If you ate 2 pounds of broccoli per day, you would get about 2 grams of PUFA. For these reasons, unless you start early in life, by the time you are an adult even the best conventional diet will not provide you with enough EFAs.

D.   The USDA Food Pyramid

You will find the food pyramid in almost every nutrition publication published after 1993. It is part of the official government recommendations for nutrition. With minor differences, it is similar to the recommendations of the American Heart Association and the National Institutes of Health (see below). Oils, fats and sweets are grouped together, as if they were equivalent or similar in their undesirable properties. They are to be used sparingly. We can expect other useful advice from the same bureaucrats, to wit: When driving at night (or crossing a street), watch for airplanes, elephants and other cars. Eat few foods containing engine oil, rat poison, pesticides and sugar (it is OK to criticize sugar because Cuba grows lots of it).

My research has shown that the diet recommended by the USDA will most likely increase rather than decrease heart disease. Oils high in EFAs are essential for adults that need to correct for years of dietary abuse and misleading recommendations by government and other public health agencies.

E.   Second Report of the Expert Panel on Detection, Evaluation, and Treatment of High Blood Cholesterol in Adults.

The National Cholesterol Education Program prepared this Second Report. Attached are key pages from its Executive Summary. These pages are from NIH Publication No. 93-3096, September, 1993. I reproduced most of them so you can understand how doctors are instructed to diagnose and treat patients with high cholesterol. There are two types of diets, Step I and Step II, for people with more severe cardiovascular disease or those who do not improve with Step I.

The Step I Diet (recommended by this report) involves an intake of saturated fat of 8% to 10% of total calories, 30% or less of calories from total fat, and cholesterol less than 300 mg/day. The Step II Diet calls for further reduction of saturated fat intake to less than 7% of total calories, and a reduction in cholesterol to less than 200 mg/day.

In NIH publication No. 93-3095, September, 1993, available to physicians, the Adult Treatment Panel II (**Panel II**) describes in greater detail the recommended treatment. The report states that in the US, people eat about 36-37% of calories as fat. This should be decreased to less than 30%. The report states that "carbohydrates can be substituted isocalorically for fat, especially saturated fat." (page II-6). For overweight individuals it recommends that saturated fats be removed from the diet without substitution.

Notice that my recommendations are very different. I recommend that people eat fewer calories from all sources, mostly fat and carbohydrates, to achieve ideal weight. It is not useful to replace calories from fat with calories from carbohydrates (quite the contrary). Moreover, individuals who consistently replace fat with carbohydrates may reduce their intake of EFAs. For most people, who do not eat enough EFAs, this recommendation could be fatal.

The Panel II also recommends that both Step I and Step II diets include up to 15% of fat from MUFAs. This consists mostly of oleic acid, the major fatty acid found in olive oil, canola oil, and high-oleic forms of sunflower seed oil and safflower oil. [**Comment**. These oils have been recently developed and are actively marketed in supermarkets and publications. Huge amounts of money are involved and are to be made by researchers who study these oils, and by the companies who develop and market them. I consider these oils hazardous. My research has shown that increasing the intake of MUFA has effects similar to increasing the intake of saturated fat. The only redeeming feature is that some of the oils high in MUFA, such as canola oil, also contain both ω3 and ω6 fatty acids. For that reason canola oil is acceptable. Olive oil contains ω6 but no ω3 fatty acids.] I wonder how much of the research and consulting fees paid to the members of the government panels comes from companies that market or produce foods high in MUFAs. Did they start receiving the money before they recommended MUFAs, or did they use their own or neutral sources of funding to study MUFAs and, after they found they were useful, decided to contact companies to obtain further funding?

Appendix

Amazingly, the Panel II report states: ". . . fish oil supplements rich in these fatty acids [ω3] are not recommended either to lower cholesterol levels or to prevent CHD" (at page II.7). I wonder how many of the members of government panels who have elevated cholesterol take fish oils to reduce it. I also wonder about the risk factors and cholesterol levels of members of these panels. Are they in excellent cardiovascular health as far as all modifiable risk factors? Has any of the panel members died at an early age because of a heart attack or stroke?

Again, there are no specific recommendations about the ratio of ω3/ω6, derivatives vs. precursors. It is as if these issues did not exist. The dietary recommendations emphasize eating fewer calories from saturated fat and more calories from MUFA, as well as eating less cholesterol. The objective of the therapy is to reduce cholesterol and LDL cholesterol.

The Panel II report states that the current American diet contains about 7% of calories as PUFA. It calls this amount a "reasonable level." I consider their data faulty and their recommendations hazardous. I doubt very much that people eat 7% of their diet as calories from PUFA in a natural form. I have reviewed carefully many of the studies and methods used to derive that magic number, "7%." Quite frequently, the number includes *trans* fatty acids. Other times it fails to consider the fact that many PUFAs are often changed or destroyed by food processing. But, most important, are the findings of my research on human blood. Whether or not people claim to eat enough or researchers tell people that they eat enough PUFAs, my research provides the ultimate proof: the analyses of what people have in their blood. My research has shown conclusively that a huge number of Americans (at least 25%) have biochemical evidence of EFA insufficiency, that is, their bodies do not contain enough EFAs. For many people, the problem is that they have too much saturated fat. But there is a significant proportion of the population who are not eating enough EFAs. Furthermore, I believe I am the only researcher in the US who has calculated the prevalence of ω3 and ω6 abnormalities using the highly sensitive methods I have developed (see tables elsewhere in this appendix). I obtained from NIH descriptions of currently funded research (as of 1993). I could not find any researchers who were studying the role of EFAs, including trans fatty acids, in the manner I did with my new methodologies. The NIH review panels have evaluated my research methods many times and stated:

Appendix

- The principal investigator [Dr. Siguel] "has considerable expertise in the area of fatty acid metabolism and is performing state-of-the-art measurements of fatty acids." (4/07/94)

- *"the applicant has provided state-of-the-art GLC methodology"; "the statistical evaluation is well thought out"; "the investigators have the necessary expertise"; "the methodology [for analysis of fatty acids] is well planned, feasible and reliable".*

- The NIH review panel of our funded grant application to analyze about 500 Framingham samples stated that *"The research has considerable merit and should give meaningful and important data." "The investigator will generate plasma fatty acid data with the described state-of-the-art gas liquid chromatography. The data reduction system is not available in the literature at this time."*

My recommendations are different. I emphasize total calories: People should eat only as many calories as they need to maintain ideal weight. They should get enough protein, carbohydrates and EFAs. The remaining calories may come from any source. Eating **more or less** SFA or MUFA is irrelevant as long as you get enough PUFA and have a balanced diet otherwise. And, of course, I recommend that *trans* fatty acids be avoided, a topic which appears to be carefully avoided by the Panel II. Is it possible that any of the panel members receives funding from the hydrogenated oil industry?

The objectives of my therapy are quite different from those of most government panels and public health organizations. Most organizations seek, as a goal, to reduce cholesterol and LDL cholesterol. My research indicates that having low or high cholesterol can be meaningless. Cholesterol decreases when people do not eat. Cholesterol can be lowered with drugs. Cholesterol levels are only rough indicator of cardiovascular health, and for many years were one of the best indicators. However, we now have the technology to look at the more fundamental substances, fatty acids.

I recommend that people have, as a goal, the attainment of a fatty acid profile similar to the one of healthy people. Cardiovascular disease and high blood pressure, among many other disorders, will improve when people get close to their ideal fatty acid profile. The reason is simple: Because optimal fatty acid profiles are fundamental to all cell and physiological processes, having a profile close to ideal would also bring human health close to the ideal.

Appendix

LIST OF TABLES AND FIGURES

The Framingham Heart Study follows several thousand people from the city of Framingham, Massachusetts. I took a random sample of approximately 5% of the subjects who participate in the study. The research was funded in part by the National Institute of Health. Based on my review of scientific literature, this is the only data of its kind, in that it describes the fatty acid composition of humans, including both the cis-isomers and TFAs in their blood.

The following describes the proposed research submitted to the federal government. When this research is funded we shall know more about the effects of EFAs and TFAs on health and disease, for both men and women. Based on my previous research, it is highly likely that this study will find that TFAs are hazardous. Furthermore, we will confirm that eating more or less saturated fat or cholesterol does not have as much an effect on heart disease as levels of EFAs. If I were a company that currently sells food low in saturated fat and EFAs and high in TFAs, I would try to delay this research as much as possible. If I were a scientist doing research on drugs to lower cholesterol, or involved in nutrition trials or studies of the role of saturated fat, or worked with industries that invest millions to market foods low in cholesterol and saturated fat, I would want to delay this research as much as possible. If most of my research evolved around saturated fat and cholesterol, I would not want this competition. If I were on the scientific review committees, I would claim that the research proposal is not sufficiently clear, that it would not provide definite answers, that it should be improved by further rewriting, and any of a number of criticisms that would delay this research for years. It takes about 3-6 months to prepare a research proposal, 6-9 months to learn that the government has rejected it, and another 3-6 months to resubmit. It is easy to postpone undesirable research for years.

We plan to study sex and age differences in relationships between 50+ cis, essential (**EFAs**), and trans fatty acids (**TFAs**) and weight, height, lipids, blood pressure, hypertension, diabetes, diet, disease states, and other variables (cross-sectional study), and incidence of cardiovascular events (longitudinal study), using plasma from 3,000+ participants in the Framingham Offspring Study, Cycle 4.

Appendix

Research has shown that high intake of saturated fatty acids is associated with increased risk of cardiovascular disease; eating mixtures of polyunsaturated fatty acids (**PUFA**) often decreases plasma lipid values; increased intake of trans fatty acids increases LDL and decreases HDL cholesterol; and plasma levels of PUFA are negatively correlated with indicators of cardiovascular disease. There are no data on sex & age differences in complex plasma fatty acid profiles from a large sample of the US population, nor are there data on how these differences relate to disease state. Primary goals are: (1) to calculate the prevalence of distributions of EFAs, TFAs, saturated, and monounsaturated fatty acids, test age & sex differences after controlling for risk factors such as weight, height, hypertension, diabetes and smoking, and measure the extent of fatty acid abnormalities and EFA deficiency; (2) to calculate the prevalence of distributions of isomer and TFAs and test differences as in (1); (3) to evaluate and test relationships between fatty acids and diet, cardiovascular risk factors, such as blood pressure, smoking, obesity indices, diabetes, and disease states such as coronary heart disease (**CHD**) (Cycle 4 cross-sectional analyses); (4) to relate fatty acid profiles and TFAs to blood lipids, especially Total/HDL cholesterol; (5) to predict from Cycle 4 EFA profiles, cardiovascular events (i.e., myocardial infarct or angina) using Cycle 5 and 6 data. We expect to characterize a high prevalence of EFA abnormalities and EFA deficiency, and to find that EFAs are negatively associated and TFAs are positively associated with Total/HDL cholesterol, and EFA levels are decreased in subjects with diabetes, hypertension, CHD, and smokers. Evidence that EFA levels are inversely associated and TFAs are directly associated with hyperlipidemia and CHD will assist understanding the mechanisms of cardiovascular disease and provide guidelines for cost-effective nutritional prevention and treatment.

We will provide estimates of the population distributions of more than 50 fatty acids, including the Essential Fatty Acids (**EFAs**), and the frequency of what we call "Absolute EFA insufficiency" (**AEFAI**), "Relative EFA insufficiency" (**REFAI**) and EFA deficiency (**EFAD**), and measure various isomers and *trans* fatty acids (**TFAs**) derived from food processing to provide estimates of their population distributions. We will seek to determine how age, sex, and various medical conditions and diseases are related to fatty acid profiles, levels of TFAs, and the prevalence of insufficiency and deficiency patterns.

Appendix

Unless otherwise stated, the tables and figures in this section are based on 200 non-hospitalized adults ages 30-69 (50% men, 50% women) participating in the Framingham Heart Study and patients with a wide range of diseases, mostly gastrointestinal disease and obesity. Patients with gastrointestinal disease usually have malabsorption. The men and women shown here are not necessarily healthy. In fact, probably more than 50% of them have either heart disease, abnormal cholesterol, high blood pressure or some other disease.

FATTY ACID DISTRIBUTIONS AND TEST RESULTS

Table 1. Fatty acid metabolic pathways and the relevant enzymes.

This table presents the most significant pathways or biochemical changes in fatty acids. From this table you can figure out which fatty acids are the derivatives of the EFAs, and can understand how some fatty acids are converted to other fatty acids. The enzymes can be inhibited by nutritional deficiencies, age, sex and other factors. When the enzymes are inhibited, the chemical reactions occur more slowly, thus fewer derivatives are made. This is not necessarily bad: The body needs an optimal mixture of precursors and derivatives. If you have enough EFAs and have a balanced nutritional diet, your body makes the best decisions for you.

Table 2. Prevalent levels (percentiles) of fatty acids and ratios.

This table presents the prevalent levels of different types of fatty acids. For example, if we look at the row that has linoleic acid, the 25% column states that 25% of the population have a lesser amount in their blood than the value indicated. The 75 % column states that 75% have less than the value shown, or in other words, that 25% have more than the value shown. If you have a fatty acid profile done, you can determine whether your are closer to the 25%, 50% or 75% mark.

This is how to use this information: If your cholesterol, triglycerides, or blood pressure are elevated, look at this table, in particular at the total values for ω3 and ω6. If you find that your values for ω3 or ω6 are below 75% of the population, then you should eat more and bring them above the 75% mark. The reason for this is that lower levels of EFAs are associated with high cholesterol, high triglycerides and high blood pressure. I will soon be publishing more sophisticated tables that will allow your doctor to be even more precise on the mixture of fatty acids that you should take. Knowing the results of your fatty acid profile, the ideal fatty acid profile, and what values people usually have, you can plan your diet and also determine how far you have to go to correct your imbalance of EFAs.

Table 3.   Fatty acid profile EFA-SR for a patient with Crohn's disease.

Patients with Inflammatory Bowel Disease have fat malabsorption. This patient has very low levels of linoleic acid (ω6). (How low? Look at Table 2 to compare with other people). If you look at linolenic acid, you will also find that the patient has low levels. They are not extremely low, but they are still low when compared with most other people. The patient has increased levels of ω7 and ω9. This is the shift towards production of MUFAs which was discussed in chapter I.3. The patient has high levels of 16:1ω7 and 20:3ω9/20:4ω6, which indicate EFA insufficiency, that is, some cells do not receive enough EFAs.

Table 4.   Fatty acid profile EFA-SR for a patient with hypertension and overweight.

In this patient the situation is different. If we look at the total concentrations of fatty acids, we will see that they are much higher than the corresponding ones for the patient with inflammatory bowel disease. He has too many lipids in his blood (hyperlipidemia). We can also look at the EPA/AA ratio. Most people have around 0.07-0.10. His ratio is 0.06. A desirable target for a patient who is at risk of developing too many clots is about 0.20, or even higher. Therefore, he is well below his target level. See the figures to get an idea of values in the general population. He also has elevated *trans* fatty acids. His ω3 fatty acids (about 2.7%), although not below the 95% to qualify as "low" in the printed report, are quite low compared to desirable levels above 4%. He has elevated 16:1ω7 (2.8%), indicating EFAI. The treatment involves losing weight, increase intake of ω3 and ω6.

Appendix

Figure 1. Indicators of Essential Fatty Acid Status.

On the Y-axis we have the ratio $20:3\omega9/20:4\omega6$. The higher this number, the greater the deficiency of EFAs. On the X-axis we have a measure of how many EFAs the person has in his or her body. You can look at your own test results and compare them with sick patients or with the average men and women in America. Remember that this "average" man or woman is not necessarily healthy. However, it helps to know whether you are far better or worse than the average person. Ideally, you want to be as far as possible to the right.

Figure 2. Indicators of Essential Fatty Acid Status.

This figure is similar to Figure 1. However, the Y-axis shows $16:1\omega7$. It presents different indicators of EFA status. Ideally, you want to be as far as possible to the right.

Figure 3. Index of coagulation vs. EFA Status.

The Y-axis is EPA/AA, a measure of platelet aggregation or clot formation. The higher the number, the less likely that the body will form clots. You can see that most people have values between 0.07 and 0.10. If you have a tendency to bleed, you want to be at or below average. If you have a tendency to form clots, you want to be far above average. As the graph indicates, if you eat more $\omega3$ compared with $\omega6$, the ratio will increase.

Figure 4. Relative vs. absolute EFA insufficiency.

The purpose of this graph is to illustrate the differences between relative and absolute insufficiency. Healthy subjects, shown on the graph as the REF group (Reference subjects without disease), have about "average" values of concentrations of fat in the blood, and high levels of EFAs. People with high levels of EFAs have low levels of T/T = $20:3\omega9/20:4\omega6$. Thus, the healthy reference group is at the left, towards the middle. Patients with Coronary Artery Disease have higher values of T/T indicating insufficient levels of EFAs. Many have too much fat in their blood, which means that they are high on the Y-axis. Finally, patients with gastrointestinal disease have low amounts of fat in their blood and high levels of T/T. This is what we call Absolute EFA insufficiency.

GI = Patients with gastrointestinal disease. CAD = patients with
Coronary Artery Disease. REF = Reference subjects without disease.

Figure 5. Different types of fatty acids

This figure illustrates what a cis (natural) and *trans* fatty acid look like.
See how an unsaturated cis (natural) fatty acid has kinks and how the
trans fatty acid is straight, like a saturated fatty acid.

BLOOD AND URINE TESTS

Tests are ordered in sequence depending on results

To preserve your blood and you as a patient, your doctor has to decide
what tests to order. If you go to your doctor and say: "Doctor, I do not
feel well, but I do not know what the problem is," and you are unable to
identify specific and objective symptoms, then your doctor must guess
what is wrong with you. Because there are tens of thousands of
possible diagnostic tests and he/she can only do a few, he/she is not
likely to find the reason for your problem. It is therefore critical that
you help your physician find what is wrong with you. When you do not
feel well, keep a diary. What are your symptoms; what pain or other
physical changes do you feel? What are the signs which you can see
and measure? When do they occur (at what time of day and after any
particular activity)? What makes then better or worse? Your accurate
description helps the doctor determine the best diagnostic strategy.
Remember that something which happened to you three days ago may
have an effect on you today. Do not necessarily associate something
you did yesterday with how you feel today.

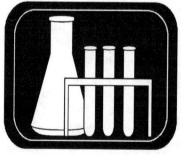

I hear many patients complain about
unspecified "illness," "allergies,"
"infections" or some other strange, ill-
defined cause for their disease. Usually
somebody gave them a name or diagnosis
long ago, and they repeat it, or else they
repeat something they read without fully
understanding its entire meaning.
Instead of describing their symptoms, they
repeat somebody else's diagnosis, which is

quite often incorrect. Every illness, if it makes you feel sick, must cause you some well-defined repetitive and reproducible symptoms. Otherwise it is merely the usual fluctuation in well being that we all have from day to day. Even very healthy people have ups and downs during the day. Sometimes they feel tired, sometimes they feel full of energy; sometimes depressed, sometimes euphoric. Unfortunately, sometimes symptoms of illness are very diffuse and one may be forced to wait until they become severe and the disease has progressed to the point that it can be identified. Otherwise, trying to treat a problem blindly may do more harm than good.

To be effective, a physician must have a tentative diagnosis or idea about what may be wrong. He/she orders those tests which will allow confirmation of the diagnosis, and subsequent determination of what therapy to use. Sometimes your doctor will order some blood tests today and more tests one week later.

You may wonder: Why did my doctor not order all the tests at the same time? The reason is that he/she did not know which tests he/she was going to order the following week. For example, a blood test may show anemia. Then the doctor will order tests to determine what type of anemia you have. You may have iron deficiency, or Vitamin B12 deficiency, or you may have another problem. But if you do not have anemia you would not need those tests. Suppose that instead of anemia you have too much glucose (too much "sugar") in your blood. The doctor will then order tests different than the ones used for anemia.

When a doctor is dealing with a person who cannot communicate (i.e., a child) or someone with poorly defined symptoms, the doctor will rely primarily on the physical exam to identify the problem, and can order a set of "baseline" tests that test the function of major organs of the body (see below). It is for this reason that several office visits are frequently needed before a diagnosis can be obtained. Your doctor cannot possibly order all likely tests during your first visit because you do not have enough blood (or money) for them.

A doctor rarely depends on one test result. Repeated test results vary at least 10% due to normal variations in diet, day to day changes in your body, changes in the water content of your blood, humidity, whether or not you drink liquids before the blood test (your blood may be diluted or concentrated), instrument calibration, etc. It is not unusual for 1% of samples to be improperly labeled due to human error, or for the sample to be lost or damaged in transit. It is impossible to

Appendix

prevent all possible errors. Clinical laboratories have one of the smallest error rates possible in human activities, but there are still errors. When you realize that millions of blood tests are done every month, you can understand why hundreds of errors will occur. Thus, a physician looks for a trend consistent with your clinical symptoms.

For example, a healthy 25 year old woman may have a cholesterol of 120 (mg/dl) indicating that she is in good health. If a 45 year old man, who two months ago had a cholesterol level of 250, now has a level of 120, a little detective work is required to determine why this is so. If he has not followed an amazing diet, there could have been an error in the test or he could have been ill and unable to eat for several days which caused his cholesterol to temporarily decline. Triglycerides can vary drastically according to the size of the last meal before blood testing and the number of hours spent fasting (not eating) before the test. If you fast more than 12 hours, the differences are small. But if you fast only 10 hours, the fat composition of the previous meal has a large impact on the amount of triglycerides in the body.

It takes brilliance, education, training and luck to select a small set of tests that will identify your problem. Therefore, you should be patient when a doctor fails to order the "ideal" test: The doctor is constrained by the amount of your blood, the side effects of doing too many tests, and the costs of all these tests. And nearby hovers the lawyer and others who expect to make a quick buck from the suffering of others.

Baseline or common tests

There are two groups of tests that a physician orders for practically all patients. One is called "Complete Blood Count" or **CBC**. This test counts your red cells, white cells and platelets. Most modern equipment also studies the size and type of red cells to detect gross abnormalities, and also counts the different types of white cells that assist to diagnose a disease. This test is pretty much the same everywhere, although laboratories with sophisticated equipment can provide better analyses of the status of red and white cells. Ordering the CBC does not mean that the doctor has ordered all blood tests.

Another group of tests is known as the "chemistry profile." This group of tests varies from one laboratory to another. It usually includes about 20 measures of different chemicals in the body that assess the function of the liver, kidney, muscle, heart, and basic minerals needed to make all cells work better.

Appendix

Indications applicable to all tests

♦ You want to compare results from the same laboratory. If you must change laboratories, remember that small variations in the results could be due to the change in laboratory. You change laboratories usually when you change physicians or when you go to a hospital. There are several large commercial laboratories in the USA. They provide excellent results for routine tests. Large commercial laboratories have excellent quality control and can afford to check their instruments every day, and to run your test again if there was a mistake. They use automated instruments that minimize the possibility of human error. This is one instance where bigger is usually better. However, your doctor may have had a better experience with another laboratory. He or she usually knows best.

♦ Highly specialized tests are often done exclusively by small laboratories which have the necessary equipment and personnel.

♦ Modern automated equipment usually produces better results than older manual equipment. As a general rule, try to get a laboratory with the most modern equipment.

♦ Inquire about medications and other supplements. As a general rule, you should stop taking any vitamins and minerals for at least two days before the test, sometimes even longer. This will give enough time for the excess vitamins and minerals to clear from the blood. Otherwise the test results could be affected. In fact, if you are going to have a test done to measure your vitamins and minerals, it may be better not to take any for at least one week. This will help because your blood will then reflect your body's stores. To measure a deficiency we need to know what your body has, not what you ate at your last meal. Be sure to discuss these issues with your doctor; otherwise your test results may be incorrect.

♦ Interrupt medications if they interfere with test results. For example, some pain medication may alter test results. Ask your laboratory to see if you should interrupt it before the tests.

♦ Aspirin and similar drugs have lasting effects. If you are going to have blood tests to measure how well your blood coagulates (see next chapter), such as a Bleeding Time, you MUST avoid any aspirin, antiinflammatory agents and related pain killers. If it is essential for you to take them, you may be able to take Tylenol or an

---

Appendix

equivalent generic drug. PLEASE ask your doctor. You should not take any of these drugs for at least 10 days before your blood test, or even longer if possible.

Urine tests: general indications

Ask your physician if you will be required to provide a urine sample. Urine samples require special preparation for each type of urine tests.

How to collect urine for 24 hours

You frequently must collect your urine for 24 hours. Different tests require different containers. In general, it is better to keep the urine refrigerated. The urine will not hurt you or the food in the refrigerator.

How to collect the urine is as important as having the right container. Many people do it the wrong way. Let us say that you decide to start urine collection at 7 AM (a usual recommended time). Then at 7 AM you urinate and THROW AWAY that urine. From 7 AM until 7 AM the next day you save all the urine. At 7 AM the next day you urinate again. This time, however, you SAVE that urine. The trick is to throw away the first urine when you start, and keep the last urine when you quit. In this way you will have collected the urine *formed* during 24 hours. If you make a mistake, start all over again. However, if you throw away the last urine or collect for a longer period, or you cannot start again, tell the laboratory. They can make an adjustment if you explain what you did. For example, if the last urine was saved at 6 AM, and you threw away the 7 AM urine, then you have collected urine for 23 hr. instead of 24 hours. The laboratory may be able to adjust for your error. Careful records are the best way to prevent or correct errors. One last thing: Do not collect urine the day before you will be having your blood drawn: You will skip dinner and your drugs, and your urine will be different. Ask your physician for advice.

Spot urine first void

This means that you urinate and save the first thing that comes out. Sometimes you save part of it, sometimes all of it. This reflects the urine accumulated for several hours.

Spot urine second void

You urinate, but the first part that comes out is not saved. You save the rest. This reflects your most recent urine.

Appendix

Spot urine second void after a drink

This is a variation of the spot urine second void. You urinate, and throw it away. Then you drink water and about 20 minutes later you urinate again; this time you save it.

Further comments and examples

Sometimes you will have to take your drugs; other times you will not. Suppose you are hypertensive and take a drug which may affect your potassium. Your doctor wants to measure your urine for 24 hours WHILE you take your drug to see if you lose too much potassium in the urine. If you do, he will then give you a potassium supplement.

You are diabetic. The doctor may use a 24 hours urine to see how well you are doing during a day. He/she may use a FIRST VOID in the morning to see what kind of urine you accumulated during the night. The results of these tests help your doctor and you determine the amount and type of insulin and food to take during the day and night.

How blood tests work

Injury or disease causes damage to tissues and cells. As a result, the membranes of the cells are weakened and cells release some of their content into the body fluids, including blood. Different organs release different mixtures of chemicals. By analyzing the mixture of chemicals in the blood physicians can often tell what organ is damaged: whether it is the liver, the kidney, or the heart. Due to costs, we often rely on a small number of chemicals, about 10 to 20. The technology is available for more precise diagnosis, but we would need to spend more money for this precision.

Laboratory tests measure chemicals (substances) in the blood. When the body is healthy and the cells are healthy, only a small amount of the contents inside the cells leaks into the blood. These are "normal" leaks. Scientists have measured the chemicals in the blood of healthy people and established a range of "healthy values". These amounts are called "normal levels" or "reference levels." Over the years, laboratories and researchers have measured thousands of chemicals, and thus established healthy reference values for them.

When the blood of a patient is analyzed, the results are compared with reference values. When the values are different from those of the

Appendix

reference population, we suspect cell injury or disease.

Why we use blood for nutritional tests

Ideally we would like to study the body composition to determine if
there is a whole body deficiency of certain nutrients, such as a vitamin
or a mineral. When we analyze foods for chemical composition, we put
the food in a blender, we mix it well, and take a small part to analyze.
For obvious reasons, people are reluctant to be mixed in a blender.
They also refuse to allow scientists to take parts of their body and blend
them. Instead, we use a small amount of blood and use the blood test
results as "*indicators*" of what is going on in the body. However, these
"indicators" can sometimes produce misleading results. Many factors
alter blood test results. For example, you may not have enough
potassium in your body, but there may be enough in your blood. The
blood test results are influenced by your previous meals, drugs, fasting,
weight, etc. To minimize these effects, we ask people to fast for 14
hours to allow the blood to "equilibrate" with the rest of the body. We
also compare blood test results for patients with blood test results of
healthy subjects, in order to have comparable test results and establish
an "ideal" blood profile.

OTHER BLOOD AND URINE TESTS
FOR CARDIOVASCULAR DISEASE

"Other commonly used tests"

Topics: Chemistry profile. The complete blood count (CBC). Protein
electrophoresis

Summary

There are several common tests used to judge your overall health
status. The Chemistry profile measures about 20 different chemicals
in your blood used to evaluate each major organ. The complete blood
count (CBC) measures the status of your red cells, white cells and
platelets. Protein electrophoresis provides an overall evaluation of
your immune system.

Appendix

Introduction

Blood testing is one of the most efficient areas in health care. Over the last ten years the cost of blood testing has declined while the quality of testing has improved. There is probably no other area of medicine with lower error rates. Even so, with thousands of tests performed daily at most institutions, some test results are likely to be in error due to unpredictable factors, such as changes in humidity, sample evaporation, etc.

Chemistry Profile

This is a group of blood tests that include the chemicals most often tested by physicians. The test is done using **serum**. Serum is the liquid part left when blood coagulates in a tube. (Plasma is the liquid part before blood coagulates.) Plasma and serum are similar, but when the blood coagulates (forms a big clot), many of the chemicals in the blood are altered.

Different laboratories give the chemistry profile different but similar names such as Chemistry Profile or Basic Chemistry Set. Some doctors still know it as the "SMAC20" in recognition of the 20 tests done by one of the most popular machines (old models). These blood tests include tests of your electrolytes (the common minerals sodium, potassium, etc.), enzymes that indicate how well liver, heart, and kidneys work, and often tests for other minerals like calcium, iron or magnesium. When there are EFA abnormalities, the cells "leak" enzymes and minerals into the blood and urine. This increased "leak" is harmful and can be reduced by correction of the EFA abnormality. Numerous tests measure the substances that leak out of cells.

Complete Blood Count

This test counts the different types of blood cells that you have. It is not a "complete" set of tests, merely a complete count of the types of common cells in your blood. The test includes one or more of the following:

A count of your Red Cells. An analysis of the structure of your Red Cells. If you have a problem with your blood, the size and shape of the cells provides a clue to the problem. A deficiency of iron usually

---

produces small cells. A deficiency of B_{12} produces large cells. Most nutritional deficiencies produce fewer cells.

A count of your White Cells and the type of cell. This helps to identify an infection and the structure of your immune system. When you have an infection, this number increases. When you have an immune deficiency, this number frequently decreases.

Differential (optional): analyzes the different types of white cells. There are many different types of white cells and the relative presence or absence of some types helps to diagnose an infection or a blood cancer.

A count of platelets. People with few platelets may not form clots when they need them, for example, when they cut their skin.

Size of cells

Some laboratories now have instruments that study the size of each type of cell and print a report. Some physicians are not aware of these tests and the laboratories throw them away. You may ask your physician to request the laboratory to send a copy of the cell size distributions. They are quite helpful in evaluating nutritional disorders. Unfortunately, most laboratories have not decided what to charge for this procedure. I find these graphs complex but useful. This is not for people with weak mathematical training.

Cell reproduction: reticulocyte count

This test counts the number of young, developing red cells. You have too many young cells when your body is replenishing red cells at a rate faster than normal. The average life of a red cell is 120 days. If your cells live only 60 days, something is killing them. This test is very important and simple to do, yet it is rarely done even though it is very inexpensive. It helps to determine the cause of anemia and also to find out if your cells are dying prematurely. In the past the test was not accurate because it required manual counting of cells and many laboratories count only 1000 cells. At least 2000 cells must be counted for accurate results. Some laboratories now have automated equipment and can count over 10,000 cells. This produces a more accurate test. Many physicians do not order the test because they are unaware that modern technology produces highly accurate and useful results.

If you have a normal count of red cells and no "anemia", but an elevated reticulocyte count, there is a high probability that something is prematurely killing your red cells, probably some nutritional abnormality or another disorder. A deficiency of EFAs makes the red cell membranes unstable and the cells die at a young age. If you have normal counts of red cells, no other disease, but an elevated reticulocyte count, you can suspect an EFA abnormality. This is an early sign of future disease. If you fail to correct this problem, as you get older your body will not be able to produce as many red cells as it needs to compensate for their premature death. You may then develop anemia.

If you have a decreased count of red cells ("anemia") but only normal levels of reticulocytes, it means that the body is not producing enough red cells to compensate. The cause is likely to be a nutritional deficiency, frequently not enough iron, B_{12} or folate, or it could be a combination of various factors, including EFA deficiency. When you start eating a balanced diet, your reticulocyte count goes up. This can also be seen if your doctor orders a graph with the distribution of sizes of cells (mentioned above). In my experience I have found that patients with heart disease have increased reticulocyte counts and no anemia. This finding indicates insufficient levels of EFAs.

Protein Electrophoresis (serum)

This test requires very little blood and produces a report which, when properly interpreted, can provide significant information regarding the proteins (such as enzymes) in your blood. Some laboratories have the modern technology required to produce a comprehensive report and a clear graph or curve that helps to characterize a multitude of chemical processes inside your body, such as the presence of an inflammation or infection, and the status of your immune system. The test indicates that you may be ill but is not specific about the cause of the disease. I use it as an indicator of health status or progress: Is the patient getting better? Often an EFA abnormality manifests itself as a defective immune system.

More specific studies can be done for patients with suspected immune deficiencies. It is now possible to analyze the amount of each type of immunoglobulin (structures that fight foreign bodies) and the activity of each type of white cell. However, such tests are expensive and do not help to tell you what to do next.

Appendix

Fatty acid analysis of adipose fat

A fatty acid analysis can be done on your fat tissue (adipose fat) to measure the type of fat in your adipose fat instead of your blood.[1] This test measures your life history: what you have accumulated in your body (as far as fat is concerned). The technician takes a small syringe and gets a very tiny amount of fat from your buttocks or your abdomen. The amount is so small that it is usually invisible to the naked eye. It doesn't hurt and the only side effect it ever produces (and even this is rare) is a tiny bruise. It feels like a subcutaneous injection and it is done the same way. Adipose tissue analysis is important when you must know your total fat composition. This occurs with severe fat malabsorption, such as in cystic fibrosis, severe heart disease, unusual immune disorders and various rare conditions.

Blood tests, pricing and insurance reimbursement

The following information may assist you in deciding when to have blood tests done and how to minimize your expenses. This is one of the most complex areas of medicine because reimbursement procedures are constantly changing and each insurance organization has different rules. Therefore, you must find the rules applicable to your own situation.

In general, Medicare requires uniform pricing across the USA. Tests done for Medicare patients must be billed by the laboratory, who directly bills Medicare (rather than the doctor, the hospital or the patient). Tests ordered by a Health Maintenance Organization ("**HMO**") or similar pre-paid group plans must be ordered and approved by a "provider" authorized by the organization. Otherwise, the patient may be responsible for the bill or the laboratory does not get paid. If you think that a test is needed for your care, the HMO must provide it or it could be liable for injuries that follow from failure to order the test. It is best to discuss these issues amiably with your personal physician, who will most likely order what is best for you. However, many tests have "false positive" results, meaning results that appear to indicate an abnormality when none is present. For example, if a test indicates prostate cancer, you should not necessarily rush to have biopsies or

Appendix

other complex procedures: Sometimes you have "abnormal" test results
as a result of normal biological variation.

Frequently physicians order tests for patients without the patient
understanding the tests ordered. However, the patient may be
responsible for paying for them. I strongly urge all readers to
understand what tests and diagnostic procedures are ordered,
particularly with invasive procedures. *You should be told how the
test will change your treatment.* You should request that risks be
minimized. For example, the smallest possible tube should be used to
draw blood; the largest possible protector should be used for X-rays.

Diagnostic blood tests needed to diagnose a disease, rather than merely
prevent a disease, are covered by most insurance programs. You may
have a co-payment or deductible. When the physician or hospital
orders the test, the laboratory bills the physician or hospital, often at a
professional discount. Discounts are usually illegal to patients because
there must be only one list price for all patients. If a discount is offered,
the insurance company may consider that the discounted price is the
real "list price" and pay only a percent of that price. If these absurd
rules were changed, patients could obtain significant discounts from
laboratories by prepayment. At least 30% of the expenses of most tests
are due to collection and billing expenses and regulatory paperwork.

Laboratories, like physicians, are required to attempt to collect all the
money owed by the patient. Failure to attempt to collect is interpreted
by the insurance company as an official discount in the list price. If you
are not covered by insurance, you can save money by offering the
physician his actual price (list - professional discount). If you are
covered by insurance, your best approach for quick service is to offer to
prepay a portion of the test, pay the rest when you receive the total bill,
and then submit the bill for insurance reimbursement.

Appendix

NUTRITIONAL TESTS

"It is your blood and urine: Know why they are taken."

Topics: Nutritional testing. Blood vs. urine. Vitamin and mineral tests. Common deficiencies. Calcium, Magnesium, Potassium, Manganese, Iron, Vitamins A, C, E.

Summary

Nutritional testing is quite complex. Even specialists are often puzzled by the results. Tests are usually done using blood or urine samples. Nutrients are not stored in the blood or urine but in other parts of the body. They are released into the blood to be carried to the organs that need them. Because the body stores large quantities of most nutrients, deficiencies and excesses are difficult to detect unless they are quite severe. The blood usually carries the normal amount of nutrients even when the total body stores are quite low. Therefore, physicians use urine tests to determine whether the body is preserving nutrients or discarding them. Nutrients are preserved when they are deficient, and discarded when they are present in excess or when there is a body disease that affects the maintenance of nutrition. However, with disease, the kidneys often do not work well, and the concentration of nutrients in the urine may increase even though the body ought to be conserving them. Interpretation of blood and urine tests is quite difficult and constitutes a specialty of medicine.

Your blood does not always reflect body stores

Nutritional testing is quite complex. Test results are not the same as test scores or scores at games. A result may appear abnormal, but be a "normal" physiological variation; a result may appear "normal," but in the context of other test results and clinical condition, it indicates disease. Proper test interpretation is a very difficult science.

This discussion is limited to common tests done with blood or urine which are relevant to the diagnosis of cardiovascular disease and EFA abnormalities. Nutrients are not stored in the blood or urine, but rather in other parts of the body. They are released into the blood to be carried to the organs that need them. Because the body stores large quantities of most nutrients, deficiencies and excesses are difficult to detect unless they are quite severe. Quite often the blood carries the normal amount of nutrients even when the total body stores are quite low. The reason is that the body carefully regulates your nutrient levels and always tries to carry approximately the same amount of nutrients in the blood. If a person does not eat enough, the body releases nutrients from its storage areas. If a person eats too much, the body discards the excess in the urine or saves the excess in a storage area for future use.

To identify a nutritional deficiency we really want to know how much of it the body stores. This can rarely be done because it would necessitate cutting out small parts of the body and potentially harming the person. Instead, doctors study the blood and urine and draw inferences about the composition of the body. Studies have shown what a healthy person usually has in the blood. When the values of a patient differ from the values of a group of healthy people used as "reference" or "normal" values, a doctor tries to determine the reason for the difference. Sometimes the difference is due to normal physiological variation, that is, differences from one person to another. Other times the differences reflect a disease, or a deficiency or excess.

The use of blood vs. urine

An analysis of a patient's urine helps to determine whether the body is in balance: Is the person eating what the body needs to maintain itself? When a person has the proper balance of nutrients, the amount of nutrients consumed by the body and discarded in the urine are approximately the same as the total amount eaten in the food. Studies have shown what an average healthy person discards in the urine. When the urine contains too much of a chemical, it means that either the body is discarding excessive intake or there is some disease that is causing bodily destruction. When the urine contains small quantities, it indicates that the body is preserving the nutrient, often because one does not eat enough. Thus, urine analysis is particularly useful to identify excessive intake or deficiencies of vitamins and minerals.

Tests for common deficiencies

Calcium

A very common blood and urine test. This blood test is often done as part of the chemical profile mentioned in the previous chapter. Because calcium is very important to the body, the body carefully regulates the amount of calcium in the blood and, except in unusual cases, such as cancer or another disease that destroys the bones, blood calcium levels are usually normal. Several approaches can be used to identify a nutritional calcium deficiency. A hormone, Parathyroid Hormone (PTH), is elevated in the blood of people who do not eat enough calcium. When this hormone is elevated, calcium is released from the bones into the cells. In addition, the kidneys of healthy people regulate and maintain appropriate calcium levels in blood. When healthy people eat too much calcium, within limits, the kidneys excrete it. When they do not eat enough, the kidneys preserve calcium and the calcium in urine is quite low. When there is not enough calcium in the diet, the body destroys the bone to provide enough calcium to other organs that need it most. Therefore, an elevated PTH together with little calcium in urine suggests insufficient intake of calcium. After eating adequate calcium for several weeks, urinary calcium should increase and PTH decrease, suggesting that the problem has been corrected. For complicated cases, bone studies determine whether the bones have enough calcium in them.

Iron, Vitamin B$_{12}$ and Folate

These are common blood tests to diagnose anemia. They are usually done in conjunction with other studies of the shape and size of blood cells to determine whether the problem is insufficient iron, B$_{12}$ or folate intake, or an inability of the body to utilize these nutrients. Besides ordering iron, B$_{12}$ or folate, a doctor orders tests for other chemicals that indicate how the body uses them. The combination of the shape of the red cells and the test results helps the doctor to find if there is a deficiency or excess, or an inability of the body to use the vitamins and minerals it has.

Magnesium and Potassium

These are also routine blood tests to evaluate overall health status. Healthy people have normal levels; abnormal levels usually indicate some disease. However, because the body has large stores of potassium and magnesium inside the cells, blood tests are usually normal except when the deficiency is very severe. A practical approach combines blood tests with urine collected during 24 hours. The kidneys of a healthy person preserve potassium and magnesium when the person does not eat enough. Therefore, a decreased level in blood (even if within the normal range) together with low urine levels suggests that the body needs more. As a general rule, healthy people should eat more rather than less: Any excess is usually discarded by the body. But people with bad kidneys or those taking medication that inhibits kidney function should be careful: Too much potassium or magnesium can very quickly stop the heart and kill a person.

Although potassium is easily obtained in capsules, most people rarely need them unless they take drugs that make them lose potassium. Some diuretics cause potassium and magnesium loss in the urine. Vegetables, fruits, meat and fish are rich in potassium and magnesium. Magnesium acts as a laxative and eating too many magnesium supplements could cause diarrhea.

Insufficient levels of EFAs make the cell membranes more leaky and cause them to lose potassium, magnesium, manganese and calcium from the cells to the blood and then the urine. This is one case where, paradoxically, we find increased urine loss of potassium, magnesium or calcium even though the body needs to preserve them. Patients with significant EFA abnormalities often need potassium, magnesium, calcium, and manganese supplements. However, before taking the supplement, the doctor should test for blood levels due to the danger associated with excesses of potassium and magnesium. One such danger is that the heart can stop working! Deficiencies of potassium or magnesium often cause muscle weakness and cramps.

Manganese

Manganese is similar to Magnesium, but it is not common to test for a deficiency of manganese. It is found mostly inside cells. Deficiencies of manganese are very rarely found, because the test is almost never done. Patients who have significant deficiencies of magnesium may also have manganese deficiency. Patients with malabsorption of nutrients due to gastrointestinal disease may have manganese deficiency. A deficiency causes muscle weakness and other problems yet to be determined. The test is commercially available and doctors can order it in the same way they order magnesium. However, because the concentrations in blood are very low, special, very clean tubes are required.

Selenium and Vitamin E.

These tests are not common. For Vitamin E, an analysis of the blood is usually adequate; for Selenium a combination of blood and urine tests similar to the ones used for potassium is recommended. Specially cleaned containers are required to study selenium because very small amounts of extraneous materials can contaminate the test results.

Vitamin E and Selenium are antioxidants and deficiencies may accelerate the aging process. Several studies praised the benefits of Vitamin E. I rarely suggest that people take more than 100 I.U./day on average (or take 2 capsules of 400 I.U. each week, which are cheaper than 7 of 100 I.U.). Patients who need to eat more EFAs often need to eat more vitamin E and selenium to prevent the oxidation of EFAs. Before starting on a diet very high in EFAs, I often get a baseline level of vitamin E and selenium to determine how much to provide as a supplement, particularly in patients with fat malabsorption.

Vitamin C

This is not a common test. Blood must be drawn in a special tube for vitamin C analysis. In the past blood and urine tests were adequate to identify vitamin C deficiency. However, since many people are now taking vitamin C supplements and many foods are fortified with vitamin C, test results are often misleading. When a person takes large doses of vitamin C for prolonged periods of time, his body metabolizes (destroys) the excessive vitamin C. After a while the body adapts to the high intake of vitamin C. If this person reduces the vitamin C intake to a more "normal" level, the body acts as if it is not getting enough. Eventually, it may adapt again. Thus, people who eat large doses of vitamin C on and off may trick their bodies into creating artificial deficiencies and excesses. The solution, of course, is not to take excessive doses of vitamin C. If you are taking too much, you must withdraw slowly, as if you are addicted to a drug. Patients who increase their intake of EFAs should eat enough vitamin C because it helps to maintain optimal levels of fats in the blood. Vitamin C deficiency contributes to elevated cholesterol in the blood and future heart disease. If a patient cannot tell me how much vitamin C he/she has taken, I suggest a change to a moderate intake of about 200-400

Appendix

mg/day from all sources (supplements and food). If necessary, I will
then do a blood test and establish the daily intake.

Carnitine

Carnitine is not usually required in the diet. However, people who have
malabsorption due to gastrointestinal disease, may have a deficiency of
carnitine. Carnitine deficiency impairs the ability of the body to use
fatty acids. Because fatty acids are used by muscles as energy, people
with carnitine deficiency have muscle weakness and get tired very
quickly. There is a blood test to check your carnitine levels. In
addition, the blood test for essential fatty acids, the **EFA-SR**, indicates
whether you have abnormal metabolism of the fatty acids used for
energy by the muscle cells.

Nutritional deficiencies vs. disease

Many people think that nutritional disease usually means a nutritional
deficiency which must be corrected with vitamin and mineral
supplements. In fact, in the USA and many well developed countries,
the major nutritional disease is due to excessive eating of calories from
saturated fat and carbohydrates, and eating too much protein. Eating
too much food and the wrong food is the major problem, not eating too
few vitamins or minerals! In future years we may see the harmful
effects of indiscriminate, excessive intake of vitamins and minerals
which no responsible doctor or nutritionist advocates. These excesses,
encouraged by misunderstood publicity about research studies, and the
widespread availability of vitamins and minerals in high doses, require
many years before they produce noticeable disease. The food industry
is aware of these problems and has worked to prepare rational
recommendations to assist people in eating only what they need.
Although "blind" taking of large doses of vitamins and minerals is not
recommended, there are millions of people who have selective
deficiencies and ought to take supplements tailored to their needs.

---

[1] London SJ Sacks FM, Caesar J, Stampfer MJ, Siguel, EN, Willett, WC. Fatty
Acid Composition of Subcutaneous Adipose Tissue and Diet Among
Postmenopausal US Women. *Am. J. Clin. Nutr* 1991; 54:340-5.

Table 1

Major Fatty Acids and Their Pathways

From Diet: Saturated fat, proteins, carbohydrates

18:0 <———16:0

Palmitic   Stearic

Delta 9 desaturase   ⇓   ⇓

	Essential (EFAs)		Nonessential (NoEFAs)	
FAMILY:	ω3	ω6	ω9	ω7
Parent	linolenic	linoleic	oleic	palmitoleic
Precursor = PFA	18:3ω3	18:2ω6	18:1ω9	16:1ω7

Derivatives = DFA

	ω3	ω6	ω9	ω7
Delta 6 desaturase	⇓	⇓	⇓	⇓
	18:4ω3*	18:3ω6 GLA	18:2ω9	16:2ω7
Elongase enzyme	⇓	⇓	⇓	⇓
	20:4ω3*	20:3ω6 DGLA	20:2ω9	18:2ω7
Delta 5 Desaturase	⇓	⇓	⇓	⇓
	20:5ω3* EPA	20:4ω6 Arachidonic	20:3ω9 Mead	18:3ω7
Elongase enzyme	⇓	⇓	⇓	⇓
	22:5ω3*	22:4ω6 Adrenic	22:3ω9	20:3ω7
Delta 4 Desaturase	⇓	⇓	⇓	⇓
	22:6ω3* DHA	22:5ω6	22:4ω9	

Other pathways

20:2ω6   18:1ω7

Through elongations: 16:0 –> 18:0 –> 20:0 –> 22:0 –> 24:0

18:1ω9 –> 20:1ω9 –> 22:1ω9 –> 24:1ω9

Indicators of EFAD: 20:3ω9, 16:1ω7.

*   Fish oil fatty acids (increased after diets rich in fish oils).

Table 2   Percentile Distributions for Fatty Acids

Fatty Acids	25%	50%	75%
Saturated fat		Percent	
14:0 Myristic	0.65	0.81	1.04
16:0 Palmitic	19.42	20.32	21.73
18:0 Stearic	6.76	7.14	7.47
20:0 Arachidic	0.27	0.31	0.34
22:0 Behenic	0.75	0.88	0.99
24:0 Lignoceric	0.69	0.81	0.95
Monounsaturated			
16:1w7 Palmitoleic	1.45	1.82	2.33
18:1w7 Vaccenic	1.34	1.44	1.57
18:1w9 Oleic	15.71	17.49	18.94
20:1w9	0.13	0.14	0.16
20:3w9 Mead	0.10	0.13	0.17
24:1w9 Nervonic	0.85	0.98	1.13
Omega-6			
18:2w6 Linoleic	27.43	30.19	32.97
18:3w6 GLA	0.39	0.49	0.61
20:2w6	0.19	0.21	0.23
20:3w6 DGLA	1.35	1.55	1.77
20:4w6 AA, Arachidonic	6.44	7.21	8.27

22:4w6	0.25	0.29	0.34
22:5w6	0.19	0.24	0.29
Derivatives DFA6	9.24	10.14	11.14
Omega-3			
18:3w3 Linolenic	0.38	0.48	0.57
20:5w3 EPA	0.43	0.52	0.64
22:5w3	0.47	0.53	0.61
22:6w3 DHA	1.33	1.66	1.92
Derivatives DFA3	2.32	2.69	3.17
Trans Fatty Acids			
16:1w7T palmitelaidic	0.07	0.08	0.09
18:1 Trans	1.44	1.73	2.05
18:2 Trans	0.30	0.35	0.43
Total by category			
Saturated	29.32	30.37	31.53
Monounsaturated	20.07	22.02	23.98
Omega-6	37.95	40.94	43.49
Omega-3	2.78	3.16	3.66

Table 2   Percentile Distributions for Fatty Acids

Miscellaneous Fatty Acids	25%	50%	75%
18:1w5 food isomer	0.02	0.03	0.04
14:1w5 Myristoleic	0.05	0.07	0.09

Indicators of EFA Status	Ratios	Ratios	Ratios
PUFA/NoPUFA	0.76	0.84	0.93
16:1w7/18:2w6	0.05	0.06	0.08
20:3w9/20:4w6 ("T/T" ratio)	0.014	0.018	0.022
20:3w9/20:2w6	0.47	0.61	0.82
22:5w6/22:6w3	0.11	0.15	0.21
18:3w3/18:2w6	0.01	0.02	0.02
omega-3/omega-6	0.07	0.08	0.09

Derivative/Precursors			
Derivatives/Precursor-w9	0.06	0.07	0.09
Derivatives/Precursor-w6	0.29	0.34	0.38
Derivatives/Precursor-w3	4.53	5.76	7.55
Derivatives omega-3/omega-6	0.22	0.26	0.31

Eicosanoid Precursors (ratio series S1, S2 and S3)			
20:5w3/20:4w6 S3/S2	0.06	0.07	0.09
20:4w6/20:3w6 S2/S1	3.83	4.83	5.77

The percentiles were calculated for each value independent of the others.

Boston University Medical Center, University Diagnostic Services
Clinical Laboratory, Fatty Acid Analysis
88 E. Newton St.,   Bldg. Evans 312, Boston, MA 02118-2393

Essential Fatty Acid Status Report EFA-SR

Patient		Condition		ID: 1234	
Physician	Dr. D	Inflammatory Bowel Disease	Dateblood	6/13/94	
			Lab ID	999	

Fatty Acids	Percent	High/Low
Saturated fat		
14:0 Myristic	0.58	
16:0 Palmitic	24.35	High
18:0 Stearic	6.42	
20:0 Arachidic L/H not reported	0.41	
22:0 Behenic L/H not reported	0.58	
24:0 Lignoceric L/H not reported	0.45	
Monounsaturated		
16:1w7 Palmitoleic EFA status	5.31	High
18:1w7 Vaccenic	3.93	High
18:1w9 Oleic	22.46	High
20:1w9 L/H not reported	0.22	
20:3w9 Mead EFA status L/H not reported	0.39	High
24:1w9 Nervonic L/H not reported	1.79	
Omega-6		
18:2w6 Linoleic	16.85	Low
18:3w6 GLA L/H not reported	0.51	
20:2w6 L/H not reported	0.23	

Clinical Laboratory, Fatty Acid Analysis
88 E. Newton St.,   Bldg. Evans 312, Boston, MA 02118-2393

20:3w6 DGLA		1.63
20:4w6 AA, Arachidonic		8.61
22:4w6	L/H not reported	0.43
22:5w6	L/H not reported	0.25
Derivatives DFA6		11.66

Omega-3		
18:3w3 Linolenic		0.50
20:5w3 EPA	L/H not reported	0.51
22:5w3	L/H not reported	0.66
22:6w3 DHA		1.49
Derivatives DFA3		2.66

Trans Fatty Acids	Percent	**H if > Mean Pop.
16:1w7T palmitelaidic	0.03	Low
18:1 Trans	0.35	Low
18:2 Trans	0.08	Low

Total by category	Percent	High/Low	Concentration	High/Low
Saturated	32.78	High	86.29	Not reported
Monounsaturated	34.11	High	89.78	Not reported
Omega-6	28.51	Low	75.03	Not reported
Omega-3	3.16	Low	8.32	Not reported

Boston University Medical Center, University Diagnostic Services
Clinical Laboratory, Fatty Acid Analysis
88 E. Newton St.,   Bldg. Evans 312, Boston, MA 02118-2393

Essential Fatty Acid Status Report/ Fatty Acid Profile

Patient   0   0   Condition   0   ID: 1234

Lab ID   999

Miscellaneous Fatty Acids	Percent	High/Low
15:0 odd	0.09	Ranges not established; compare with 5th, 95th % prevalence
18:1w6 food isomer	0.03	Ranges not established; compare with 5th, 95th % prevalence
18:1w5 food isomer	0.15	Ranges not established; compare with 5th, 95th % prevalence
16:2w9 up with EFAI	0.09	Ranges not established; compare with 5th, 95th % prevalence
14:1w5 Myristoleic	0.07	Ranges not established; compare with 5th, 95th % prevalence
Cholesterol estimated		mg/dl
Triglyceride estimated		mg/dl Large Trig. suggests patient not fasting

Indicators of EFA Status		Ratios (no units)	High/Low
PUFA/NoPUFA		0.47	Low
16:1w7/18:2w6		0.32	High
20:3w9/20:4w6 ("T/T" ratio)		0.046	High
20:3w9/20:2w6		1.75	High
22:5w6/22:6w3	L/H not reported	0.17	
18:3w3/18:2w6	L/H not reported	0.03	
w-3/w-6	L/H not reported	0.11	
(24:0+24:1w9)/18:0	L/H not reported	0.35	

Derivative/Precursors (beware: very high variability)			
Derivatives/Precursor-w9	L/H not reported	0.11	

Clinical Laboratory, Fatty Acid Analysis

88 E. Newton St., Bldg. Evans 312, Boston, MA 02118-2393

Essential Fatty Acid Status Report EFA-SR

Patient			Condition		ID: **1234**
Physician	Dr. D		Obesity, Hypertension	Dateblood	**3/1/94**
				Lab ID	888

Fatty Acids		Percent	High/Low
Saturated fat			
14:0 Myristic		0.67	
16:0 Palmitic		21.98	
18:0 Stearic		6.69	
20:0 Arachidic	L/H not reported	0.26	
22:0 Behenic	L/H not reported	0.48	
24:0 Lignoceric	L/H not reported	0.38	
Monounsaturated			
16:1w7 Palmitoleic EFA status		2.82	High
18:1w7 Vaccenic		1.92	High
18:1w9 Oleic		19.82	
20:1w9	L/H not reported	0.17	
20:3w9 Mead EFA status		0.10	
24:1w9 Nervonic	L/H not reported	1.12	
Omega-6			
18:2w6 Linoleic		27.50	Low
18:3w6 GLA	L/H not reported	0.39	
20:2w6	L/H not reported	0.25	

Boston University Medical Center, University Diagnostic Services
Clinical Laboratory, Fatty Acid Analysis
88 E. Newton St.,   Bldg. Evans 312, Boston, MA 02118-2393

20:3w6 DGLA	2.68	High
20:4w6 AA, Arachidonic	6.49	
22:4w6 L/H not reported	0.27	
22:5w6 L/H not reported	0.20	
Derivatives DFA6	10.26	

Omega-3		
18:3w3 Linolenic	0.82	
20:5w3 EPA L/H not reported	0.39	
22:5w3 L/H not reported	0.42	
22:6w3 DHA	1.11	Low
Derivatives DFA3	1.92	Low

Trans Fatty Acids	Percent	**H if > Mean Pop.
16:1w7T palmitelaidic	0.15	High
18:1 Trans	1.67	High
18:2 Trans	0.26	

Total by category	Percent	High/Low	Concentration	High/Low
Saturated	30.46		135.42	Not reported
Monounsaturated	25.95	High	115.34	Not reported
Omega-6	37.76	Low	167.84	Not reported
Omega-3	2.74		12.19	Not reported

Clinical Laboratory, Fatty Acid Analysis
88 E. Newton St.,   Bldg. Evans 312, Boston, MA 02118-2393

Essential Fatty Acid Status Report/ Fatty Acid Profile

Patient	0	Condition	Obesity, Hypertens	ID:	1234
Indicators of EFA Status			**Ratios (no units)**		**High/Low**
PUFA/NoPUFA			0.72		Low
16:1w7/18:2w6			0.10		High
20:3w9/20:4w6 ("T/T" ratio)			0.015		
20:3w9/20:2w6			0.40		
22:5w6/22:6w3	L/H not reported		0.18		
18:3w3/18:2w6	L/H not reported		0.03		
w-3/w-6	L/H not reported		0.07		

Derivative/Precursors (beware: very high variability)					
Derivatives/Precursor-w9	L/H not reported		0.07		
Derivatives/Precursor-w6	L/H not reported		0.37		
Derivatives/Precursor-w3	L/H not reported		2.35		
Derivatives w-3/w-6	L/H not reported		0.19		

Eicosanoid Precursors (ratio series S1, S2 and S3)					
20:5w3/20:4w6 S3/S2			0.06		
20:4w6/20:3w6 S2/S1			2.42		Low

EFA Insufficiency ? =*	Likely

* Insufficiency = T/T High, or 16:1w7 High, or 18:2w6 Low

18:2w6 =	Low	DFA6 =
18:3w3 =		DFA3 =	Low

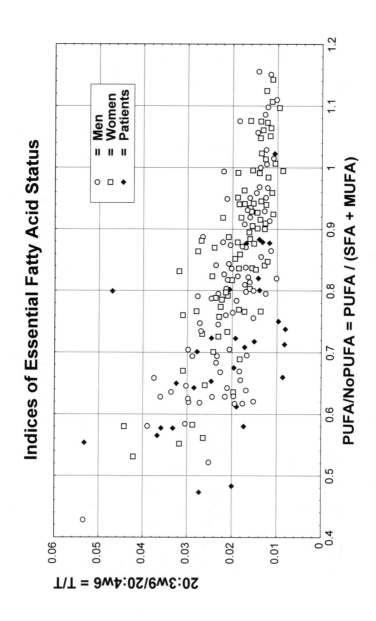

Indices of Essential Fatty Acid Status

Legend:
○ = Men
□ = Women
◆ = Patients

x-axis: PUFA/NoPUFA = PUFA / (SFA + MUFA)

y-axis: 20:3w9/20:4w6 = T/T

Indicators of Essential Fatty Acid Insufficiency

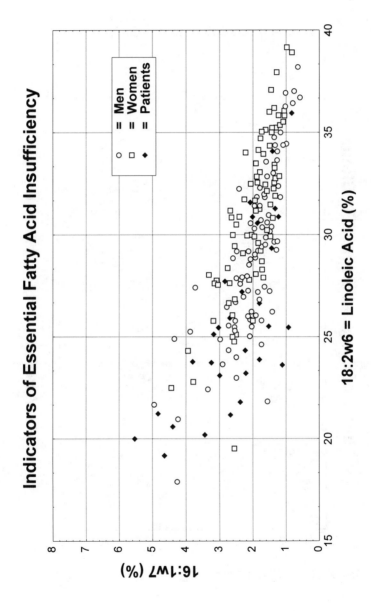

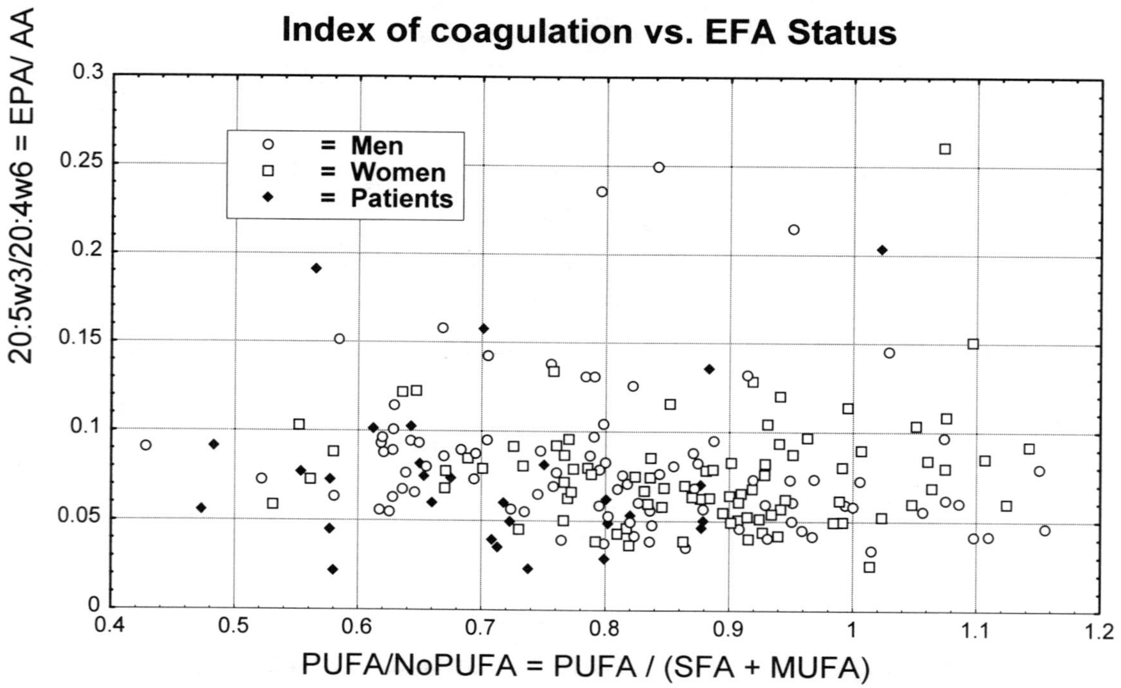

Index of coagulation vs. EFA Status

PUFA/NoPUFA = PUFA / (SFA + MUFA)

20:5w3/20:4w6 = EPA/ AA

o = Men
□ = Women
♦ = Patients

Relative (normal/ up conc., CAD data) vs Absolute EFAI (low conc., GI data)

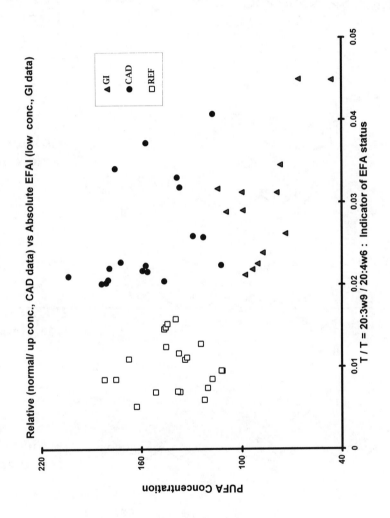

T / T = 20:3w9 / 20:4w6 : Indicator of EFA status

PUFA Concentration

▲ GI
● CAD
□ REF

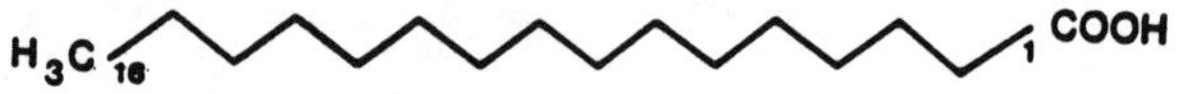

16:0
palmitic acid

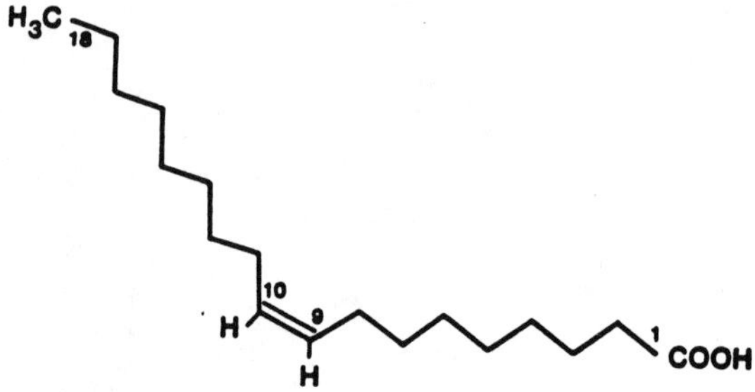

18:1ω9c
oleic acid

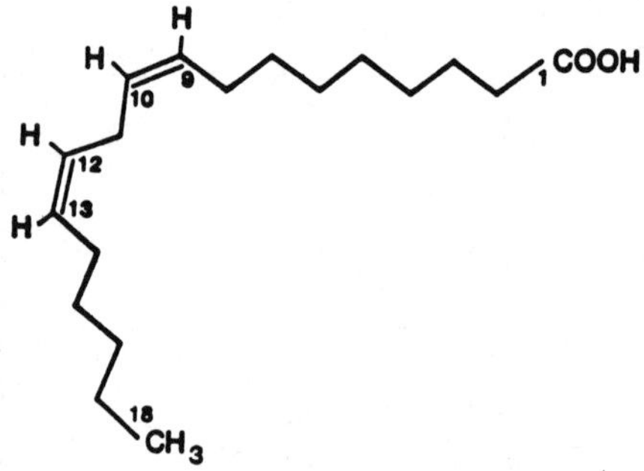

18:2ω6c
linoleic acid

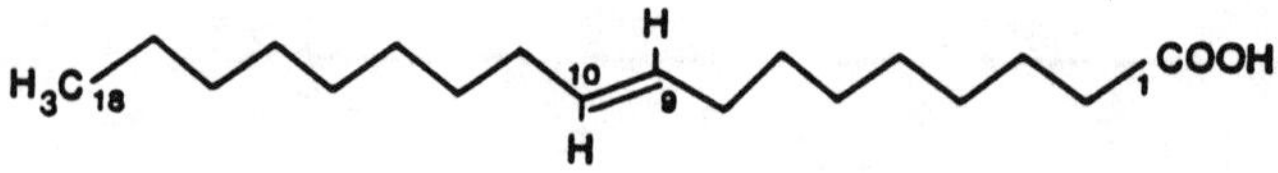

18:1ω9t
elaidic acid

H₃C –   methyl
– COOH   carboxyl

Provisional Table on the Content of Omega-3 Fatty Acids and Other Fat Components in Selected Fc

Dashes (—) denote lack of reliable data for nutrient known to be present.
Tr = trace (less than 0.05 grams per 100 grams of food.)

Food item	Total fat	Total satu- rated	Total monoun- saturated	Total polyun- saturated	18:3	20:5	22:6	Choles- terol
	g	g	g	g	g	g	g	mg
Finfish								
Anchovy, European........	4.8	1.3	1.2	1.6	--	0.5	0.9	--
Bass, freshwater	2.0	.4	.7	.7	Tr	.1	.2	59
Bass, striped	2.3	.5	.7	.8	Tr	.2	.6	80
Bluefish	6.5	1.4	2.9	1.6	--	.4	.8	59
Burbot	.8	.2	.1	.3	--	.1	.1	60
Capelin	8.2	1.5	3.8	1.5	.1	.6	.5	--
Carp	5.6	1.1	2.3	1.4	.3	.2	.1	67
Catfish, brown bullhead ...	2.7	.6	1.0	.8	.1	.2	.2	75
Catfish, channel	4.3	1.0	1.6	1.0	Tr	.1	.2	58
Cisco	1.9	.4	.5	.6	.1	.1	.3	--
Cod, Atlantic	.7	.1	.1	.3	Tr	.1	.2	43
Cod, Pacific	.6	.1	.1	.2	Tr	.1	.1	37
Croaker, Atlantic	3.2	1.1	1.2	.5	Tr	.1	.1	61
Dogfish, spiny	10.2	2.2	4.2	2.7	.1	.7	1.2	52
Dolphinfish	.7	.2	.1	.2	Tr	Tr	.1	--
Drum, black..............	2.5	.7	.8	.5	Tr	.1	.1	--
Drum, freshwater.........	4.9	1.1	2.2	1.2	.1	.2	.3	64
Eel, European	18.8	3.5	10.9	1.4	.7	.1	.1	108
Flounder, unspecified	1.0	.2	.3	.3	Tr	.1	.1	46
Flounder, yellowtail	1.2	.3	.2	.3	Tr	.1	.1	--
Grouper, jewfish	1.3	.3	.3	.4	Tr	Tr	.3	49
Grouper, red..............	.8	.2	.1	.2	--	Tr	.2	--
Haddock..................	.7	.1	.1	.2	Tr	.1	.1	63
Hake, Atlantic	.6	.2	.2	.1	Tr	Tr	Tr	--
Hake, Pacific.............	1.6	.3	.3	.6	Tr	.2	.2	--
Hake, red................	.9	.2	.3	.3	--	.1	.1	--
Hake, silver	2.6	.5	.7	.9	.1	.2	.3	--
Hake, unspecified	1.9	.5	.6	.5	--	.1	.4	--
Halibut, Greenland	13.8	2.4	8.4	1.4	Tr	.5	.4	46
Halibut, Pacific	2.3	.3	.8	.7	.1	.1	.3	32
Herring, Atlantic	9.0	2.0	3.7	2.1	.1	.7	.9	60
Herring, Pacific	13.9	3.3	6.9	2.4	.1	1.0	.7	77
Herring, round...........	4.4	1.3	.8	1.5	.1	.4	.8	28
Mackerel, Atlantic	13.9	3.6	5.4	3.7	.1	.9	1.6	80
Mackerel, chub	11.5	3.0	4.7	3.0	.3	.9	1.0	52
Mackerel, horse	4.1	1.2	1.4	.9	Tr	.3	.3	41
Mackerel, Japanese horse..	7.8	2.5	2.4	2.3	.1	.5	1.3	48
Mackerel, king	13.0	2.5	5.9	3.2	--	1.0	1.2	53
Mullet, striped	3.7	1.2	1.1	1.1	.1	.3	.2	49
Mullet, unspecified	4.4	.3	1.3	1.5	Tr	.5	.6	34
Ocean perch..............	1.6	.3	.6	.5	Tr	.1	.1	42
Perch, white	2.5	.6	.9	.7	.1	.2	.1	80
Perch, yellow	.9	.2	.1	.4	Tr	.1	.2	90
Pike, northern	.7	.1	.2	.2	Tr	Tr	.1	39
Pike, walleye	1.2	.2	.3	.4	Tr	.1	.2	86
Plaice, European	1.5	.3	.5	.4	Tr	.1	.1	70
Pollock	1.0	.1	.1	.5	--	.1	.4	71
Pompano, Florida	9.5	3.5	2.6	1.1	--	.2	.4	50

d Foods (100 Grams Edible Portion, Raw)

Food item	Total fat	Total satu- rated	Total monoun- saturated	Total polyun- saturated	18:3	20:5	22:6	Choles- terol
	g	g	g	g	g	g	g	mg
Finfish—Con.								
Ratfish	1.2	0.3	0.4	0.1	Tr	Tr	0.1	--
Rockfish, brown	3.3	.8	.8	1.0	Tr	.3	.4	--
Rockfish, canary	1.8	.4	.5	.6	Tr	.2	.3	34
Rockfish, unspecified	1.4	.2	.3	.6	Tr	.2	.3	--
Sablefish	15.3	3.2	8.1	2.0	.1	.7	.7	49
Salmon, Atlantic	5.4	.8	1.8	2.1	.2	.3	.9	--
Salmon, chinook	10.4	2.5	4.5	2.1	.1	.8	.6	--
Salmon, chum..............	6.6	1.5	2.9	1.5	.1	.4	.6	74
Salmon, coho	6.0	1.1	2.1	1.7	.2	.3	.5	--
Salmon, pink..............	3.4	.6	.9	1.4	Tr	.4	.6	--
Salmon, sockeye	8.6	1.5	4.1	1.9	.1	.5	.7	--
Saury....................	9.2	1.6	4.8	1.8	.1	.5	.8	19
Scad, Muroaji	8.7	2.8	2.2	2.6	.1	.5	1.5	47
Scad, other	.5	.1	.1	.1	--	Tr	Tr	27
Sea bass, Japanese	1.5	.4	.3	.5	Tr	.1	.3	41
Seatrout, sand	2.3	.7	.8	.4	Tr	.1	.2	--
Seatrout, spotted	1.7	.5	.4	.3	Tr	.1	.1	--
Shark, unspecified	1.9	.3	.4	.8	--	Tr	.5	44
Sheepshead	2.4	.6	.7	.5	Tr	.1	.1	--
Smelt, pond	.7	.2	.1	.3	--	.1	.2	72
Smelt, rainbow	2.6	.5	.7	.9	.1	.3	.4	70
Smelt, sweet	4.6	1.6	1.2	1.0	.3	.2	.1	25
Snapper, red	1.2	.2	.2	.4	Tr	Tr	.2	--
Sole, European	1.2	.3	.4	.2	Tr	Tr	.1	50
Sprat	5.8	1.4	2.0	1.5	--	.5	.8	38
Sturgeon, Atlantic	6.0	1.2	1.7	2.1	Tr	1.0	.5	--
Sturgeon, common	3.3	.8	1.6	.5	.1	.2	.1	--
Sunfish, pumpkinseed	.7	.1	.1	.2	Tr	Tr	.1	67
Swordfish	2.1	.6	.8	.2	--	.1	.1	39
Trout, arctic char	7.7	1.6	4.6	.9	Tr	.1	.5	--
Trout, brook	2.7	.7	.8	.9	.2	.2	.2	68
Trout, lake	9.7	1.7	3.6	3.4	.4	.5	1.1	48
Trout, rainbow	3.4	.6	1.0	1.2	.1	.1	.4	57
Tuna, albacore	4.9	1.2	1.2	1.8	.2	.3	1.0	54
Tuna, bluefin	6.6	1.7	2.2	2.0	--	.4	1.2	38
Tuna, skipjack	1.9	.7	.4	.6	--	.1	.3	47
Tuna, unspecified	2.5	.9	.6	.5	--	.1	.4	--
Whitefish, lake	6.0	.9	2.0	2.2	.2	.3	1.0	60
Whiting, European	.5	.1	.1	.1	Tr	Tr	.1	31
Wolffish, Atlantic	2.4	.4	.8	.8	Tr	.3	.3	--
Crustaceans								
Crab, Alaska king	.8	.1	.1	.3	Tr	.2	.1	--
Crab, blue	1.3	.2	.2	.5	Tr	.2	.2	78
Crab, Dungeness..........	1.0	.1	.2	.3	--	.2	.1	59
Crab, queen	1.1	.1	.2	.4	Tr	.2	.1	127

Food item	Total fat	Total satu- rated	Total monoun- saturated	Total polyun- saturated	18:3	20:5	22:6	Choles- terol
	g	g	g	g	g	g	g	mg
Crustaceans—Con.								
Crayfish, unspecified........	1.4	0.3	0.4	0.3	Tr	0.1	Tr	158
Lobster, European..........	.8	.1	.2	.2	--	.1	.1	129
Lobster, northern	.9	.2	.2	.2	--	.1	.1	95
Shrimp, Atlantic brown......	1.5	.3	.3	.5	Tr	.2	.1	142
Shrimp, Atlantic white.......	1.5	.2	.2	.6	Tr	.2	.2	182
Shrimp, Japanese (kuruma) prawn........	2.5	.5	.5	1.0	Tr	.3	.2	58
Shrimp, northern	1.5	.2	.3	.6	Tr	.3	.2	125
Shrimp, other	1.3	.4	.3	.3	Tr	.1	.1	128
Shrimp, unspecified	1.1	.2	.1	.4	Tr	.2	.1	147
Spiny lobster, Caribbean	1.4	.2	.2	.6	Tr	.2	.1	140
Spiny lobster, southern rock	1.0	.1	.2	.3	Tr	.2	.1	--
Mollusks								
Abalone, New Zealand	1.0	.2	.2	.2	Tr	Tr	--	--
Abalone, South African......	1.1	.3	.3	.2	Tr	Tr	Tr	--
Clam, hardshell	.6	Tr	Tr	.1	Tr	Tr	Tr	31
Clam, hen..................	.7	.2	.1	.1	--	Tr	Tr	--
Clam, littleneck	.8	.1	.1	.1	Tr	Tr	Tr	--
Clam, Japanese hardshell	.8	.1	.1	.2	--	.1	.1	--
Clam, softshell	2.0	.3	.2	.6	Tr	.2	.2	--
Clam, surf	.8	.1	.1	.2	Tr	.1	.1	--
Conch, unspecified	2.7	.6	.5	1.1	Tr	.6	.4	141
Cuttlefish, unspecified	.6	.1	.1	.1	Tr	Tr	Tr	--
Mussel, blue	2.2	.4	.5	.6	Tr	.2	.3	38
Mussel, Mediterranean	1.5	.4	.4	.3	--	.1	.1	--
Octopus, common	1.0	.3	.1	.3	--	.1	.1	--
Oyster, eastern	2.5	.6	.2	.7	Tr	.2	.2	47
Oyster, European	2.0	.4	.2	.7	.1	.3	.2	30
Oyster, Pacific	2.3	.5	.4	.9	Tr	.4	.2	--
Periwinkle, common..........	3.3	.6	.6	1.1	.2	.5	Tr	101
Scallop, Atlantic deepsea	.8	.1	.1	.3	Tr	.1	.1	37
Scallop, calico	.7	.1	--	.2	Tr	.1	.1	--
Scallop, unspecified	.8	.1	.1	.3	Tr	.1	.1	45
Squid, Atlantic	1.2	.3	.1	.5	Tr	.1	.3	--
Squid, short-finned	2.0	.4	.4	.7	Tr	.2	.4	--
Squid, unspecified	1.1	.3	.1	.4	Tr	.1	.2	--
Fish Oils								
Cod liver oil	100	17.6	51.2	25.8	0.7	9.0	9.5	570
Herring oil	100	19.2	60.3	16.1	0.6	7.1	4.3	766
Menhaden oil	100	33.6	32.5	29.5	1.1	12.7	7.9	521
MaxEPA™, concentrated fish body oils	100	25.4	28.3	41.1	0	17.8	11.6	600
Salmon oil	100	23.8	39.7	29.9	1.0	8.8	11.1	485

Provisional Table on the Content of Omega-3 Fatty Acids and Other Fat Components in Selected

Dashes (—) denote lack of reliable data for nutrient known to be present.
Tr = trace (less than 0.05 grams per 100 grams of food.)

Food item	Total fat	Total saturated	Total monoun-saturated	Total polyun-saturated	18:3	Choles-terol
	g	g	g	g	g	mg
Beef						
Chuck, blade roast, all grades, separable lean & fat, raw	23.6	10.0	10.8	0.9	0.3	73
Ground, regular, raw	27.0	10.8	11.6	1.0	.2	85
Round, full cut, choice grade, separable lean & fat, raw	17.5	7.4	7.8	.7	.2	66
Separable fat from retail cuts, raw	70.9	31.0	32.4	2.6	1.0	99
T-Bone steak, choice grade, lean only, raw	8.0	3.2	3.4	.3	Tr	60
T-Bone steak, choice grade, separable lean & fat, raw	26.1	11.2	11.7	1.0	.3	71
Cereal Grains						
Barley, bran	5.3	1.0	.6	2.7	.3	0
Corn, germ	30.8	3.9	7.6	18.0	.3	0
Oats, germ	30.7	5.6	11.1	12.4	1.4	0
Rice, bran	19.2	3.6	7.3	6.6	.2	0
Wheat, bran	4.6	.7	.7	2.4	.2	0
Wheat, germ	10.9	1.9	1.6	6.6	.7	0
Wheat, hard red winter	2.5	.4	.3	1.2	.1	0
Dairy and Egg Products						
Cheese, Cheddar	33.1	21.1	9.0	.9	.4	105
Cheese, Roquefort	30.6	19.3	8.5	1.3	.7	90
Cream, heavy whipping	37.0	23.0	10.7	1.4	.5	137
Milk, whole	3.3	2.1	1.0	.1	.1	14
Egg yolk, chicken, raw	32.9	9.9	13.2	4.3	.1	1,281
Fats and Oils						
Butter	81.1	50.5	23.4	3.0	1.2	219
Butter oil	99.5	61.9	28.7	3.7	1.5	256
Chicken fat	99.8	29.8	44.7	20.9	1.0	85
Duck fat	99.8	33.2	49.3	12.9	1.0	100
Lard	100	39.2	45.1	11.2	1.0	95
Linseed oil	100	9.4	20.2	66.0	53.3	0
Margarine, hard, soybean	80.5	16.7	39.3	20.9	1.5	0
Margarine, hard, soybean and soybean (hydrog.)	80.5	13.1	37.6	26.2	1.9	0
Margarine, hard, soybean (hydrog.) & palm	80.5	17.5	31.2	28.2	2.3	0
Margarine, hard, soybean (hydrog.) & cottonseed	80.5	15.6	36.1	25.3	2.8	0
Margarine, hard, soybean (hydrog.) & palm (hydrog.)	80.5	15.1	32.0	29.8	3.0	0
Margarine, liquid, soybean (hydrog.), soybean, & cottonseed	80.6	13.2	28.1	35.8	2.4	0
Margarine, soft, soybean (hydrog.) & cottonseed	80.4	16.5	31.3	29.1	1.6	0
Margarine, soft, soybean (hydrog.) & palm	80.4	17.1	25.2	34.6	1.9	0
Margarine, soft, soybean, soybean (hydrog.) & cottonseed (hydrog.)	80.4	16.1	30.7	30.1	2.8	0

Foods (100 Grams Edible Portion)

Food item	Total fat	Total satu- rated	Total monoun- saturated	Total polyun- saturated	18:3	Choles- terol
	g	g	g	g	g	mg
Fats and Oils—Con.						
Mutton tallow	100	47.3	40.6	7.8	2.3	102
Rapeseed oil (Canola)	100	6.8	55.5	33.3	11.1	0
Rice bran oil	100	19.7	39.3	35.0	1.6	0
Salad dressing, comm., blue cheese, reg.	52.3	9.9	12.3	27.8	3.7	17
Salad dressing, comm., Italian, reg. ...	48.3	7.0	11.2	28.0	3.3	0
Salad dressing, comm., mayonnaise, imitation, soybean, w/o cholesterol ...	47.7	7.5	10.5	27.6	4.6	0
Salad dressing, comm., mayonnaise, safflower & soybean	79.4	8.6	13.0	55.0	3.0	59
Salad dressing, comm., mayonnaise, soybean	79.4	11.8	22.7	41.3	4.2	59
Salad dressing, comm., mayonnaise-type	33.4	4.7	9.0	18.0	2.0	26
Salad dressing, comm., Thousand Island, reg.	35.7	6.0	8.3	19.8	2.5	0
Salad dressing, home recipe, French....	70.2	12.6	20.7	33.7	1.9	0
Salad dressing, home recipe, vinegar & soybean oil	50.1	9.1	14.8	24.1	1.4	0
Shortening, household, lard & veg. oil	100	40.3	44.4	10.9	1.1	56
Shortening, household, soybean (hydrog.) & cottonseed (hydrog.)....	100	25.0	44.5	26.1	1.6	0
Shortening, special-purpose, for bread, soy (hydrog.) & cottonseed ...	100	22.0	33.0	40.6	4.0	0
Shortening, special-purpose, for cake mixes, soybean (hydrog.) & cottonseed (hydrog.)..............	100	27.2	54.2	14.1	1.1	0
Shortening, special-purpose, heavy- duty, frying, soybean (hydrog.).....	100	18.4	43.7	33.5	2.4	0
Soybean lecithin	100	15.3	10.9	45.1	5.1	0
Soybean oil	100	14.4	23.3	57.9	6.8	0
Soybean oil (hydrog.) & cottonseed oil..	100	14.9	43.0	37.6	2.8	0
Soybean oil (partially-hydrog.)	100	14.9	43.0	37.6	2.6	0
Spread, margarine-like, about 60% fat, soybean (hydrog.) & palm (hydrog.)	60.8	14.1	26.0	18.1	1.6	0
Spread, margarine-like, about 60% fat, soybean (hydrog.), palm (hydrog.), & palm	60.8	13.5	24.1	20.4	1.6	0
Tomatoseed oil	100	19.7	22.8	53.1	2.3	0
Walnut oil	100	9.1	22.8	63.3	10.4	0
Wheat germ oil	100	18.8	15.1	61.7	6.9	0
Fruits						
Avocados, California, raw	17.3	2.6	11.2	2.0	.1	0
Raspberries, raw.......................	.6	Tr	Tr	.3	.1	0
Strawberries, raw	.4	Tr	Tr	.2	.1	0
Lamb and Veal						
Lamb, leg, raw (83% lean, 17% fat)	17.6	8.1	7.1	1.0	.3	71
Lamb, loin, raw (72% lean, 28% fat)	27.4	12.8	11.2	1.6	.5	71
Veal, leg round with rump, raw (87% lean, 13% fat)	9.0	3.8	3.7	.6	.1	71

Food item	Total fat	Total satu- rated	Total monoun- saturated	Total polyun- saturated	18:3	Choles- terol
	g	g	g	g	g	mg

Legumes

Food item	Total fat	Total satu- rated	Total monoun- saturated	Total polyun- saturated	18:3	Choles- terol
Beans, common, dry.....................	1.5	0.2	0.1	0.9	0.6	0
Chickpeas, dry.........................	5.0	.5	1.1	2.3	.1	0
Cowpeas, dry	1.9	.6	.1	.8	.3	0
Lentils, dry...........................	1.2	.2	.2	.5	.1	0
Lima beans, dry........................	1.4	.3	.1	.7	.2	0
Peas, garden, dry	2.4	.4	.1	.4	.2	0
Soybeans, dry	21.3	3.1	4.4	12.3	1.6	0

Nuts and Seeds

Food item	Total fat	Total satu- rated	Total monoun- saturated	Total polyun- saturated	18:3	Choles- terol
Beechnuts, dried	50.0	5.7	21.9	20.1	1.7	0
Butternuts, dried	57.0	1.3	10.4	42.7	8.7	0
Chia seeds, dried	26.3	10.5	7.3	7.3	3.9	0
Hickory nuts, dried	64.4	7.0	32.6	21.9	1.0	0
Soybean kernels, roasted & toasted.....	24.0	3.2	5.6	12.7	1.5	0
Walnuts, black	56.6	3.6	12.7	37.5	3.3	0
Walnuts, English/Persian	61.9	5.6	14.2	39.1	6.8	0

Pork

Food item	Total fat	Total satu- rated	Total monoun- saturated	Total polyun- saturated	18:3	Choles- terol
Pork, cured, bacon, raw...............	57.5	21.3	26.3	6.8	.8	67
Pork, cured, breakfast strips, raw.....	37.1	12.9	16.9	5.6	.9	69
Pork, cured salt pork, raw.............	80.5	29.4	38.0	9.4	.7	86
Pork, fresh, ham, raw	20.8	7.5	9.7	2.2	.2	74
Pork, fresh, jowl, raw	69.6	25.3	32.9	8.1	.6	90
Pork, fresh, leaf fat, raw	94.2	45.2	37.2	7.3	.9	110
Pork, fresh, separable fat, raw	76.7	27.9	35.7	8.2	.7	93

Poultry

Food item	Total fat	Total satu- rated	Total monoun- saturated	Total polyun- saturated	18:3	Choles- terol
Chicken, broiler fryers, flesh & skin, giblets, neck, raw*	14.8	4.2	6.1	3.2	.1	90
Chicken, dark meat, w/o skin, raw*....	4.3	1.1	1.3	1.0	Tr	80
Chicken, light meat, w/o skin, raw*....	1.7	.4	.4	.4	Tr	58
Chicken, skin only, raw*...............	32.4	9.1	13.5	6.8	.3	109
Turkey, flesh, with skin, roasted*	9.7	2.8	3.2	2.5	.1	82

Vegetables

Food item	Total fat	Total satu- rated	Total monoun- saturated	Total polyun- saturated	18:3	Choles- terol
Beans, Navy, sprouted, cooked	.8	Tr	Tr	.5	.3	0
Beans, pinto, sprouted, cooked	.9	.1	Tr	.5	.3	0
Broccoli, raw	.4	Tr	Tr	.2	.1	0
Cauliflower, raw	.2	Tr	Tr	Tr	.1	0
Kale, raw	.7	Tr	Tr	.3	.2	0
Leeks, freeze-dried, raw	2.1	.3	Tr	1.2	.7	0
Lettuce, butterhead, raw	.2	Tr	Tr	.1	.1	0
Radish seeds, sprouted, raw	2.5	.7	.4	1.1	.7	0
Seaweed, Spirulina, dried	7.7	2.6	.7	2.0	.8	0
Soybeans, green, raw	6.8	.7	.8	3.8	3.2	0
Soybeans, mature seeds, sprouted, cooked	4.5	.5	.5	2.5	2.1	0
Spinach, raw..........................	.4	Tr	Tr	.1	.1	0

* Contains trace amounts of 20:5, 22:5, and 2!:6.

U.S. GOVERNMENT PRINTING OFFICE: 1986 O—926-294

A. BACKGROUND

This report reaffirms that an increased blood cholesterol level, specifically high LDL-cholesterol, increases risk for coronary heart disease (CHD). Conversely, lowering total cholesterol and LDL-cholesterol levels reduces CHD risk. Two approaches can be taken to lower blood cholesterol levels in the American population. One is a clinical approach that identifies individuals at high risk who need intensive intervention efforts. The second is a public health (population) approach that aims to shift the distribution of cholesterol levels in the entire population to a lower range through dietary change. The two approaches are complementary and together represent a coordinated strategy for reducing coronary risk.

The first Adult Treatment Panel report published in 1988 outlined a systematic clinical approach to treatment of high blood cholesterol in adults. It was followed in 1990 by the report of the Laboratory Standardization Panel, which made recommendations for improving the accuracy of cholesterol measurement, and by the report of the Population Panel, which set forth a public health approach, and in 1991 by the Children's Panel report. Together these four reports provide the basis for the National Cholesterol Education Program's strategy for control of high blood cholesterol in Americans.

Since the first ATP report was published in 1988, several issues have emerged that receive special attention in the second report. The primary new issues will be summarized briefly in this section, and consideration will be given to the others under section E, Other Issues.

❑   CHD Risk Status as a Guide to Intensity of Therapy

The intensity of treatment of the individual patient depends on the patient's risk status. Those at higher risk for CHD should receive more aggressive intervention than patients at lower risk. There is a spectrum of risk from very high to low, and patients should be categorized into three general risk categories when a decision is made about the appropriate cholesterol-lowering therapy: these include (1) those at highest risk for future CHD events because of prior CHD or other athero-sclerotic disease (e.g., peripheral arterial disease or symptomatic carotid artery disease), (2) patients without evident CHD who are at high risk because of high blood cholesterol together with multiple other CHD risk factors, and (3) patients with high blood cholesterol but who are at low risk otherwise. The latter group especially includes young adult men (<35 years) or premenopausal women.

❏   Cholesterol Management in Patients With CHD
    and Other Atherosclerotic Diseases

Clinical trials demonstrate conclusively that serum cholesterol lowering will reduce
morbidity and mortality from CHD in patients with established CHD. In addition,
pooling of data from available clinical trials reveals a definite trend toward
decreased total mortality in these patients. Treatment of elevated LDL-cholesterol in patients with prior CHD and/or other atherosclerotic disease is called
"secondary prevention," whereas clinical management of patients without CHD
is called "primary prevention." This distinction is somewhat arbitrary, since
atherosclerosis is a long-term process and the risk status of high-risk individuals is
not fundamentally different on the day before their myocardial infarction than on
the day after it. Secondary prevention nonetheless receives increased emphasis in
this report, since a substantial proportion of new CHD events occurs in patients
with established CHD, and it appears that many CHD patients are not getting the
aggressive cholesterol-lowering therapy that is warranted.

❏   The Total Mortality Issue in Primary Prevention of CHD

Clinical trials demonstrate that serum cholesterol lowering will reduce new
CHD events and CHD mortality in primary prevention, i.e., in patients without
established CHD. An important question is whether cholesterol lowering will also
reduce total mortality in primary prevention. Individual clinical trials have not
had the size or power to evaluate the issue of total mortality and have not
provided a conclusive answer to this question. Neither individual clinical trials nor
meta-analyses of pooled data reveal a reduction in total mortality. Some analyses
of drug trials raise the possibility of increases in non-CHD mortality resulting from
drug therapy that offset the benefit of reduction in CHD mortality. However, the
causes of non-CHD mortality are different in different trials, and it is not known
whether these reported increases in non-CHD mortality are due to drug therapy
or to chance. Dietary therapy has not been found to be associated with increased
non-CHD mortality. Therefore, evidence that cholesterol lowering will reduce
CHD morbidity and mortality supports efforts to use dietary therapy in primary
prevention for patients with high cholesterol levels and to reserve drug treatment
for high-risk patients in whom the benefits outweigh the potential side effects.
The possibility of adverse effects from drug treatment as well as considerations of
cost warrant the recommendation to be cautious about drug therapy in primary
prevention for patients not at high risk from multiple risk factors or very high
LDL-cholesterol levels. Cholesterol lowering through dietary means and physical
activity is safer, and these should be the major form of therapy for primary
prevention. These considerations led the panel to recommend that drug treatment
be used sparingly in young adult men and premenopausal women.

❏   Low HDL-Cholesterol

There is growing evidence that a low HDL-cholesterol level imparts increased risk
for CHD. Therefore, a low HDL-cholesterol (<35 mg/dL) is classified as a major
risk factor for CHD, and HDL-cholesterol should be measured in initial risk
assessment when accurate testing is available. A high HDL-cholesterol also
appears to be protective against CHD, and levels ≥60 mg/dL can be called a
"negative" risk factor. LDL-cholesterol is the primary target of cholesterol-
lowering therapy because direct clinical trial evidence for the benefit of lowering
LDL is strong, and similar evidence for raising HDL is less conclusive. However,
therapeutic decisions should take into account HDL-cholesterol levels. For low
HDL levels, hygienic therapies are the first line of treatment: physical activity,
smoking cessation, and weight loss in the overweight. If drug therapy is needed
to lower LDL levels in a patient with a high LDL who also has a low HDL, agents
that raise HDL levels should be considered.

❏   Young Adults

In young men (<35 years) and premenopausal women, elevated total and LDL-
cholesterol levels increase the long-term risk of CHD. Nevertheless, young men
and premenopausal women with moderately high LDL-cholesterol levels (160 to
220 mg/dL) are at relatively low risk for CHD in the near future unless they have
multiple other risk factors, particularly diabetes mellitus or a family history of
premature CHD. For these patients who are otherwise at low risk, cholesterol
lowering through dietary means and increased physical activity is warranted, but
drug therapy should be delayed. For most young adult men and premenopausal
women, drug therapy should be considered when LDL-cholesterol levels are very
high (≥220 mg/dL) or multiple other risk factors are also present.

❏   High Blood Cholesterol in Women

Elevated blood cholesterol levels increase the risk of CHD in women, although
after age 65 the relationship is somewhat less consistent than before that age.
In general, women are at lower risk for CHD than are men of the same age. As
indicated above, premenopausal women in particular are at low risk. Although
CHD risk in women lags behind that of men by about 10 years, risk increases
progressively after the menopause. Therefore, dietary therapy, combined with
weight reduction in the obese, and increased physical activity are indicated in
women with high cholesterol levels, but a more cautious approach in use of drugs
is warranted for women compared to men of the same age. In premenopausal
women, drug therapy for high cholesterol levels should generally be delayed. If
postmenopausal women have unusually high LDL-cholesterol levels or multiple

other risk factors, they can be considered for drug therapy; h   any
women with high LDL-cholesterol levels, use of estrogen repl   ːrapy
may obviate the need for drug treatment.

❑   Age

CHD rates are much higher in elderly patients than in younger groups. As a result,
despite the fact that the relative risk of CHD conferred by an elevated cholesterol
is weaker in the elderly than in young or middle-age adults, a high cholesterol
level leads to more events in the elderly. A high proportion of all CHD events
occurs in the elderly. While there are limited clinical trial data available in the
elderly population, extrapolation of data from trials showing reduction in CHD
risk in middle-age patients seems reasonable. Angiographic studies show that even
advanced coronary atherosclerosis responds to cholesterol-lowering treatment.
These considerations suggest that substantial benefit in CHD risk reduction for
the elderly may be achieved by cholesterol lowering. In spite of these general-
izations, many elderly patients will not be suitable candidates for aggressive
cholesterol lowering. These include patients of advanced physiologic or chrono-
logic age or those with severe competing illnesses (e.g., chronic congestive heart
failure, dementia, advanced cerebrovascular disease, or active malignancy). On
the other hand, elderly patients who are otherwise in good health and who can
expect a reasonably long life in the absence of CHD should not be excluded from
cholesterol-lowering therapy. The level of aggressiveness in cholesterol lowering
depends on the assessment of CHD risk. Patients with established CHD or with
multiple risk factors may warrant drug therapy, in addition to dietary therapy,
whereas those at lower risk should be treated prudently with diet and exercise.

Consideration of all the above issues led the panel to make two changes in the
guidelines. (1) The presence of CHD now places a patient in a separate category
in which the goal for LDL-cholesterol lowering is set lower than before. (2) As
in the first ATP report, determination of the risk status in patients without CHD
depends not only on LDL-cholesterol levels but on other CHD risk factors as well.
However, ATP II identifies and defines the risk factors that modify the target goal
for LDL-cholesterol (see **table 1**) somewhat differently from ATP I. These now
include age ($\geq$45 years in men and $\geq$55 years in women), a family history of
premature CHD, cigarette smoking, hypertension, low levels of HDL-cholesterol
(<35 mg/dL), and diabetes mellitus. A high level of HDL-cholesterol ($\geq$60 mg/dL)
is called a "negative" risk factor. In addition to these listed risk factors, obesity and
physical inactivity are important CHD risk factors which physicians should treat
as targets of intervention.

Table 1

Risk Status Based on Presence of CHD Risk Factors Other Than LDL-Cholesterol

Positive Risk Factors

❑ Age
　　Male:　 ≥45 years
　　Female: ≥55 years, or premature menopause without estrogen
　　　　　　 replacement therapy

❑ Family history of premature CHD (definite myocardial infarction or sudden death before 55 years of age in father or other male first-degree relative, or before 65 years of age in mother or other female first-degree relative)

❑ Current cigarette smoking

❑ Hypertension (≥140/90 mmHg,* or on antihypertensive medication)

❑ Low HDL-cholesterol (<35 mg/dL*)

❑ Diabetes mellitus

Negative Risk Factor**

❑ High HDL-cholesterol (≥60 mg/dL)

High risk, defined as a net of two or more CHD risk factors, leads to more vigorous intervention in figures 1 and 2. Age (defined differently for men and for women) is treated as a risk factor because rates of CHD are higher in the elderly than in the young, and in men than in women of the same age. Obesity is not listed as a risk factor because it operates through other risk factors that are included (hypertension, hyperlipidemia, decreased HDL-cholesterol, and diabetes mellitus), but it should be considered a target for intervention. Physical inactivity is similarly not listed as a risk factor, but it too should be considered a target for intervention, and physical activity is recommended as desirable for everyone. High risk due to coronary or peripheral atherosclerosis is addressed directly in figure 3.

* Confirmed by measurements on several occasions.
** If the HDL-cholesterol level is ≥60 mg/dL, subtract one risk factor (because high HDL-cholesterol levels decrease CHD risk).

Food Guide Pyramid

A Guide to Daily Food Choices

Fats, Oils, & Sweets
USE SPARINGLY

The small tip of the Pyramid shows fats, oils, and sweets.
These are foods such as salad dressings and oils, cream,
butter, margarine, sugars, soft drinks, candies, and sweet
desserts. These foods provide calories and little else
nutritionally. Most people should use them sparingly.

KEY
□ Fat (naturally occurring   ☑ Sugars
and added)   (added)

These symbols show that fat and added
sugars come mostly from fats, oils, and
sweets, but can be part of or added to
foods from the other food groups as well.

Milk, Yogurt,
& Cheese
Group
2-3 SERVINGS

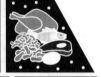

Meat, Poultry, Fish,
Dry Beans, Eggs,
& Nuts Group
2-3 SERVINGS

Vegetable
Group
3-5 SERVINGS

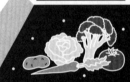

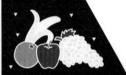

Fruit
Group
2-4 SERVINGS

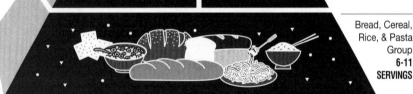

Bread, Cereal,
Rice, & Pasta
Group
**6-11
SERVINGS**

SOURCE: U.S. Department of Agriculture/U.S. Department of Health and Human Services

Use the Food Guide Pyramid to help you eat better
every day. . .the Dietary Guidelines way. Start with
plenty of Breads, Cereals, Rice, and Pasta; Vegetables;
and Fruits. Add two to three servings from the Milk
group and two to three servings from the Meat group.

Each of these food groups provides some, but not all,
of the nutrients you need. No one food group is more
important than another — for good health you need
them all. Go easy on fats, oils, and sweets, the foods in
the small tip of the Pyramid.

Appendix

INDEX

A

Absolute EFAD · 45
Absolute EFAI · 45
Adrenoleukodystrophy · 282
Adult Onset Diabetes · 115
AIDS · 281
alcohol · 137
Allergies · 263
Alzheimer's · 269
American Diet · 151
American Heart Association, **AHA**
 · 303
Amino acids · 58
Anemia · 208, 299
angina · 110
Antibodies · 262
antioxidants · 37, 268
Apoproteins · 103
arachidonic acid · 32
arteriosclerosis · 107
arthritis · 261
Asthma · 263
atherosclerosis · 108

B

behaviors · 150
bleeding time · 44, 102, 206
blood cells · 208
blood circulation · 111, 251
Boston Egg White Diet · 189
Brown fat · 197
Brown sugar · 328
burns · 299

butter · 39

C

calcium · 253
Calories · 2, 83
Cancer · 266
carbohydrates · 56
Cardiac insufficiency · 112
cell membranes · 6
Cells · 6
chocolate · 331
Cholesterol · 73
Cholesterol-esters · 22
choline · 71
clot · 103, 206
Clot formation · 108, 249
Cold water fish · 224
Complex Carbohydrates · 148
Coronary insufficiency · 112
Crohn's disease · 269
crude fiber · 69
Cystic Fibrosis · 280

D

daughters · 24
derivatives · 24, 25
desaturation · 42
DHA · 26, 221
Diabetes · 115, 260
Diarrhea · 271
diet · 2
dietary fiber · 69
Disease · 7, 208
docosahexaenoic, **DHA** · 221
dyslipidemia · 256
dyslipoproteinemia · 94

E

Eating out · 333
EFA insufficiency, EFAI · 45
eicosanoids · 43, 44
eicosapentaenoic acid, EPA · 32, 221
elongation · 42
energy · 2, 20
Enzymes · 6
EPA · 26, 221
EPA/AA · 221, 239
EPA/AA ratio · 32, 213
essential fat · 24
Essential oils · 17

F

familial diseases · 257
fasting glucose · 207
fat cells · 185
Fat replacements · 329
Fatty Acid Profile · 104
fish oils · 206, 221, 249
fluidity · 75
Food Guide Pyramid · 39
Food preparation · 330
Free fatty acids · 37
Free radicals · 37
Fructose · 57

G

genes · 139
glucose · 57, 115, 136, 207
glucose regulation · 146

H

HDL Cholesterol · 94, 99, 256
headache · 110
health hints · 150
Healthy foods · 150

Healthy levels · 81
heart attack · 110
hidden fat · 152
High blood pressure · 108
High Density Lipoproteins, **HDL** · 81
Hydrogenation · 32, 33
hyperaggregatory · 249
hypercholesterolemia · 22
hypercoagulable · 113
Hyperlipidemia · 256, 258
hyperlipoproteinemia · 94
Hypertension · 113, 135, 252
hypertriglyceridemia · 21
hypolipoproteinemia · 94

I

IDL · 256
immune · 262
infant formulas · 47
Inflammation · 262, 271
inflammatory bowel disease, **IBD** · 269
insufficiency, EFA · 171
Insulin Dependent Diabetics · 115
intravenous feedings · 230
isomers · 34, 147

K

Kidney disease · 261
kink · 32, 165

L

Lactoovovegetarian · 307
LDL cholesterol · 94,100, 256
Lecithin · 71
Linoleic · 24
Linolenic · 24
Lipids · 17

lipoproteins · 94
Living Foods · 310
long chain fatty acids · 282
Lp(a) · 105

M
Macrobiotic · 308
magnesium · 253
Malabsorption · 271
malnutrition · 185, 271
margarine · 39
mayonnaise · 218, 331
Medium chain · 49
Medium Chain Triglicerides · 201
membrane fluidity · 165
mitochondria · 197
Molasses · 328
monounsaturated fatty acids,
MUFA · 164
MUFAs · 164
Multiple Sclerosis · 269

N
natural · 10
natural carbohydrates · 164
New American Diet · 316
Normal levels · 78
Nutrients · 7
Nutrition · 3
Nutritional status · 3

O
Obstruction · 273
Oil quality · 217
ω3 deficiency · 31
ω6 deficiency · 30
ω7, ω9 · 42
organs · 6
Overweight · 136, 185

Ovo vegetarian · 307
Oxidation · 37

P
Pancreas · 115
Parent · 24
Partial Obstruction · 271
peptides · 60
PFAi · 42
pharmacological dose · 12, 230
phospholipid · 21
physical activity · 299
physiological · 230
physiological doses · 11
Phytochemicals · 71
plasma · 93
Platelet aggregation · 44, 103
platelets · 93
**Polyunsaturated Fatty Acid,
PUFA** · 24
Poor circulation · 251
potassium · 253
Precursor · 24, 25
Pregnant women · 298
Premenstrual syndrome · 297
Prevention · 231
prevention program · 142
preventive approach · 230
Pritikin Program · 317
PUFA · 24
pumps · 252
Pyramid · 305

R
RDA · 85
Red cells · 93
red wine · 137
reference levels · 79

relative EFA insufficiency · 171
Relative EFAI · 45
reticulocyte count · 208

S

salt · 146
salt substitutes · 253
satiety signal · 200
Scarsdale Diet · 317
season · 147
Setpoint Diet · 318
Saturated fat, SFAs · 164
short bowel syndrome · 279
Short chain · 49
sickle cell · 283
Side effects · 222
skin · 264
Smoking · 135
sodium · 253
solidify · 217
Stress · 137
stroke · 110, 114, 255
sucrose · 57
sudden death · 113
Sugar · 57
symptoms · 208

T

temperature · 197

tests · 89
TFAs · 33
thin · 114
thrombosis · 109
thrombus · 109
Total/HDL · 101
trans fatty acids, TFAs · 32, 33, 147
Treatment · 231
Triglyceride · 21, 101

U

Ulcerative Colitis · 269
uncoupling protein · 197
USDA · 148

V

Vegetable oils · 215
vegetarian diet · 153, 306
Very Long chain · 49
VLDL · 94, 256

W

Water · 70
weight loss · 179
Weight Watchers · 315
white cells · 93
women · 295

REF: FATTY ACID ANALYSIS/ FATTY ACID PROFILES

March 12, 1994

Dear Colleague:

Plasma fatty acids are established risk factors for cardiovascular disease, diabetes, hypertension, hyperlipidemia, and other disorders. These conditions can now be treated with diets rich in specific fatty acids (but not high in total fat or calories).
With more than 10 years experience in the diagnosis of disorders of fatty acid metabolism., we are available to fulfill a clinical need to assess fatty acid status. Using High Resolution Capillary Column Gas Liquid Chromatography (GLC), our method quantifies plasma levels of the major fatty acids, including the essential fatty acids (EFAs), linoleic and linolenic acid. The EFA Status Report (EFA-SR), documents fatty acids of chain length C14 up to C24, including the EFAs, arachidonic acid, eicosapentaenoic acid (EPA), docosahexaenoic acid (DHA), the eicosanoid precursors and key *trans* fatty acids . Our results have been published in peer review medical journals and our methods, based upon Patent No. 5075101, were used to analyze samples from the Framingham Heart Study.

The **EFA-SR** will assist you in diagnosing abnormalities of fatty acid metabolism and in optimizing nutritional treatment. With the aid of the **EFA-SR**, you may improve management of altered plasma lipid levels and hypertension. The **EFA-SR** will also assist in monitoring blood coagulation, in preventing cardiovascular disease and the complications of diabetes mellitus, and in improving the overall health status of your patients.   Not only do our reports identify the amounts of each fatty acid, but also they include an interpretative diagnosis together with treatment suggestions.   Because EFAs are essential nutrients, deficiencies diagnosed by the **EFA-SR** may be corrected with enteral or parenteral lipid or oil supplements. The enclosed brochure describes conditions where the EFA-SR is useful.
We routinely analyze whole plasma, but we can also analyze other tissues. If you are interested in collaborative research, please FAX/mail a brief description to 617-638-8603 and a researcher will contact you at your convenience. We can partially subsidize collaborative research. Prices depend on the analyses requested, the type of sample, and whether it is for clinical or research purposes.

We provide different types of analyses to match your clinical needs:

The **"Fatty Acid Status Profile (FASP)"** consists of more than 25 fatty acids used to assess the health status of a patient.   The set includes the major fatty acids, saturated, monounsaturated (*w*7 and *w*9), the EFAs (linoleic and linolenic), EFA derivatives, total *w*6 and *w*3, including 20:5*w*3 (EPA), 22:5*w*3 and 22:6*w*3 (DHA).

The **"Fatty Acid Metabolic Profile (FAMP)"** includes the Fatty Acid Status Profile, 16:1*w*7T and a group of *trans* fatty acids with 18 carbons in length. *This is the initial profile we recommend for most patients..* We have shown that *trans* and EFAs are major risk factors for coronary artery disease. If *trans* are normal, patients may be monitored with the **FASP** listed above.

We welcome suggestions for other profiles that may interest physicians or researchers.

Cordially yours,

Francisco R Velazquez, M.D.
Medical Director, Clinical Chemistry, Department of Laboratory Medicine

Attachments: (1) Fatty acid metabolism brochure; (2) Example of a patient EFA-SR report;
(3) Reference values; (4) Guidelines to interpret fatty acids; (5) Instruction to submit samples; (6) Physician Request Form (patient clinical information and insurance/billing).

Test Submission Form

Laboratory performing test: Boston University Medical Center Hospital, Laboratory Medicine
Address   Room H-305, 3rd Floor,   88 E Newton St.,   Boston,   MA 02118-2393
Individual to contact: Francisco R. Velazquez, M.D. c/o Fatty Acid Laboratory.
Title of Contact Person   Medical Director, Clinical Chemistry, Department of Laboratory Medicine.
Telephone number (specimen handling):   617-638-7859;   FAX: 617-638-4556
Technical questions: 617 638-8604 (leave specific message with questions);   FAX 617-638-8603

Name of Tests: The "Fatty Acid Status Profile (FASP)" consists of more than 25 fatty acids used to assess the health status of a patient. The set includes the major fatty acids, saturated, monounsatured ($w7$ and $w9$), the EFAs (linoleic and linolenic), EFA derivatives, total $w6$ and $w3$, including 20:5$w3$ (EPA), 22:5$w3$ and 22:6$w3$ (DHA).

The "Fatty Acid Metabolic Profile (FAMP)" includes the **FASP**, 16:1$w7$T and a group of *trans* fatty acids with 18 carbons in length. ***This is the initial profile we recommend for most patients.*** If trans are normal, patients may be monitored with cis profile **FASP**.
Other profiles are available upon request from a set of 100+ peaks.
Notice: This is NOT a Free Fatty Acid analysis test.

Test Includes: Panels and profiles, percents and ratios of 30+ cis and *trans* fatty acids and calculated indices. Diagnostic consultation report available upon request; 2-page report with individual values compared with a reference population, a proposed diagnosis (supplemented, if requested, by a written interpretative report), additional tables and graphs, and metabolic pathway activity. Data on spreadsheet, magnetic media. Diagnostic graphs available.
Reporting results: Typically two weeks; longer for an individual diagnostic report.

Specimen: Whole plasma is best. **Advance Notice required** for new clients, for unique samples, to obtain instructions, for Red cells, fat biopsies, platelets, tissue, culture cells.
Volume: 0.4-1.0 mL plasma or 0.5 mg tissue. Minimum 0.4 mL plasma, but for children and infants can be done on 0.2 mL. For tissue culture, cells, need the number of cells in 0.020 ml packed RBCs.

Specimen collection: Plasma: Collect in lavender top tube. Centrifuge at 5° C. Refrigerate tube before/after specimen collection. Separate and freeze plasma and red cells, discard intermediate (buffy) layer. Store at lowest available temperature. Protect from light (cover with tape). Do not freeze or ship whole blood (hemolysis). Request instructions for other specimens.

Specimen Shipping :   Ship frozen specimens, under N_2 or in a small vial with little air. Ship in dry ice, next day OK. Ship early in the week so that it arrives no later than Friday morning.

Patient Preparation: Patient should fast for 14 hrs; last meal low in fat/calories. Avoid alcohol, aspirin and anti-inflammatory drugs for at least 24 hrs. TPN patients should be off TPN as close to 12 hrs as possible. Patient to follow his/her usual diet for one week, avoid oral oil supplements.

Fee: Depends on number and type of specimens submitted and whether it is for research or patient care purposes ($99 to $1,200). Collaborative research can be arranged.

Patient Requisition Form must be submitted with billing, insurance, and patient information. Volume discounts available to health care providers and referring laboratories. Health care providers are billed directly and are requested to make agreements pertaining to fees. Please call to establish an account. Insurance information not needed if there is a billing agreement.

Methodology   Fatty Acid Methyl Esters separated by high resolution long column. GLC optimized for cis-trans separation using 100 m column unless otherwise indicated. See Siguel EN et al. Criteria for EFA Deficiency in Plasma as assessed by Capillary Column Gas Liquid Chromatography. Clin Chem 33:1869-1873, 1987; Siguel, EN, Maclure, M. Relative enzyme activity of unsaturated fatty acid metabolic pathways in humans, Metabolism, 36: 664-669, 1987

Brochure and detailed information indicating types of profiles available and appropriate use available upon request. Send Self Addressed Stamped Envelope (9 x 12) + $5. Fatty Acid Profiles are used to diagnose EFA abnormalities in patients with GI disease, hyperlipidemia, DM, hypertension, coronary artery disease, atherosclerotic disease,cystic fibrosis, obesity, low EFA diets, and other conditions.

Revised FAME Lab Instructions 3/07/94

FOR YOUR INFORMATION

Send me your proposed book cover

In my next printing I plan to have a different book cover. I would appreciate your suggestions. Anyone is eligible to submit book covers to me. I will select the best cover for my book. I am looking preferably for 4-color covers. Entries will be welcomed at any time until I complete my new version. We will not accept postage-due mail. You should clearly write your name, address, and phone number. All the material submitted becomes the property of E. Siguel and Nutrek, Inc. Entries will not be acknowledged or returned. You must include a statement transferring all copyrights to E. Siguel and Nutrek, Inc., and a statement indicating that the work is your original work. My determination about which cover to use is final and cannot be appealed or opposed. If your cover is selected, you will be required to complete appropriate transfer forms not otherwise submitted, and assume responsibility for the fact that you created the design. In turn, I will give you a copy of the book and acknowledge your work in print.

Send me your comments and note any errors you find

I want to receive your comments and questions. Please indicate: Sections that you think are not clear, including statements you think are erroneous. Why and what can be done to improve them. What questions you have. Topics that should be expanded. Please include the page number and paragraph or section that you are writing about.

If you would like to purchase 5 or more copies of this book, mail a check or money order for $15.95 per book. This price includes shipping and handling. Send to **NUTREK, Inc. c/o EFABOOK Purchase. INCLUDE a label with your correct name and address. All orders non-refundable at this price.**

Thank you!

NUTREK, Inc. c/o EFABOOK Comments

PO BOX 1269, Brookline, MA 02146-0022

Your physician may order a profile **EFA-SR** with an interpretative report to assist in the diagnosis of EFA abnormalities, available from

NUTREK, Inc., or Boston University Medical Center Hospital, Fatty Acid Laboratory, Clinical Chemistry, Third Floor, Department of Laboratory Medicine. Boston University Medical Center Hospital. 88 East Newton St., Boston, MA 02118-2393 (note that the address may be changed by the time you read this book).

For answers to questions and to receive copies of scientific articles, write to:

EFA-SR, c/o NUTREK, Inc., P.O. BOX 1269, Brookline, MA 02146-0022

Include an 8 1/2 x 11 envelope with postage for 5 ounces and $4 for copying and handling. All orders are non-refundable due to high processing costs. Physicians may FAX questions to (617) 638-8603, or a voice mail system to be operational soon at (617) 638-8604. Watch the computer bulletin boards at Prodigy or Internet or other services that may establish special "forums" on EFAs.

For technical information on blood testing call the voice mail/Fax on demand at (617) 638-8604 (late in 1994/5).

You may be able to find corrections and updates on Forums on Nutrition on Internet, Prodigy, and others. Search for the word **EFABOOK.** We plan to have a **forum or bulletin board or newsgroup** with updated information on EFAs. Professionals may want to submit through internet their electronic address and $10//year to have them included in an internet **mailing list**. We plan to send information on EFA research and meetings.

THESE TOPICS AND MORE ARE COVERED

The US Surgeon General's report identifies the type of fat that people eat as one of the most significant factors in health and disease. Fats called **Essential Fatty Acids (EFAs)** are critical to good nutrition because humans cannot make them. Just as humans must consume vitamins, they must also get EFAs from food, but in far greater quantities than vitamins. Failure to eat enough EFAs is a cause of hardening of the arteries, abnormal clot formation, coronary heart disease, high cholesterol and high blood pressure.

Balance is the key to healthy nutrition. Linolenic acid (*Omega*-3) and linoleic acid (*Omega*-6) are essential fatty acids (**EFAs**). A balance of oils and foods rich in the "soft" EFAs help prevent and treat disease.

How to prevent and treat certain diseases, including cardiovascular disease, blocked arteries, hypertension and stroke. How to lower your cholesterol, and how to lower your blood levels of undesirable *trans* fatty acids (**TFAs**). Simple changes in your meals, supplemented with the essential fats, can reduce your chances of a heart attack or stroke due to elevated cholesterol and saturated fat. At the same time, these changes can lower blood pressure, improve or prevent arthritis, prevent the complications of diabetes, and increase mental ability and overall sense of well being. They can also make skin softer, "younger," and moist without dryness or itching.

Fish and vegetable oils: Which oils to use and when. Correcting deficiencies of essential fats with supplementation. A comparison of the medical and biochemical characteristics of major dietary oils, including canola, soybean, walnut and flax seed oil.

Warning signs of heart disease or stroke. Case histories. Guidelines for eating so your blood clots quickly enough to prevent bleeding but slowly enough to avoid obstructing an artery. How to correct for years of neglect using individualized mixtures of EFAs.

Dietary modifications for children, adults; middle aged and elderly people; pregnant women; people who want to lose weight, athletes. Unique risks for women and children.

The key to weight control. How to lose two or more pounds per week without going hungry. A weight loss diet, scientifically designed to make people lose fat, not just water. Foods and snacks that curb the appetite.

ABOUT THE AUTHOR

Dr. Siguel has researched the effects of fats on health and disease for more than 15 years. He has developed a state of the art blood test to diagnose abnormalities of essential fatty acids and lipid metabolism, for which he was awarded the only US Patent of its kind. Dr. Siguel studies the relationship between fat consumption and cardiovascular disease, hypertension, high cholesterol, elevated triglycerides, dermatitis, complications of diabetes mellitus, and delaying aging. He personally has done the research that others speak or write about.

Dr. Siguel has shown that a diet deficient in essential fatty acids is probably the most significant nutritional factor in cardiovascular disease. Dr. Siguel also has shown that fats from hydrogenated and processed oils ("*trans* fatty acids") are associated with heart disease and abnormal cholesterol levels. His research, including his new blood test to measure EFA deficiencies, has been presented to the scientific community at professional meetings and in scientific journals.

Dr. Siguel has been interviewed by CNN, Boston TV, National Public Radio and other news media. His articles have appeared in *Natural Health Journal, Cardiovascular World News, American Journal of Cardiology, Clinical Chemistry, Metabolism, Clinical Nutrition, Archives of Pathology and Lab Medicine, Nutrition and Cancer, Nutrition Support Services, American Journal of Clinical Nutrition*, and many more. Dr. Siguel is a member of the American Medical Association and a *Fellow* of the American Association for the Advancement of Science, publishers of the journal *Science*. His research on the role of EFAs in HDL and total cholesterol was the subject of a press conference called by the American College of Cardiology (3/14/94). He was the featured Clinician of the month (2/94) in Preventive Medicine Update.

In addition to his medical degree, Dr. Siguel has a Ph.D. with expertise in experimental design and data analysis, which qualifies him to understand complex statistical methods. He has received one of the highest US Public Health Service awards for his work in health statistics and other commendations for his work for the Public Health Service. He has supervised the evaluation of Health Maintenance Organizations, drug abuse treatment programs, and alternative health care reform proposals. In his spare time, he writes articles for Medical Laboratory Observer on the applications of computers to laboratory medicine, reads MAD magazine and rides a bicycle around town.

Author